Pulmonary Embolism

Editors

PETER S. MARSHALL
WASSIM H. FARES

CLINICS IN
CHEST MEDICINE

www.chestmed.theclinics.com

September 2018 • Volume 39 • Number 3

ELSEVIER

1600 John F. Kennedy Boulevard • Suite 1800 • Philadelphia, Pennsylvania, 19103-2899

http://www.theclinics.com

CLINICS IN CHEST MEDICINE Volume 39, Number 3
September 2018 ISSN 0272-5231, ISBN-13: 978-0-323-61376-7

Editor: Colleen Dietzler
Developmental Editor: Casey Potter

Clinics in Chest Medicine (ISSN 0272-5231) is published quarterly by Elsevier Inc., 360 Park Avenue South, New York, NY 10010-1710. Months of issue are March, June, September, and December. Periodicals postage paid at New York, NY and additional mailing offices. Subscription prices are $366.00 per year (domestic individuals), $691.00 per year (domestic institutions), $100.00 per year (domestic students/residents), $419.00 per year (Canadian individuals), $858.00 per year (Canadian institutions), $479.00 per year (international individuals), $858.00 per year (international institutions), and $230.00 per year (international and Canadian students/residents). International air speed delivery is included in all Clinics subscription prices. All prices are subject to change without notice. **POSTMASTER:** Send address changes to Clinics in Chest Medicine, Elsevier Health Sciences Division, Subscription Customer Service, 3251 Riverport Lane, Maryland Heights, MO 63043. **Customer Service: Telephone: 1-800-654-2452** (U.S. and Canada); **1-314-447-8871** (outside U.S. and Canada). **Fax: 1-314-447-8029. E-mail: journalscustomerservice-usa@elsevier.com (for print support); journalsonlinesupport-usa@elsevier.com (for online support).**

Reprints. For copies of 100 or more of articles in this publication, please contact the Commercial Reprints Department, Elsevier Inc., 360 Park Avenue South, New York, NY 10010-1710. Tel.: 212-633-3874; Fax: 212-633-3820; E-mail: reprints@elsevier.com.

Clinics in Chest Medicine is covered in *MEDLINE/PubMed (Index Medicus), Current Contents/Clinical Medicine, EMBASE/Excerpta Medica, Science Citation Index,* and *ISI/BIOMED.*

Contributors

EDITORS

PETER S. MARSHALL, MD, MPH
Assistant Professor, Section of Pulmonary,
Critical Care and Sleep Medicine,
Department of Internal Medicine,
Yale School of Medicine, New Haven,
Connecticut, USA

WASSIM H. FARES, MD, MSC
Director Yale Pulmonary Vascular Disease
Center, Section of Pulmonary, Critical Care
and Sleep Medicine, Associate Professor,
Department of Internal Medicine, Yale School
of Medicine, New Haven, Connecticut,
USA

AUTHORS

WILLIAM R. AUGER, MD, FCCP
Professor of Clinical Medicine, Director,
CTEPH Program, UC San Diego Health,
University of California, San Diego, La Jolla,
California, USA

AFSHA AURSHINA, MBBS
Postdoctoral Research Fellow of Surgery,
Section of Vascular Surgery, Department of
Surgery, Yale School of Medicine, New Haven,
Connecticut, USA

DEBABRATA BANDYOPADHYAY, MD
Associate Professor of Medicine, Pulmonary
and Critical Care Medicine, Geisinger, Danville,
Pennsylvania, USA

ISABEL S. BAZAN, MD
Section of Pulmonary, Critical Care and Sleep
Medicine, Yale School of Medicine, New
Haven, Connecticut, USA

BEHNOOD BIKDELI, MD
Division of Cardiology, Department of
Medicine, Columbia University Medical
Center, NewYork-Presbyterian Hospital,
New York, New York, USA; Center for
Outcomes Research and Evaluation (CORE),
Yale School of Medicine, New Haven,
Connecticut, USA

JORGE BORGES, MD
Division of Cardiology, Section of Vascular
Medicine and Intervention, Department of
Medicine, Massachusetts Hospital, Boston,
Massachusetts, USA

GHADA BOURJEILY, MD
Associate Professor of Medicine, The Miriam
Hospital, The Warren Alpert Medical School of
Brown University, Providence, Rhode Island,
USA

CHRISTOPHER DEEB DADO, MD
Pulmonary and Critical Care Fellowship, Rhode
Island Hospital, The Warren Alpert Medical
School of Brown University, Providence,
Rhode Island, USA

OMKAR DESAI, MD
Section of Pulmonary, Critical Care and Sleep
Medicine, Department of Medicine, Yale
School of Medicine, New Haven, Connecticut,
USA

MIA DJULBEGOVIC, MD
Resident, Traditional Internal Medicine
Residency Program, Department of Internal
Medicine, Yale School of Medicine, New
Haven, Connecticut, USA

JEAN M. ELWING, MD, FCCP
Professor of Medicine, Director, Pulmonary
Hypertension Program, Division of Pulmonary,
Critical Care and Sleep Medicine, University of
Cincinnati College of Medicine, Cincinnati,
Ohio, USA

WASSIM H. FARES, MD, MSC
Director Yale Pulmonary Vascular Disease
Center, Section of Pulmonary, Critical Care and
Sleep Medicine, Associate Professor,
Department of Internal Medicine, Yale School
of Medicine, New Haven, Connecticut, USA

HUBERT JAMES FORD III, MD
Division of Pulmonary and Critical Care
Medicine, University of North Carolina at
Chapel Hill, Chapel Hill, North Carolina,
USA

BRIAN FUNAKI, MD
Professor and Chief, Vascular and
Interventional Radiology, Department of
Radiology, The University of Chicago
Medicine, Chicago, Illinois, USA

KAVITHA GOPALRATNAM, MBBS
Division of Pulmonology, Yale New Haven
Health, Bridgeport Hospital, Bridgeport,
Connecticut, USA

EILEEN M. HARDER, MD
Department of Internal Medicine, Yale School
of Medicine, New Haven, Connecticut,
USA

GUSTAVO A. HERESI, MD, MS
Director Pulmonary Vascular and
CTEPH Program, Department of Pulmonary
and Critical Care Medicine, Respiratory
Institute, Cleveland Clinic, Cleveland, Ohio,
USA

BRIAN P. HOLLY, MD
Assistant Professor, Vascular and
Interventional Radiology, Johns Hopkins
Hospital, Interventional Radiology Center,
Baltimore, Maryland, USA

EBTESAM ATTAYA ISLAM, MD, PhD
Assistant Professor, Department of
Internal Medicine, Division of Pulmonary
and Critical Care Medicine, Texas Tech
University Health Sciences Center, Lubbock,
Texas, USA

DAVID JIMENEZ, MD, PhD
Respiratory Department, Hospital Ramón y
Cajal and Medicine Department, Universidad
de Alcalá (IRYCIS), Madrid, Spain

CHRISTOPHER KABRHEL, MD, MPH
Department of Emergency Medicine, Center
for Vascular Emergencies, Massachusetts
General Hospital, Boston, Massachusetts,
USA

CYRUS KHOLDANI, MD
Division of Pulmonary and Critical Care
Medicine, Stanford University School of
Medicine, Palo Alto, California, USA

ALFRED IAN LEE, MD, PhD
Associate Professor of Medicine, Section of
Hematology, Department of Internal Medicine,
Yale School of Medicine, New Haven,
Connecticut, USA

DAVID W. LEE, MD
Division of Cardiology, University of North
Carolina at Chapel Hill, Chapel Hill, North
Carolina, USA

MARK L. LESSNE, MD
Vascular & Interventional Specialists,
Charlotte Radiology, Charlotte, North Carolina,
USA

BARBARA L. LeVARGE, MD
Assistant Professor, Division of Pulmonary
Diseases and Critical Care Medicine,
Department of Medicine, University of North
Carolina at Chapel Hill, Chapel Hill, North
Carolina, USA

ANDREW TOBIAS LEVINSON, MD, MPH
Assistant Professor of Medicine, The Miriam
Hospital, The Warren Alpert Medical School of
Brown University, Providence, Rhode Island,
USA

RACHEL LIU, MD
Assistant Professor, Department of Emergency
Medicine, Yale School of Medicine,
New Haven, Connecticut, USA

PETER S. MARSHALL, MD, MPH
Assistant Professor, Section of Pulmonary,
Critical Care and Sleep Medicine, Department
of Internal Medicine, Yale School of Medicine,
New Haven, Connecticut, USA

MEGAN McCULLOUGH, MD
Department of Internal Medicine, Yale
School of Medicine, New Haven, Connecticut,
USA

KATELYN McNAMARA
Research Assistant, Department of Emergency
Medicine, Yale School of Medicine, New
Haven, Connecticut, USA

JASLEEN KAUR MINHAS, MD
Chief Resident, Department of Medicine, North
Shore Medical Center, Salem, Massachusetts,
USA

CHRIS MOORE, MD
Associate Professor, Department of
Emergency Medicine, Yale School of Medicine,
New Haven, Connecticut, USA

QUYEN NGUYEN, MD
Instructor in Medicine, Division of Pulmonary,
Allergy and Critical Care Medicine, University
of Pittsburgh, UPMC, Pittsburgh,
Pennsylvania, USA

**CASSIUS IYAD OCHOA CHAAR, MD, MS,
FACS**
Assistant Professor, Section of Vascular
Surgery, Department of Surgery, Yale School
of Medicine, New Haven, Connecticut,
USA

JEFFREY S. POLLAK, MD
Robert I. White Jr. Professor of Interventional
Radiology, Department of Radiology
and Biomedical Imaging, Section of
Vascular and Interventional Radiology, Yale
School of Medicine, New Haven, Connecticut,
USA

FARBOD NICHOLAS RAHAGHI, MD, PhD
Instructor, Pulmonary and Critical Care
Medicine, Brigham and Women's Hospital,
Harvard Medical School. Boston,
Massachusetts, USA

**BELINDA N. RIVERA-LEBRON, MD, MS,
FCCP**
Assistant Professor of Medicine, Division of
Pulmonary, Allergy and Critical Care Medicine,
University of Pittsburgh, UPMC, Pittsburgh,
Pennsylvania, USA

JOSANNA M. RODRIGUEZ-LOPEZ, MD
Instructor in Medicine, Division of Pulmonary
and Critical Care Medicine, Department of
Medicine, Massachusetts General Hospital,
Harvard Medical School, Boston,
Massachusetts, USA

LISA J. ROSE-JONES, MD
Division of Cardiology, University of North
Carolina at Chapel Hill, Chapel Hill, North
Carolina, USA

KENNETH ROSENFIELD, MD
Division of Cardiology, Section of Vascular
Medicine and Intervention, Department of
Medicine, Massachusetts Hospital, Boston,
Massachusetts, USA

RACHEL ROSOVSKY, MD, MPH
Division of Hematology and Oncology,
Department of Medicine, Massachusetts
Hospital, Boston, Massachusetts, USA

ANASTASIIA A. RUDKOVSKAIA, MD
Fellow, Pulmonary and Critical Care Medicine,
Geisinger, Danville, Pennsylvania,
USA

VICTOR TAPSON, MD
Cedars-Sinai Medical Center, Los Angeles,
California, USA

VICTOR TEST, MD
Professor of Medicine, Division Chief,
Pulmonary and Critical Care Medicine, Texas
Tech University Health Sciences Center,
Lubbock, Texas, USA

ANJALI VAIDYA, MD, FACC, FASE, FACP
Associate Professor of Medicine,
Associate Director, Pulmonary Hypertension,
Right Heart Failure, and Pulmonary
Thromboendarterectomy Program, Advanced
Heart Failure and Cardiac Transplant, Temple
University Lewis Katz School of Medicine,
Temple University Hospital, Philadelphia,
Pennsylvania, USA

RICHARD E. WINN, MD, MS
Professor of Medicine, Immunology and
Medical Microbiology, Division Chief,
Infectious Diseases, Staff, Pulmonary
Medicine Division, Texas Tech University
Health Sciences Center, Lubbock, Texas,
USA

CAMERON D. WRIGHT, MD
Mathisen Family Professor of Surgery, Division of Thoracic Surgery, Department of Surgery, Massachusetts General Hospital, Harvard Medical School, Boston, Massachusetts, USA

ROHAM T. ZAMANIAN, MD
Associate Professor of Medicine, Division of Pulmonary and Critical Care Medicine, Stanford University School of Medicine, Palo Alto, California, USA

Contents

> Overdiagnosis of venous thromboembolism is associated with increasing numbers of patient complications and health care burden. Multiple clinical tools exist to estimate the probability of pulmonary embolism and deep venous thrombosis. When used with D-dimer testing, these can further stratify venous thromboembolism risk to help inform the use of additional diagnostic testing. Although there are similar tools to estimate bleeding risk, these are not as well validated and lack reliability.

> Venous thromboembolism accounts for significant morbidity and mortality in patients with acute medical illnesses requiring hospital admission. American College of Chest Physicians guidelines recommend prophylaxis with heparins as first line and mechanical methods as second line. The risk of major bleeding with anticoagulants is less than 1% and not significantly different between agents. Although data support the use of all heparins, there is a trend toward superiority of low-molecular-weight heparins (LMWHs). Because acute illness and immobility do not end at hospital discharge, extended-duration therapy with LMWHs and direct oral anticoagulants remains under investigation.

> Imaging continues to be the modality of choice for the diagnosis of venous thromboembolic disease, particularly when incorporated into diagnostic algorithms. Improvement in imaging techniques as well as new imaging modalities and processing methods has improved diagnostic accuracy and additionally are being leveraged in prognostication and decision-making for choice of intervention. In this article, the authors review the role of imaging in diagnosis and prognostication of venous thromboembolism. They also discuss emerging imaging approaches that may in the near future find clinical usefulness in improving diagnosis and prognostication as well as differentiating disease phenotypes.

> Pulmonary artery filling defects can be observed in various pathologic processes other than pulmonary embolism, for example, nonthrombotic pulmonary embolism with biological and nonbiological materials and intrinsic pulmonary artery lesions. They have also been described in rare conditions, such as fibrosing mediastinitis

and congenital absence or stenosis of pulmonary artery, and some pulmonary parenchymal and airway malignancies. Misdiagnosis is common owing to the relative rarity of these conditions. Correct diagnosis is based on the appropriate clinical suspicion considering the unique clinical features, laboratory findings, and additional radiologic clues inferring a pathology other than pulmonary embolism.

Venous thromboembolism (VTE) is a common cause of morbidity and mortality. Presence of preexisting conditions, such as cardiopulmonary diseases, cirrhosis, renal dysfunction, and asplenia, commonly occurs in patients with VTE. Moreover, these conditions often are risk factors for developing VTE. These preexisting conditions make VTE diagnosis and treatment challenging and worsen outcomes. Current guidelines do not include detailed features in the diagnosis and management of patients with preexisting conditions. This article discusses presence of VTE in patients with preexisting cardiopulmonary diseases, cirrhosis, renal dysfunction, and asplenia.

Venous thromboembolism (VTE), referring to both deep vein thrombosis and pulmonary embolism, is a leading cause of death in the developed world during pregnancy. This increased risk is attributed to the Virchow triad, inherited thrombophilias, along with other standard risk factors, and continues for up to 6 to 12 weeks postpartum. During the peripartum period, women should be risk stratified and preventive measures should be initiated based on their risk. Diagnostic tests and treatment strategies commonly used in VTE differ in pregnancy. An understanding of these differences is imperative to diagnose with confidence and to treat appropriately.

 Video content accompanies this article at http://www.chestmed.theclinics.com.

The diagnosis and treatment of pulmonary embolism (PE) remains one of the great challenges of emergency medicine. The symptoms of PE are myriad, common, and nonspecific. Undertesting risks missing a potentially life-threatening illness, whereas overtesting adds cost, false-positive diagnoses, incidental findings, and potential adverse impacts from contrast and radiation. Once diagnosed, the severity of PE can range from truly insignificant to deadly, and treatment must be tailored appropriately to the situation. This article discusses basic tenets of emergency department diagnosis and management while highlighting current challenges and recent changes to PE treatment.

Echocardiography is valuable in the evaluation and risk stratification of patients with acute and chronic pulmonary embolism (PE). Patients with acute PE who have echocardiographic evidence of right ventricular dilatation and/or right ventricular dysfunction have a worse prognosis. A minority of patients with acute PE can develop chronic thromboembolic pulmonary hypertension. Patients with chronic thromboembolic pulmonary hypertension often have echocardiographic evidence of elevated pulmonary arterial pressures, right ventricular hypertrophy, right ventricular dysfunction, and/or left ventricular impaired relaxation.

potentially fatal disease characterized by a vasoconstrictive, proliferative, and thrombotic phenotype, which leads to increased pulmonary artery pressure, right heart failure, and death. Pathologically, in situ thromboses are found in the small distal pulmonary arteries. Dysregulation of coagulation, platelet function, and endothelial cells may contribute to a prothrombotic state. There is mixed evidence for the use of anticoagulation or antiplatelet therapy in patients with PAH.

Chronic thromboembolic pulmonary hypertension (CTEPH) is a progressive pulmonary vascular disease with significant morbidity. It is a result of an alternate natural history in which there is limited resolution of thromboemboli with pulmonary artery obstruction leading to pulmonary hypertension (PH). CTEPH requires a thorough clinical assessment, including pulmonary hemodynamics and radiologic evaluation, in addition to consultation with an expert center. Surgical intervention remains the optimal management strategy. Select patients may be candidates for catheter-based intervention with balloon pulmonary angioplasty in centers with clinical expertise. Inoperable patients or those with postintervention PH are treated with pulmonary hypertension-targeted medical therapy.

Pulmonary Embolism Response Teams (PERTs) are being created around the United States to immediately and simultaneously bring together multiple specialists to determine the best course of action and coordinate clinical care for patients with severe pulmonary embolism (PE). The organization and structure of each PERT will depend on local clinical demands and resources. Creating a follow-up clinic for patients with PE after discharge from the hospital is an essential component of any PERT program. PERT programs, which have come together to form the PERT Consortium, are changing the landscape of PE treatment and may represent a new standard of care.

The surgical treatment of deep venous thrombosis (DVT) has significantly evolved and is focused on different strategies of early thrombus removal in the acute phase and deep venous recanalization or bypass in the chronic phase. Along with the use of anticoagulation agents, endovascular techniques based on catheter-directed thrombolysis and pharmacomechanical thrombectomy have been increasingly used in patients with acute extensive DVT. Patient selection is crucial to provide optimal outcomes and minimize complications.

Vena cava filters are implantable devices that are placed to trap thrombus originating in the lower extremities and prevent it from migrating to the lungs. In general, inferior vena cava (IVC) filters are indicated for patients who cannot receive anticoagulation. Other indications for IVC filtration are less clear, and guidelines vary. All patients who have a retrievable IVC filter should be followed, and the removal of the IVC filter should be considered once its indication is lost.

Catheter-Based Therapies for Pulmonary Emboli

Jeffrey S. Pollak

More aggressive therapy for acute pulmonary embolism beyond anticoagulation is indicated in patients at higher risk for mortality and morbidity, namely, those suffering from massive and possibly submassive disease. Catheter-based thrombolysis, catheter-based mechanical thrombus debulking, or combinations of these offer opportunities for rapid clot reduction and clinical improvement with a lower bleeding risk than systemic thrombolysis and perhaps greater efficacy. Optimal low-dose regimens for direct thrombolysis have not been defined just as optimal techniques and devices for mechanical therapy have not been developed, underscoring the need for further work.

Surgical Management of Acute and Chronic Pulmonary Embolism

Barbara L. LeVarge, Cameron D. Wright, and Josanna M. Rodriguez-Lopez

Surgical pulmonary embolectomy and pulmonary thromboendarterectomy are well-established treatment strategies for patients with acute and chronic pulmonary embolism, respectively. For both procedures, techniques and outcomes have evolved considerably over the past decades. Patients with massive and submassive acute pulmonary embolism are at risk for rapid decline owing to right ventricular failure and shock. When thrombus is proximal, embolectomy can rapidly restore cardiac function. Chronic thromboembolic pulmonary hypertension is a more complex disease that requires skilled, careful dissection of the arterial wall, including vascular intima. When successful, surgery leads to clinical cure of the associated pulmonary hypertension, with excellent long-term outcomes.

PROGRAM OBJECTIVE

The goal of the *Clinics in Chest Medicine* is to provide provide practitioners with state-of-the-art information that is clinically useful, concise, well referenced, and comprehensive.

TARGET AUDIENCE

All practicing physicians and healthcare professionals who provide patient care utilizing findings from *Chest Medicine Clinics of North America*.

LEARNING OBJECTIVES

Upon completion of this activity, participants will be able to:
1. Review new imaging tools & modalities for diagnosis of deep vein thrombosis and pulmonary embolism
2. Discuss surgical management of acute and chronic pulmonary embolism
3. Recognize challenges and changes to the management of pulmonary embolism in the emergency department

ACCREDITATION

The Elsevier Office of Continuing Medical Education (EOCME) is accredited by the Accreditation Council for Continuing Medical Education (ACCME) to provide continuing medical education for physicians.

The EOCME designates this enduring material for a maximum of 15 *AMA PRA Category 1 Credit*(s)™. Physicians should claim only the credit commensurate with the extent of their participation in the activity.

All other health care professionals requesting continuing education credit for this enduring material will be issued a certificate of participation.

DISCLOSURE OF CONFLICTS OF INTEREST

The EOCME assesses conflict of interest with its instructors, faculty, planners, and other individuals who are in a position to control the content of CME activities. All relevant conflicts of interest that are identified are thoroughly vetted by EOCME for fair balance, scientific objectivity, and patient care recommendations. EOCME is committed to providing its learners with CME activities that promote improvements or quality in healthcare and not a specific proprietary business or a commercial interest.

The planning committee, staff, authors and editors listed below have identified no financial relationships or relationships to products or devices they or their spouse/life partner have with commercial interest related to the content of this CME activity:

Afsha Aurshina, MBBS; Debabrata Bandyopadhyay, MD; Isabel S. Bazan, MD; Behnood Bikdeli, MD; Jorge Borges, MD; Ghada Bourjeily, MD; Cassius Iyad Ochoa Chaar, MD, MS, FACS; Christopher Deeb Dado, MD; Omkar Desai, MD; Colleen Dietzler; Mia Djulbegovic, MD; Wassim H. Fares, MD, MSC; Hubert James Ford III, MD; Brian Funaki, MD; Kavitha Gopalratnam, MBBS; Eileen M. Harder, MD; Gustavo A. Heresi, MD, MS; Brian P. Holly, MD; David Jimenez, MD, PhD; Alison Kemp; Cyrus Kholdani, MD; David W. Lee, MD; Alfred Ian Lee, MD, PhD; Barbara L. LeVarge, MD; Andrew Tobias Levinson, MD, MPH; Rachel Liu, MD; Peter S. Marshall, MD, MPH; Rajkumar Mayakrishnan; Megan McCullough, MD; Katelyn McNamara; Chris Moore, MD; Quyen Nguyen, MD; Jeffrey S. Pollak, MD; Farbod Nicholas Rahaghi, MD, PhD; Belinda Rivera-Lebron, MD, MS, FCCP; Josanna M. Rodriguez-Lopez, MD; Lisa J. Rose-Jones, MD; Anastasiia A. Rudkovskaia, MD; Victor F. Tapson, MD; Victor Test, MD; Richard E. Winn, MD, MS; Cameron D. Wright, MD; Roham T. Zamanian, MD.

The planning committee, staff, authors and editors listed below have identified financial relationships or relationships to products or devices they or their spouse/life partner have with commercial interest related to the content of this CME activity:

William R. Auger, MD, FCCP: receives research support and is a consultant/advisor for Bayer AG.
Jean M. Elwing, MD, FCCP: receives research support from Actelion Pharmaceuticals US, Inc., Arena Pharmaceuticals, Inc., Bayer AG, Reata Pharmaceuticals, Inc., Bellerophon Therapeutics, Eiger BioPharmaceuticals, Akros Pharma Inc., and Liquidia Technologies; receives research support and is a consultant/advisor for United Therapeutics Corporation.
Ebtesam Attaya Islam, MD, PhD: spouse serves as a speaker for Salix Pharmaceuticals, ReShape LifeSciences, Inc., and EndoGastric Solutions, Inc.
Christopher Kabrhel, MD, MPH: receives research support from and is a consultant/advisor for Diagnostica Stago, Inc., Janssen Pharmaceuticals, Inc., and Siemens Medical Solutions, USA, Inc.; is a consultant/advisor for Pfizer, Inc. and Portola Pharmaceuticals, Inc. and receives research support from Boehringer-Ingelheim International GmbH.
Mark L. Lessne, MD: serves as a speaker for Cook Medical LLC.
Jasleen Kaur Minhas, MD: serves as a speaker and a consultant/advisor for Bayer AG.
Kenneth Rosenfield, MD: Is a consultant/advisor for Abbott, Cardinal Health, Cook, Surmodics, Inc., Koninklijke Philips N.V., and Amgen, Inc.; he is a consultant/advisor and owns stock for Silk Road Medical; Dr. Rosenfield is also a consultant/advisor for, owns stock and/or holds patents or receives royalties with Capture Vascular, Inc., Contego Medical, LLC, Cruzar Medsystems, Inc., Endospan Ltd., Eximo Medical Ltd., MD Insider, Micell Technologies, Inc., Shockwave Medical, Inc., Thrombolex, Inc., and Valcare Medical; receives research support from Atrium Medical Corporation, Inari Medial, and C.R. Bard, Inc.

Rachel Rosovsky, MD, MPH: receives research support from Janssen Pharmaceuticals, Inc. and Bristol-Myers Squibb Company and is a consultant/advisor for Bayer AG.

Anjali Vaidya, MD: is a consultant/advisor and participates on speaker's bureau for Actelion Pharmaceuticals US, Inc., Bayer AG, and United Therapeutics Corporation and participates on a speaker's bureau for Gilead.

UNAPPROVED/OFF-LABEL USE DISCLOSURE

The EOCME requires CME faculty to disclose to the participants:

1. When products or procedures being discussed are off-label, unlabelled, experimental, and/or investigational (not US Food and Drug Administration [FDA] approved); and
2. Any limitations on the information presented, such as data that are preliminary or that represent ongoing research, interim analyses, and/or unsupported opinions. Faculty may discuss information about pharmaceutical agents that is outside of FDA-approved labelling. This information is intended solely for CME and is not intended to promote off-label use of these medications. If you have any questions, contact the medical affairs department of the manufacturer for the most recent prescribing information.

TO ENROLL

To enroll in the *Chest Medicine Clinics* Continuing Medical Education program, call customer service at 1-800-654-2452 or sign up online at https://www.theclinics.com/cme. The CME program is available to subscribers for an additional annual fee of USD $225.

METHOD OF PARTICIPATION

In order to claim credit, participants must complete the following:

1. Complete enrolment as indicated above.
2. Read the activity.
3. Complete the CME Test and Evaluation. Participants must achieve a score of 70% on the test. All CME Tests and Evaluations must be completed online.

CME INQUIRIES/SPECIAL NEEDS

For all CME inquiries or special needs, please contact elsevierCME@elsevier.com.

CLINICS IN CHEST MEDICINE

RELATED INTEREST

Surgical Clinics of North America, Volume 98, Issue 2 (April 2018)
Vascular Surgery: Current Concepts and Treatments for Venous Disease
Marc A. Passman, *Editor*

THE CLINICS ARE AVAILABLE ONLINE!
Access your subscription at:
www.theclinics.com

Preface
Venous Thromboembolism: An Evolving Entity

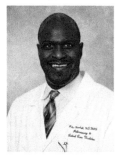 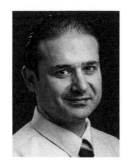

Peter S. Marshall, MD, MPH   Wassim H. Fares, MD, MSC

Editors

Recent advances in the diagnosis and treatment of venous thromboembolism (VTE) have been significant. These changes have resulted in a reduction in mortality and increased cost of caring for patients with (and suspected of) VTE. Increasingly there is recognition that certain VTE patients require special consideration. This issue discusses these and other evolving topics in the diagnosis and treatment of VTE.

Clinical tools that allow estimation of pretest probability for lower-extremity deep vein thrombosis (DVT) and pulmonary embolus (PE) are in widespread use. These tools have been combined with the D-dimer to further improve their utility, thereby informing further diagnostics. The computed-tomographic (CT) angiogram for PE is the first-line diagnostic test for PE, and it is also recognized as a validated method of classifying severity of PE in hemodynamically stable patients. Other diagnostic modalities, such as magnetic resonance angiography/magnetic resonance venography and CT contrast venography, are being given consideration.

The first step of VTE prevention in the acute care setting is to estimate the risk of occurrence in an individual and institute appropriate prophylactic measures. Management of DVT prophylaxis is changing. Evidence regarding the benefits of extending prophylaxis beyond the acute hospital setting is growing. In addition, the choice of agents available for prophylaxis has increased.

PE may present with three levels of severity. Low-risk patients lack evidence of hemodynamic compromise due to their PE and have low mortality. Clinicians are coming to realize that the risks of extended anticoagulation may outweigh the risk of no treatment: some low-risk PE patients may not require exposure to full-dose anticoagulation. Intermediate-risk PE (sub-massive PE) has a variable prognosis. These patients have evidence of right ventricular (RV) dysfunction or RV strain, as defined by imaging, echocardiography, biomarkers, or EKG, but no overt evidence of hemodynamic compromise. Controversy regarding the management of intermediate-risk patients exists. No single strategy is best for this heterogeneous group. Advances in supportive measures, catheter-directed therapies, and even surgical therapies now offer alternatives to anticoagulation in this group.

High-risk PE (massive PE) displays overt hemodynamic compromise or shock and has the poorest prognosis. The cornerstone of definitive treatment in high-risk patients has been systemic thrombolytics, and this continues. Research into alternative dosing of thrombolytic agents, use of catheter-directed therapies, and expanded use of improving surgical interventions now offers greater choice when faced with these unstable patients.

Other areas in evolution include the diagnosis and management of VTE in pregnancy, liver

Clin Chest Med 39 (2018) xv–xvi

https://doi.org/10.1016/j.ccm.2018.06.001

0272-5231/18/© 2018 Published by Elsevier Inc.

disease, preexisting cardiopulmonary disease, and end-stage renal disease. The role of inferior vena cava filters in all patients with VTE is being redefined. The use of newer oral anticoagulants (direct thrombin inhibitors and Factor Xa inhibitors) is gaining acceptance, but their use in certain populations with VTE has yet to be defined. The interaction between thrombosis and pulmonary hypertension is an area of active research, not only as it relates to chronic thromboembolic pulmonary hypertension.

The growing complexity of VTE management has inspired a multispecialty team approach with regards to PE. The PE Response Team approach to complicated patients is viewed as useful because management (in the setting of growing treatment options) requires the input of those with a wide range of expertise.

A broad range of topics was reviewed in this issue, and the increasing complexity in the diagnosis and management of VTE was highlighted. It is hoped the compilation will serve as a comprehensive resource on the topic. We would like to thank the contributors for high-quality articles and our editorial staff for expert guidance in the preparation of this issue.

Peter S. Marshall, MD, MPH
Section of Pulmonary, Critical Care &
Sleep Medicine
Department of Internal Medicine
Yale University School of Medicine
15 York Street, LCI 101
PO Box 208057
New Haven, CT 06520-8057, USA

Wassim H. Fares, MD, MSC
Yale Pulmonary Vascular Disease Center
Section of Pulmonary, Critical Care &
Sleep Medicine
Department of Internal Medicine
Yale University School of Medicine
300 Cedar Street
PO Box 208057
New Haven, CT 06520-8057, USA

E-mail addresses:
peter.marshall@yale.edu (P.S. Marshall)
wassim_fares@hotmail.com (W.H. Fares)

Clinical Probability Tools for Deep Venous Thrombosis, Pulmonary Embolism, and Bleeding

Eileen M. Harder, MD[a], Omkar Desai, MD[b],
Peter S. Marshall, MD, MPH[b],*

KEYWORDS

- Pulmonary embolus • Diagnosis • Pretest probability • Clinical decision tools
- Deep vein thrombosis • Bleeding • Venous thromboembolism

KEY POINTS

- Several validated clinical tools exist to estimate pretest probability for venous thromboembolism and bleeding.
- Pretest probability tools for venous thromboembolism can be combined with the D-dimer to further improve venous thromboembolism probability assessment.
- There are drawbacks to overevaluation and overdiagnosis for pulmonary embolism.
- The clinical probability tools for venous thromboembolism are only validated in certain populations.
- Clinical probability tools for bleeding risk cannot reliably predict major bleeding events but can place patients in a low-risk bleeding category.

INTRODUCTION

Venous thromboembolism (VTE), which includes both deep venous thrombosis (DVT) and pulmonary embolism (PE), is the third most common cardiovascular disease after acute coronary syndrome and stroke. VTE affects up to 900,000 Americans annually.[1,2] It is a significant contributor to mortality—studies suggest that it causes up to 300,000 fatalities, and it is often cited as the most common cause of in-hospital preventable death.[2–4]

VTE can present a diagnostic challenge to clinicians. Despite its high incidence and potential severity, presenting symptoms are often nonspecific or even absent, and this creates a low threshold for evaluation. As the availability and sensitivity of noninvasive diagnostic methods has increased, this has culminated in a phenomenon of overdiagnosis.[5]

Although there are multiple clinical tools to estimate VTE pretest probability, they are underused—in 1 study, only 45.5% of 3500 computed tomography pulmonary angiography scans followed Prospective Investigation of Pulmonary Embolism Diagnosis (PIOPED) II recommendations to commence evaluation with a clinical score and D-dimer.[6] Given the risks of imaging and overdiagnosis, the thoughtful workup of VTE is essential, beginning with clinical tools to estimate probability and guide management.

Disclosure Statement: The authors have no conflicts of interest. There were no funding sources for this article.
[a] Department of Internal Medicine, Yale University School of Medicine, 15 York Street, LCI 101, New Haven, CT 06520, USA; [b] Section of Pulmonary, Critical Care and Sleep Medicine, Department of Medicine, Yale University School of Medicine, 15 York Street, LCI 101, New Haven, CT 06520, USA
* Corresponding author.
E-mail address: peter.marshall@yale.edu

Clin Chest Med 39 (2018) 473–482
https://doi.org/10.1016/j.ccm.2018.04.001
0272-5231/18/

CLINICAL PROBABILITY TOOLS FOR DEEP VENOUS THROMBOSIS

A DVT usually forms in the lower legs. Given its multiple risk factors, nonspecific presentation, and potentially significant risk (up to 40% may cause PEs), it is a commonly suspected diagnosis.[7] To decrease the use of ultrasound examination and false-positive results, guidelines recommend assessment of clinical pretest probability before imaging.[8,9]

The Wells Scores for Deep Venous Thrombosis

The Wells Score is the best known and most widely used DVT pretest probability tool. The original model incorporated 9 predictors with 1 point given to each: active cancer; lower extremity immobility, paralysis, or paresis; recent immobility for more than 3 days or major surgery within 4 weeks; entire leg edema; localized tenderness along deep venous system; calf circumference difference of greater than 3 cm (measured 10 cm below the tibial tuberosity); unilateral pitting edema; and collateral nonvaricose superficial veins.[10] Two points were subtracted for the last factor, alternative diagnosis as likely or greater than DVT. Three risk groups were defined—low ($\leq$0 points), moderate (1–2), high ($\geq$3)—and in their 2006 metaanalysis, Wells and colleagues[11] observed DVT rates of 5%, 17%, and 53%, respectively.

In 2003, this model was revised into the modified Wells. Three changes were made: a tenth predictor for previous documented DVT was added and assigned 1 point, the length of time from major surgery was increased from 4 to 12 weeks, and probability was grouped into DVT unlikely (<2 points) or likely ($\geq$2).[12] In their unlikely populations, DVT rates were 0.4% (with normal D-dimer testing) and 1.4% (controls; underwent ultrasound examination alone without D-dimer testing). This rule was validated in a metaanalysis of 13 studies; an unlikely score with negative D-dimer testing was associated with a 1.2% failure rate.[13]

Management after Clinical Deep Venous Thrombosis Probability Assessment

Pretest probability guides subsequent evaluation. In the unlikely or low-risk groups, most guidelines suggest D-dimer testing—if negative, no further testing is required; if positive, leg ultrasound examination should be performed.[2,9] Multiple studies have validated this approach.[14] In the intermediate group, either high sensitivity D-dimer or leg ultrasound examination (complete venous vs proximal) should be done. High-probability patients should proceed immediately to imaging.

Limitations of the Wells Score for Deep Venous Thrombosis

Notably, the individual Wells elements are not useful in diagnosing DVT, nor does the score work as well in those who had distal DVT, were older, and had prior DVT.[13,15] Importantly, the Wells Scores have mixed accuracy in the hospital, with Silveira and colleagues[16] noting a 5.9% failure rate in 1135 inpatients.

Alternate Deep Venous Thrombosis Probability Scores

The Oudega rule was created after a high failure rate was noted in low-risk Wells patients with normal D-dimer.[17] This score assigns 6 points to elevated D-dimer, 2 to calf circumference difference of greater than 3 cm, and 1 each to male gender, oral contraceptive use, cancer, recent surgery, absence of leg trauma, and vein distension.[18] With a cutoff of less than 4 as low risk, the failure rate was less than 1.5%. The Hamilton index is another alternative—although its criteria are similar to the Wells Score, it includes gender and weights immobility, cancer, and DVT suspicion more highly.[19] Notably, although studies show similar failure rates between the Wells, Oudega, and Hamilton, these latter 2 systems have not been as widely validated.[20,21]

CLINICAL PROBABILITY TOOLS FOR PULMONARY EMBOLISM

PEs can present with a wide variety of symptoms, ranging from dyspnea, tachypnea, and pleuritic chest pain to circulatory collapse or death in a small number of patients.[22] Given the nonspecificity of presenting symptoms and the potential severity of a missed PE, it is often at the top of a differential list. As such, overdiagnosis is particularly evident in PE—incidence has increased but severity and mortality have improved. Furthermore, treatment of less severe disease has caused higher admission rates, charges, and anticoagulation complications.[23–27]

To prevent overdiagnosis, guidelines outline diagnostic algorithms for PE evaluation. Before any laboratory testing or imaging in hemodynamically stable patients, pretest probability of PE should be assessed with clinical scores.[28–31]

The Wells Scores

The original and modified Wells Scores

The Wells Scores are perhaps the most widely used PE probability tools. Originally developed in 1998 from literature review, the first model predicted PE well but was fairly complex with multiple potential outcomes.[32] In 2000, Wells and colleagues[33] reexamined their initial cohort to identify 7 variables that were significantly associated with PE (points in parentheses): clinical signs/symptoms of DVT (3), alternative diagnosis less likely than PE (3), heart rate greater than 100 bpm (1.5), immobilization for 3 days or more or surgery within 4 weeks (1.5), previous DVT or PE (1.5), hemoptysis (1), and active malignancy (1). Two probability grading systems were designated. The first, or the original Wells, split patients into low (<2 points), moderate (2–6), and high (>6) probability groups. The second was the modified Wells Score, which classified patients as PE likely (>4 points) or unlikely (≤4).

Multiple analyses have demonstrated the usefulness of the combined Wells Score and D-dimer approach. In a prospective cohort of 3306 patients, van Belle and colleagues[34] observed a 12.1% PE rate in unlikely patients by the modified Wells Score, but this decreased to 0.4% with the addition of a normal D-dimer. Furthermore, 23.2% of unlikely patients with an abnormal D-dimer had a PE. Additional analyses have also demonstrated low failure rates with Wells Score and normal D-dimer (**Table 1**).[35–37] Limitations of the Wells criteria are shown in **Table 1**. Notably, although its use is controversial in the hospitalized population, a recent metaanalysis of 3942 PE unlikely patients revealed a sensitivity of 99.7% with D-dimer testing (with a failure rate of 0.1%).[38]

The simplified Wells Score

In 2008, Gibson and colleagues[39] revised the Wells Score into a simplified version to improve ease of use. They maintained the original 7 criteria but assigned each only 1 point; PE was unlikely if the total score was 1 or less. With a negative D-dimer, unlikely modified and simplified Wells Score cohorts had similar 3-month VTE rates (0.3% vs 0.5%). Using the simplified Wells, Gibson and colleagues estimated that 30% of suspected PE patients would not require spiral computed tomography.

The Geneva Scores

The original Geneva Score

The Geneva Score was developed as a more objective alternative to the Wells system. In 1090 patients with suspected PE, Wicki and colleagues[40] identified factors significantly associated with PE: age (≥60 years), heart rate greater than 100 bpm, surgery within 4 weeks, previous DVT/PE, platelike atelectasis or hemidiaphragm elevation on chest radiography, arterial blood partial pressure of CO_2 of 39 mm Hg or less, and arterial blood partial pressure of O_2 of 82 mm Hg or

less. Each was weighted and probabilities were defined as low (<5 points), moderate (5–8), or high (>8).

The revised Geneva Score

Given the original score's requirement for chest radiographs and arterial blood gas testing , Le Gal and colleagues[41] created the revised Geneva (rGeneva) criteria: age greater than 65 years, heart rate 75 bpm or greater, pain on lower limb deep palpation and unilateral edema, hemoptysis, unilateral lower limb pain, previous DVT/PE, surgery or lower limb fracture within 4 weeks, and active cancer. PE probability was assigned as low (0–3 points), intermediate (4–10), and high (≥11). In their validation cohort, the rate of PE in the low probability group was 8% (vs 74% with high).

The simplified revised Geneva Score

In 2008, the Simplified Revised Geneva Score (SRGS) was created to further improve ease of use. All 8 original rGeneva factors were included but each was assigned only 1 point, except for heart rate OF 95 bpm or greater, which was given 2.[42] Two grading systems were assigned: a 2-level score with PE unlikely (0–2 points) or likely (≥3) and a 3-level with low (0–1 points), intermediate (2–4), or high (≥5). The rates of PE in the unlikely and low groups were 11.5% and 8%, respectively; both decreased to 0% when combined with a normal D-dimer.

Comparison of the Wells and Geneva Scores

Although many studies have attempted to identify the best model, there is no consensus. It is generally accepted that the Wells and Geneva systems perform at least equally well—in a metaanalysis of 29 studies, Ceriani and colleagues[43] showed that the Geneva (original, revised) and Wells (original, modified) scores had similar accuracies, although validation strength differed. Douma and colleagues[44] also demonstrated no difference in failure rates and accuracies between the Wells (original, simplified) and Geneva (original, revised) scores.

Notably, some analyses have even suggested that the Wells Scores are even more effective than either Geneva model. Hendriksen and colleagues[45] validated the 3 Wells Scores with the rGeneva and SRGS in 598 outpatients—when combined with a normal D-dimer, failure rates were higher with the Geneva Scores than the Wells Scores (2.7%–3.1% vs 1.2%–1.5%, respectively). Similarly, Penaloza and colleagues[46] showed that original Wells classified more patients as low probability than the SRGS (46% vs 34%) and was more accurate, with a PE prevalence of 2% (vs 4%).

Table 1
Comparison between the Wells Scores, Geneva Criteria, and clinical gestalt

	Wells Score			Geneva		Gestalt
	Original	Modified	Simplified	Revised	SRGS	
Subjective variables	• 'PE most likely diagnosis' requires judgment, is highly weighted, and has only moderate interobserver reliability[69]			• Uses only objective variables		• Relies solely on clinical experience and training
Ease of use	• Fewer variables than Geneva criteria • Simplified Wells easiest to use, but not as widely validated as original scores			• Fully standardized (no reliance on clinician experience)		• No required data or calculator
Accuracy[a]	0.62–0.85[37,39,46,70]	0.74–0.80[39,45,71]	0.72–0.79[39,44,45]	0.65–0.75[42,70,72]	0.69–0.76[42,44–46]	0.77–0.89[71,73]
Failure rate (%)	0.0–1.5[35,45,46]	0.0–1.5[37,45,46]	0.5–1.2[39,44,45]	0.0–2.7[45,72]	0.0–3.1[45,46]	0.7–1.3[57,71]
PPV (%)	19.8–21[37,45]	21[17,37,45]	21[45]	20[45]	21[45]	17–25[74]
NPV (%)[b]	99–99.5[37,44,45]	99[37,45]	99[44,45]	97–99.5[44,45]	97–99.5[42,45]	89–96[74]
Nonapplicable groups	• Pregnancy • Upper limb DVT • Life expectancy <3 mo • No PE symptoms >3 d before presentation • Anticoagulation for >72 h (or low-molecular weight heparin for >24 h in simplified)[39] • Age <18 y • CTPA contraindication[10,32,33]			• Pregnancy • High-risk PE • CTPA contraindication • Life expectancy <3 mo • Current anticoagulation[41,42] • Hospitalized patients		• No absolute contraindications • Accuracy increases with increasing clinical experience[74]

Abbreviations: CTPA, computed tomography pulmonary angiography; DVT, deep venous thrombosis; PE, pulmonary embolism; SRGS, Simplified Revised Geneva Score.
[a] Discriminative ability (ie, area under the curve).
[b] For low-risk/'unlikely' cohort with negative D-dimer.
Data from Refs.[10,32,33,35,37,39,41,42,44–46,57,71,74]

Furthermore, in the high Wells probability group, PE prevalence was 93% compared with 56% in the high SRGS cohort (P<.05).

Evaluation of the Low or Unlikely Pulmonary Embolism Probability Patient

After clinical grading, low probability patients should be evaluated to determine if D-dimer is appropriate. The PE Rule-Out Criteria (PERC) tool was created to identify the cohort in whom D-dimer testing may complicate matters. It consists of 8 variables: age less than 50 years, pulse less than 100 bpm, oxygen saturation 95% or greater on room air, unilateral leg swelling, recent major surgery or trauma within 4 weeks, hemoptysis, prior DVT/PE, and current hormone use.[47] If all 8 factors are absent, no further evaluation for PE is needed.

In low-risk pretest probability patients, Kline and colleagues[47] showed that 1.0% with negative PERC had VTE, and a similar metaanalysis showed that the PERC missed only 0.3% of PEs in this group.[48] Some guidelines now recommend PERC scoring for patients scored as low-risk with 3-level Wells or Geneva systems—if negative, no further testing, including D-dimer, is required.[31,49] Patients with positive PERC should receive at least a D-dimer test. Of note, the PERC has been validated only in clinical and emergency department settings. It is also less accurate in populations with high PE prevalence.[50]

In the low probability cohort who do receive a D-dimer, either a moderate (latex or erythrocyte agglutination) or highly sensitive (ELISA) test can be used—if negative, no further evaluation is required.[49,51,52] The intermediate cohort should receive only a highly sensitive D-dimer. Patients with positive D-dimers should proceed to computed tomography pulmonary angiography, as should those scored as high probability. Computed tomography venography or ventilation–perfusion scans are alternatives in select patients.[29,49]

Clinical Gestalt

Clinical gestalt relies on experience and training to estimate PE probability, and its use has been validated in multiple analyses.[53] It seems to perform at least well as the Geneva and Wells systems.[53–56] In 1038 patients with suspected PE, Penaloza and colleagues[56] showed that gestalt significantly outperformed the Wells and rGeneva Scores—in the low probability group, PE rates were 7.6% with gestalt, 13.0% with rGeneva, and 12.6% with Wells; in the high group, they were 72.1%, 68.8%, and 58.1%, respectively.

Importantly, in a metaanalysis of 52 studies, Lucassen and colleagues[57] evaluated gestalt, the original and modified Wells, and the original and revised Geneva. Although sensitivities were similar, the specificity of gestalt and the rGeneva were lower, leading to more false positives and unnecessary computed tomography pulmonary angiography evaluations.

Summary

The Wells and Geneva scores have similar accuracies in predicting PE. They apply to comparable populations and should not be used in patients who are pregnant, have suspected high-risk PE, or limited life expectancy. Clinical gestalt also has similar accuracy, but is affected by operator experience. When combined with a negative D-dimer, the accuracies of gestalt, Wells scores, and Geneva criteria increase. In some low-risk patients, the D-dimer is not useful, and the PERC can help to identify this cohort.

CLINICAL PROBABILITY TOOLS FOR BLEEDING

Early anticoagulation improves survival in PE, but can be harmful, with a major bleeding rate of 7.22 per 100 patient-years and a case-fatality of 13% to 20%.[58–60] Despite this risk, there are no widely validated systems to estimate bleeding risk in VTE. This section discusses clinical bleeding risk scores and their use in this population.

The RIETE Score

The RIETE score was developed in 2008 from a prospective analysis of 13,057 treated patients with VTE with a 2.4% rate of fatal bleeding.[61] Major bleeding risk factors included anemia (hemoglobin <13 g/dL for men, <12 g/dL for women), age greater than 75 years, creatinine greater than 1.2 mg/dL, recent major bleeding, malignancy history, and clinically overt PE. All factors were assigned 1 point, apart from recent bleed (2), anemia (1.5), and creatinine (1.5). Risk categories were defined as low (0 points), intermediate (1–4), and high (>4), which had respective major bleeding rates of 0.1%, 2.8%, and 6.2%, respectively.

The Outpatient Bleeding Risk Index

The Outpatient Bleeding Risk Index was developed in 1989 and refined by Beyth and colleagues[62] in 1995. The authors assigned 1 point each to age 65 years or greater, history of gastrointestinal bleed or stroke, and 1 or more comorbidities (recent myocardial infarction, hematocrit <30%, creatinine >1.5 mg/dL, diabetes). The score was low risk if 0 points, moderate if 1 to 2, and high if 3 or greater. Although developed for the non-VTE population, Wells and colleagues[63] validated the ORBI in the VTE cohort, where it significantly distinguished between bleeding rates in the low- and moderate-risk groups (0% vs 4.3%).

Additional Bleeding Scores

The Kuijer score is based on only 3 variables (score = [1.6 × age] + [1.3 × sex] + [2.2 × malignancy]) and groups bleeding risk as low (0 points), intermediate (1–3), and high (>3).[64] In their validation cohort, major bleeding risk was 1% in the low-risk group (vs 7% in the high-risk group). The Kearon system was also developed in VTE patients and identified risk factors as age 65 years or greater, previous stroke, previous peptic ulcer or gastrointestinal bleeding, renal impairment, anemia, thrombocytopenia, liver disease, diabetes, and antiplatelet therapy.[65]

Comparison Between Bleeding Risk Scores

Unfortunately, most analyses have shown that these scores have poor predictive value for bleeding risk. In 515 adult patients, Donze and colleagues[66] observed poor discriminatory power of the Outpatient Bleeding Risk Index, Kuijer, and RIETE scores (c-statistics = 0.54–0.57), such that these scores performed as well as random

chance in predicting bleeding risk. Similarly, Scherz and colleagues[67] also showed poor discriminatory power of the ORBI, Kuijer, Kearon, and RIETE scores (c-statistic = 0.49–0.60) in a prospective study of 663 elderly patients.

Nonvenous Thromboembolism Bleeding Risk Scores in the Deep Venous Thrombosis/Pulmonary Embolism Population

Non-VTE bleeding risk scores have not been successfully extrapolated to the DVT/PE population. Klok and colleagues attempted to prospectively validate the Kuijer, RIETE, HAS-BLED, HEMOR-RHAGES, and ATRIA in 448 PE patients; however, most scores classified them as intermediate- or high-risk for bleed at 30 days with poor discriminatory values (c-statistics: Kuijer 0.57, RIETE 0.58, atrial fibrillation scores 0.59–0.64). Other analyses have suggested that, although the HAS-BLED score may best predict late events, it still poorly estimates major VTE bleeding risk.[68] Interestingly, analyses have suggested that bleeding risk factors in the first week may differ from those associated with after the initial treatment.[60]

Summary

Prospectively validated clinical tools to predict VTE bleeding risk—the RIETE, ORBI, and

---

Table 2
Complications associated with overtesting and overdiagnosis of PE

Complication	Associated Risk
Bleeding	• Major bleeding can occur in up to 12% of treated VTE patients[69,70] • Anticoagulation complications increased from 3.1 to 5.3 per 100,000 from 1998 to 2006 (P<.001)[69] • Bleeding risk may outweigh benefit in some populations, with a 5.3% major bleed rate in isolated subsegmental PE but only a 0.7% risk of recurrent VTE[71]
Cost	• Total charges for PE admission increased from $25,293 to $43,740 from 1998 to 2006[72] • Newer anticoagulants can cost $3000 annually and, although the warfarin drug itself is cheaper, the associated bridge and monitoring increase its cost[69,73,74]
Nephrotoxin exposure	• CTPA contrast nephropathy occurs in 14%–24% of patients, with higher rates in those with critical illness or renal comorbidities[75–77] • There are no protective effects from N-acetylcysteine, normal saline, or sodium bicarbonate[76]
Contrast dye allergy	• Although not studied specifically in CTPAs, it is recognized that mild contrast reactions occur in 15% of patients receiving iodinated contrast, moderate in 1%–2%, and severe in 0.2%[77]
Radiation	• Females have a significantly higher CTPA-related lifetime attributable risk of cancer death (vs males, 48.7 vs 42.1 per 100,000 for age group 20–29; P<.0001)[78] • Estimates suggest that 3 out of every 1000 20-year-old women who undergo CTPA will develop cancer[69,79]

Abbreviations: CTPA, computed tomography pulmonary angiography; PE, pulmonary embolism; VTE, venous thrmboembolism.
Data from Refs.[69,71–79]

Kuijer—can reliably identify low risk patients; however, these scores cannot reliably predict major bleeding events. This complicates the early management of moderate and high probability PE patients, making it difficult to weigh the benefits of early anticoagulation against the risk of major bleeding.

SUMMARY

Given the potential complications associated with VTE over testing and overdiagnosis (**Table 2**), pretest probability tools play an important role in directing further evaluation and minimizing unnecessary testing. Despite clear and convincing evidence that the use of these tools improves patient care they are underused. These tools can reliably identify patients at low risk for VTE and, when combined with a negative d-dimer, can essentially eliminate PE as a diagnostic consideration.

REFERENCES

1. Goldhaber SZ. Venous thromboembolism: epidemiology and magnitude of the problem. Best Pract Res Clin Haematol 2012;25(3):235–42.
2. Geerts WH, Bergqvist D, Pineo GF, et al. Prevention of venous thromboembolism: American College of Chest Physicians evidence-based clinical practice guidelines (8th Edition). Chest 2008;133(6 Suppl): 381s–453s.
3. Heit JA, Cohen AT, Anderson FA. Estimated annual number of incident and recurrent, non-fatal and fatal Venous Thromboembolism (VTE) events in the US. Blood 2005;106(11):910.
4. Anderson FA Jr, Wheeler HB, Goldberg RJ, et al. A population-based perspective of the hospital incidence and case-fatality rates of deep vein thrombosis and pulmonary embolism. The Worcester DVT Study. Arch Intern Med 1991;151(5):933–8.
5. Le Gal G, Righini M. Controversies in the diagnosis of venous thromboembolism. J Thromb Haemost 2015;13(Suppl 1):S259–65.
6. Adams DM, Stevens SM, Woller SC, et al. Adherence to PIOPED II investigators' recommendations for computed tomography pulmonary angiography. Am J Med 2013;126(1):36–42.
7. Monreal M, Ruiz J, Olazabal A, et al. Deep venous thrombosis and the risk of pulmonary embolism. A systematic study. Chest 1992;102(3):677–81.
8. Bates SM, Jaeschke R, Stevens SM, et al. Diagnosis of DVT: antithrombotic therapy and prevention of thrombosis, 9th ed: American College of Chest Physicians evidence-based clinical practice guidelines. Chest 2012;141(2 Suppl):e351S–418.
9. Mazzolai L, Aboyans V, Ageno W, et al. Diagnosis and management of acute deep vein thrombosis: a joint consensus document from the European society of cardiology working groups of aorta and peripheral circulation and pulmonary circulation and right ventricular function. Eur Heart J 2017. [Epub ahead of print].
10. Wells PS, Anderson DR, Bormanis J, et al. Value of assessment of pretest probability of deep-vein thrombosis in clinical management. Lancet 1997; 350(9094):1795–8.
11. Wells PS, Owen C, Doucette S, et al. Does this patient have deep vein thrombosis? JAMA 2006; 295(2):199–207.
12. Wells PS, Anderson DR, Rodger M, et al. Evaluation of D-dimer in the diagnosis of suspected deep-vein thrombosis. N Engl J Med 2003;349(13):1227–35.
13. Geersing GJ, Zuithoff NPA, Kearon C, et al. Exclusion of deep vein thrombosis using the Wells rule in clinically important subgroups: individual patient data meta-analysis. BMJ 2014;348:g1340.
14. Kraaijenhagen RA, Piovella F, Bernardi E, et al. Simplification of the diagnostic management of suspected deep vein thrombosis. Arch Intern Med 2002;162(8):907–11.
15. Goodacre S, Sutton AJ, Sampson FC. Meta-analysis: the value of clinical assessment in the diagnosis of deep venous thrombosis. Ann Intern Med 2005;143(2):129–39.
16. Silveira PC, Ip IK, Goldhaber SZ, et al. Performance of wells score for deep vein thrombosis in the inpatient setting. JAMA Intern Med 2015;175(7):1112–7.
17. Oudega R, Hoes AW, Moons KG. The Wells rule does not adequately rule out deep venous thrombosis in primary care patients. Ann Intern Med 2005;143(2):100–7.
18. Toll DB, Oudega R, Vergouwe Y, et al. A new diagnostic rule for deep vein thrombosis: safety and efficiency in clinically relevant subgroups. Fam Pract 2008;25(1):3–8.
19. Subramaniam RM, Chou T, Heath R, et al. Importance of pretest probability score and D-dimer assay before sonography for lower limb deep venous thrombosis. AJR Am J Roentgenol 2006;186(1): 206–12.
20. van der Velde EF, Toll DB, Ten Cate-Hoek AJ, et al. Comparing the diagnostic performance of 2 clinical decision rules to rule out deep vein thrombosis in primary care patients. Ann Fam Med 2011;9(1): 31–6.
21. Subramaniam RM, Snyder B, Heath R, et al. Diagnosis of lower limb deep venous thrombosis in emergency department patients: performance of Hamilton and modified Wells scores. Ann Emerg Med 2006;48(6):678–85.
22. Stein PD, Beemath A, Matta F, et al. Clinical characteristics of patients with acute pulmonary embolism: data from PIOPED II. Am J Med 2007; 120(10):871–9.

23. Burge AJ, Freeman KD, Klapper PJ, et al. Increased diagnosis of pulmonary embolism without a corresponding decline in mortality during the CT era. Clin Radiol 2008;63(4):381–6.

24. DeMonaco NA, Dang Q, Kapoor WN, et al. Pulmonary embolism incidence is increasing with use of spiral computed tomography. Am J Med 2008; 121(7):611–7.

25. Wiener RS, Schwartz LM, Woloshin S. Time trends in pulmonary embolism in the United States: evidence of overdiagnosis. Arch Intern Med 2011; 171(9):831–7.

26. Prologo JD, Gilkeson RC, Diaz M, et al. CT pulmonary angiography: a comparative analysis of the utilization patterns in emergency department and hospitalized patients between 1998 and 2003. AJR Am J Roentgenol 2004;183(4):1093–6.

27. Smith SB, Geske JB, Kathuria P, et al. Analysis of national trends in admissions for pulmonary embolism. Chest 2016;150(1):35–45.

28. Remy-Jardin M, Pistolesi M, Goodman LR, et al. Management of suspected acute pulmonary embolism in the era of CT angiography: a statement from the Fleischner Society. Radiology 2007;245(2): 315–29.

29. Torbicki A, Perrier A, Konstantinides S, et al. Guidelines on the diagnosis and management of acute pulmonary embolism: the task force for the diagnosis and management of acute pulmonary embolism of the European Society of Cardiology (ESC). Eur Heart J 2008;29(18):2276–315.

30. British Thoracic Society Standards of Care Committee Pulmonary Embolism Guideline Development Group. British Thoracic Society guidelines for the management of suspected acute pulmonary embolism. Thorax 2003;58(6):470–83.

31. Fesmire FM, Brown MD, Espinosa JA, et al. Critical issues in the evaluation and management of adult patients presenting to the emergency department with suspected pulmonary embolism. Ann Emerg Med 2011;57(6):628–52.e5.

32. Wells PS, Ginsberg JS, Anderson DR, et al. Use of a clinical model for safe management of patients with suspected pulmonary embolism. Ann Intern Med 1998;129(12):997–1005.

33. Wells PS, Anderson DR, Rodger M, et al. Derivation of a simple clinical model to categorize patients probability of pulmonary embolism: increasing the models utility with the SimpliRED D-dimer. Thromb Haemost 2000;83(3):416–20.

34. van Belle A, Buller HR, Huisman MV, et al. Effectiveness of managing suspected pulmonary embolism using an algorithm combining clinical probability, D-dimer testing, and computed tomography. JAMA 2006;295(2):172–9.

35. Wells PS, Anderson DR, Rodger M, et al. Excluding pulmonary embolism at the bedside without diagnostic imaging: management of patients with suspected pulmonary embolism presenting to the emergency department by using a simple clinical model and d-dimer. Ann Intern Med 2001;135(2): 98–107.

36. Kruip MJ, Slob MJ, Schijen JH, et al. Use of a clinical decision rule in combination with D-dimer concentration in diagnostic workup of patients with suspected pulmonary embolism: a prospective management study. Arch Intern Med 2002;162(14):1631–5.

37. Geersing G-J, Erkens PMG, Lucassen WAM, et al. Safe exclusion of pulmonary embolism using the Wells rule and qualitative D-dimer testing in primary care: prospective cohort study. BMJ 2012;345: e6564.

38. Bass AR, Fields KG, Goto R, et al. Clinical decision rules for pulmonary embolism in hospitalized patients: a systematic literature review and meta-analysis. Thromb Haemost 2017;117(11):2176–85.

39. Gibson NS, Sohne M, Kruip MJ, et al. Further validation and simplification of the Wells clinical decision rule in pulmonary embolism. Thromb Haemost 2008;99(1):229–34.

40. Wicki J, Perneger TV, Junod AF, et al. Assessing clinical probability of pulmonary embolism in the emergency ward: a simple score. Arch Intern Med 2001;161(1):92–7.

41. Le Gal G, Righini M, Roy PM, et al. Prediction of pulmonary embolism in the emergency department: the revised Geneva score. Ann Intern Med 2006;144(3): 165–71.

42. Klok FA, Mos IC, Nijkeuter M, et al. Simplification of the revised Geneva score for assessing clinical probability of pulmonary embolism. Arch Intern Med 2008;168(19):2131–6.

43. Ceriani E, Combescure C, Le Gal G, et al. Clinical prediction rules for pulmonary embolism: a systematic review and meta-analysis. J Thromb Haemost 2010;8(5):957–70.

44. Douma RA, Mos IC, Erkens PM, et al. Performance of 4 clinical decision rules in the diagnostic management of acute pulmonary embolism: a prospective cohort study. Ann Intern Med 2011;154(11):709–18.

45. Hendriksen JM, Geersing GJ, Lucassen WA, et al. Diagnostic prediction models for suspected pulmonary embolism: systematic review and independent external validation in primary care. BMJ 2015;351: h4438.

46. Penaloza A, Melot C, Motte S. Comparison of the Wells score with the simplified revised Geneva score for assessing pretest probability of pulmonary embolism. Thromb Res 2011;127(2):81–4.

47. Kline JA, Mitchell AM, Kabrhel C, et al. Clinical criteria to prevent unnecessary diagnostic testing in emergency department patients with suspected pulmonary embolism. J Thromb Haemost 2004; 2(8):1247–55.

48. Singh B, Mommer SK, Erwin PJ, et al. Pulmonary embolism rule-out criteria (PERC) in pulmonary embolism—revisited: a systematic review and meta-analysis. Emerg Med J 2013;30(9):701.

49. Raja AS, Greenberg JO, Qaseem A, et al. Evaluation of patients with suspected acute pulmonary embolism: best practice advice from the clinical guidelines committee of the American College of Physicians. Ann Intern Med 2015;163(9):701–11.

50. Hugli O, Righini M, Le Gal G, et al. The pulmonary embolism rule-out criteria (PERC) rule does not safely exclude pulmonary embolism. J Thromb Haemost 2011;9(2):300–4.

51. Stein PD, Woodard PK, Weg JG, et al. Diagnostic pathways in acute pulmonary embolism: recommendations of the PIOPED II Investigators. Radiology 2007;242(1):15–21.

52. Kearon C, Ginsberg JS, Douketis J, et al. An evaluation of D-dimer in the diagnosis of pulmonary embolism: a randomized trial. Ann Intern Med 2006;144(11):812–21.

53. Musset D, Parent F, Meyer G, et al. Diagnostic strategy for patients with suspected pulmonary embolism: a prospective multicentre outcome study. Lancet 2002;360(9349):1914–20.

54. Chagnon I, Bounameaux H, Aujesky D, et al. Comparison of two clinical prediction rules and implicit assessment among patients with suspected pulmonary embolism. Am J Med 2002;113(4):269–75.

55. Runyon MS, Webb WB, Jones AE, et al. Comparison of the unstructured clinician estimate of pretest probability for pulmonary embolism to the Canadian score and the Charlotte rule: a prospective observational study. Acad Emerg Med 2005;12(7):587–93.

56. Penaloza A, Verschuren F, Meyer G, et al. Comparison of the unstructured clinician gestalt, the Wells score, and the revised Geneva score to estimate pretest probability for suspected pulmonary embolism. Ann Emerg Med 2013;62:117–24.

57. Lucassen W, Geersing GJ, Erkens PM, et al. Clinical decision rules for excluding pulmonary embolism: a meta-analysis. Ann Intern Med 2011;155(7):448–60.

58. Smith SB, Geske JB, Maguire JM, et al. Early anticoagulation is associated with reduced mortality for acute pulmonary embolism. Chest 2010;137(6):1382–90.

59. Kearon C, Kahn SR, Agnelli G, et al. Antithrombotic therapy for venous thromboembolic disease: American College of Chest Physicians evidence-based clinical practice guidelines (8th Edition). Chest 2008;133(6 Suppl):454s–545s.

60. Klok FA, Niemann C, Dellas C, et al. Performance of five different bleeding-prediction scores in patients with acute pulmonary embolism. J Thromb Thrombolysis 2016;41(2):312–20.

61. Ruiz-Gimenez N, Suarez C, Gonzalez R, et al. Predictive variables for major bleeding events in patients presenting with documented acute venous thromboembolism. Findings from the RIETE Registry. Thromb Haemost 2008;100(1):26–31.

62. Beyth RJ, Quinn LM, Landefeld CS. Prospective evaluation of an index for predicting the risk of major bleeding outpatients treated with warfarin. Am J Med 1998;105:91–9.

63. Wells PS, Forgie MA, Simms M, et al. The outpatient bleeding risk index: validation of a tool for predicting bleeding rates in patients treated for deep venous thrombosis and pulmonary embolism. Arch Intern Med 2003;163(8):917–20.

64. Kuijer PM, Hutten BA, Prins MH, et al. Prediction of the risk of bleeding during anticoagulant treatment for venous thromboembolism. Arch Intern Med 1999;159(5):457–60.

65. Kearon C, Ginsberg JS, Kovacs MJ, et al. Comparison of low-intensity warfarin therapy with conventional-intensity warfarin therapy for long-term prevention of recurrent venous thromboembolism. N Engl J Med 2003;349(7):631–9.

66. Donze J, Rodondi N, Waeber G, et al. Scores to predict major bleeding risk during oral anticoagulation therapy: a prospective validation study. Am J Med 2012;125(11):1095–102.

67. Scherz N, Mean M, Limacher A, et al. Prospective, multicenter validation of prediction scores for major bleeding in elderly patients with venous thromboembolism. J Thromb Haemost 2013;11(3):435–43.

68. Riva N, Bellesini M, Di Minno MN, et al. Poor predictive value of contemporary bleeding risk scores during long-term treatment of venous thromboembolism. A multicentre retrospective cohort study. Thromb Haemost 2014;112(3):511–21.

69. Wiener RS, Schwartz LM, Woloshin S. When a test is too good: how CT pulmonary angiograms find pulmonary emboli that do not need to be found. BMJ 2013;347:f3368.

70. Spencer FA, Emery C, Joffe SW, et al. Incidence rates, clinical profile, and outcomes of patients with venous thromboembolism. The Worcester VTE Study. J Thromb Thrombolysis 2009;28(4):401–9.

71. Donato AA, Khoche S, Santora J, et al. Clinical outcomes in patients with isolated subsegmental pulmonary emboli diagnosed by multidetector CT pulmonary angiography. Thromb Res 2010;126(4):e266–70.

72. Park B, Messina L, Dargon P, et al. Recent trends in clinical outcomes and resource utilization for pulmonary embolism in the United States: findings from the nationwide inpatient sample. Chest 2009;136(4):983–90.

73. Bullano MF, Willey V, Hauch O, et al. Longitudinal evaluation of health plan cost per venous thromboembolism or bleed event in patients with a prior venous thromboembolism event during

hospitalization. J Manag Care Pharm 2005;11(8): 663–73.

74. Kahler ZP, Beam DM, Kline JA. Cost of treating venous thromboembolism with heparin and warfarin versus home treatment with rivaroxaban. Acad Emerg Med 2015;22(7):796–802.

75. Mitchell AM, Jones AE, Tumlin JA, et al. Prospective study of the incidence of contrast-induced nephropathy among patients evaluated for pulmonary embolism by contrast-enhanced computed tomography. Acad Emerg Med 2012;19(6):618–25.

76. Turedi S, Erdem E, Karaca Y, et al. The high risk of contrast-induced nephropathy in patients with suspected pulmonary embolism despite three different

prophylaxis: a randomized controlled trial. Acad Emerg Med 2016;23(10):1136–45.

77. Namasivayam S, Kalra MK, Torres WE, et al. Adverse reactions to intravenous iodinated contrast media: a primer for radiologists. Emerg Radiol 2006; 12(5):210–5.

78. Woo JKH, Chiu RYW, Thakur Y, et al. Risk-benefit analysis of pulmonary CT angiography in patients with suspected pulmonary embolus. Am J Roentgenology 2012;198(6):1332–9.

79. Smith-Bindman R, Lipson J, Marcus R, et al. Radiation dose associated with common computed tomography examinations and the associated lifetime attributable risk of cancer. Arch Intern Med 2009;169(22):2078–86.

Prevention of Deep Vein Thrombosis and Pulmonary Embolism in High-Risk Medical Patients

Megan McCullough, MD[a],*, Cyrus Kholdani, MD[b,1],
Roham T. Zamanian, MD[b,2]

KEYWORDS

- Venous thromboembolism • Deep vein thrombosis • Pulmonary embolism • Prevention and control

KEY POINTS

- Venous thromboembolism (VTE) occurs in approximately 3% to 16% of hospitalized patients on wards and 10% to 40% of those in medical intensive care units.
- American College of Chest Physician guidelines along with a growing body of literature implore the use of pharmacologic prophylaxis in high-risk patients and mechanical prophylaxis when anticoagulants are contraindicated.
- There is consistent evidence that unfractionated heparin, low-molecular-weight heparin, and fondaparinux reduce VTE events by approximately 50% to 75% in high-risk groups, with a trend toward superiority of low-molecular-weight heparin.
- The risk of major bleeding with pharmacologic prophylaxis is low and large meta-analyses show that low-molecular-weight heparin may have slightly decreased bleeding risk compared with unfractionated heparin.
- Mechanical prophylaxis with intermittent pneumatic compression devices decrease VTE in acutely ill medical adults but with lesser efficacy compared with pharmacologic prophylaxis.

INTRODUCTION

Incident venous thromboembolism (VTE), which includes deep vein thrombosis (DVT) and pulmonary embolism (PE), accounts for $7 billion to $10 billion of United States health care expenditures each year.[1] Approximately 10% of inpatient deaths are attributable to VTE, 60% of which occur in nonsurgical patients based on necroscopy examination.[2,3] Pharmacologic and mechanical modalities can decrease the rate of VTE by 50–75%, yet the rate of appropriate VTE prophylaxis in acutely ill medical patients has been reported as low as 40% in the recent past.[4] In the United States, the Joint Commission and the Centers for Medicaid & Medicare Services consider VTE prophylaxis in high-risk patients a core quality measure.[5] Features that confer higher risk are either inherited or acquired. The most common acquired risks are age, acute congestive heart failure, respiratory failure, rheumatologic disease, inflammatory bowel disease, malignancy,

Disclosure Statement: The authors do not have any financial interest in the subject matter or material discuss nor with a company making a competing product.
[a] Department of Internal Medicine, Yale University School of Medicine, 789 Howard Avenue, New Haven, CT 06510, USA; [b] Division of Pulmonary and Critical Care Medicine, Stanford University School of Medicine, Palo Alto, CA, USA
[1] 300 Pasteur Drive A251, Stanford, CA 94305.
[2] 300 Pasteur Drive A251, MC 5221, Stanford, CA 94305.
* Corresponding author.
E-mail address: megan.mccullough@yale.edu

Clin Chest Med 39 (2018) 483–492
https://doi.org/10.1016/j.ccm.2018.04.002
0272-5231/18/© 2018 Elsevier Inc. All rights reserved.

trauma, prolonged immobility, and postsurgical status.[6,7] The studies that guide VTE prophylaxis date back to the 1970s and extend through present day. Prophylaxis options range from a variety of injectable heparins to direct oral anticoagulants among medical therapies and from graduated compression stockings (GCS) to intermittent pneumatic compression (IPC) devices among mechanical ones (**Table 1**).

American College of Chest Physicians (ACCP) guidelines suggest that any form of prophylaxis can lead to reduction in VTE by 0 to 1 fewer per 1000 persons in low-risk patients and by 34 fewer per 1000 in high-risk patients.[8] In medical patients,

Table 1
Types of venous thromboembolism prophylaxis

Prophylaxis Method	Mechanism of Action	Advantages	Disadvantages	Indications for Primary Venous Thromboembolism Prophylaxis
UFH	Nonspecifically binds to ATIII to inactivate thrombin	Low cost Reversal agent	Frequent dosing Unpredictable dose response Causes HIT Nonspecific binding to plasma proteins	Hospitalized medical patients Critically ill adults
LMWH Enoxaparin Dalteparin	Specifically inactivates factor Xa via ATIII	Once-daily dosing Trend toward improved efficacy over UFH	Increased cost compared with unfractionated heparin Protamine reverses 60% of activity Causes HIT Enoxaparin requires dose adjustment in renal impairment whereas dalteparin does not	Hospitalized medical patients Critically ill adults Enoxaparin approved for extended-duration VTE prophylaxis in those with active malignancy
Pentasaccharide Fondaparinux	Specifically inactivates factor Xa via ATIII	Once-daily dosing	Increased cost compared with UFH but similar to LMWH No reversal agent	Hospitalized medical patients Critically ill adults Active malignancy
Betrixiban	Direct and selective inhibition of factor Xa	Oral agent	High cost No reversal agent Used with caution in renal impairment	Extended-duration prophylaxis in hospitalized medical patients Not endorsed by guidelines yet
GCS	Increases blood flow, decreases venous stasis	Low cost Does not increase bleeding risk	Not effective for VTE prophylaxis Skin breakdown	Not considered first line
IPC	Increases blood flow leading to release of tPA, prostacyclin, and NO	Does not increase bleeding risk	Poor efficacy when not battery powered or when low compliance Not as effective as pharmacologic prophylaxis	Immobilization due to stroke Medical patients in whom pharmacologic prophylaxis is contraindicated

Abbreviations: ATIII, antithrombin III; GCS, graduated compression stockings; HIT, heparin induced thrombocyopenia; IPC, intermittent pneumatic compression device; LMWH, low molecular weight heparin; NO, nitric oxide; tPA, tissue plasminogen activator; UFH, unfractionated heparin; VTE, venous thromboembolism.

VTE risk reduction does not translate to a mortality benefit given the prohibitive enrollment numbers needed to detect such a difference.[9] In both medical and surgical fields, experts suggest the use of risk assessment models (RAMs) to determine which patients will benefit most from VTE prophylaxis. The ACCP guidelines recommend the Padua Prediction Score to risk-stratify medical patients.[8] The largest VTE prophylaxis clinical trials use components of these RAMs in their inclusion criteria, but a single RAM has not been universally applied. Heterogeneity in study methods are limited not only to inclusion criteria but also to VTE detection methods, which include screening those with a positive D-dimer or VTE symptoms or all subjects regardless of symptoms. Although differences in seminal clinical trials have an impact on generalizability, clinical themes can be gleaned from the literature for most patient populations. When the decision lies not in whether or not to provide VTE prophylaxis but rather in which type, clinicians must appreciate the nuance that distinguishes one high-risk patient from the next. This article presents evidence to support a population-specific approach to mechanical and pharmacologic VTE prophylaxis (**Fig. 1**).

HOSPITALIZED MEDICAL PATIENTS

According to a meta-analysis performed by Kahn and colleagues[8] to develop the ACCP antithrombotic guidelines in 2012, baseline risk for all nonsurgical hospitalized patients was 0.8% for DVT and 0.4% for PE. When they calculated risk based on the Padua Prediction Score, they found a rate of 0.3% in low-risk patients and 11% in high-risk patients.[8] This rate of VTE occurrence was also demonstrated by Greene and colleagues[10] in their retrospective study of more than 60,000 admissions from a consortium of 35 hospitals in which the overall risk of VTE was 1%. In trials that screen all subjects for VTE regardless of symptoms, the incidence can be as high as 20% over the course of hospitalization.[11] The studies (described later) comprise a cannon of literature that support the use of anticoagulation to prevent DVT and PE in high-risk acutely ill medical patients.

Unfractionated Heparin Versus Placebo

Evidenced-based use of subcutaneous low-dose unfractionated heparin (UFH) for VTE prophylaxis

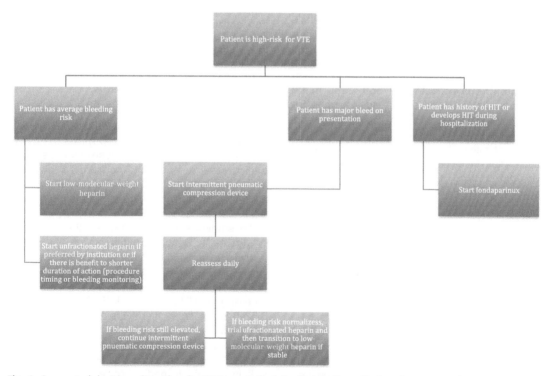

Fig. 1. Suggested decision algorithm for VTE prophylaxis in acutely ill medical patients. Consider patient's risk of VTE. Both LMWH and UFH are first-line agents, but the once-daily dosing of LMWH and trend toward greater efficacy make it preferred at some institutions. UFH may be preferred if a patient will be going for a procedure with high bleeding risk. If patient has evidence of major bleeding on presentation (life-threatening bleed, bleeding requiring transfusion of 2 or more units, or bleeding in critical organ or area), start IPC. If patient has a history of HIT or develops HIT, start fondaparinux.

dates back to a landmark trial in 1973 that found that 5000 units of subcutaneous heparin, administered 3 times a day, decreased overall VTE from 21.5% to 3.6%.[12] Critics of this study note that it was a small trial of 350 patients (22% medical) and VTE events were detected by universal screening with I-fibrinogen scanning. In 1981, a randomized control trial of 100 subjects reproduced these findings in a high-risk medical cohort. The investigators found that thrice daily heparin injections decreased VTE risk from 26% in the placebo group to 4% in the treatment group.[13] It was primarily on the basis of studies such as these along with others involving surgical populations that VTE prophylaxis became widespread on the inpatient medical wards.

Unfractionated Heparin Dosing Strategy

Whether heparin should be dosed twice daily or thrice daily is a topic of clinical interest. When data from a variety of trials are pooled, there seem to be similar event rates of VTE with twice-daily and thrice daily dosing.[8] In a meta-analysis published in 2007 that included data from 8000 subjects, however, there was a statistically significant decrease in the event rate of PE with thrice daily dosing.[14] This decrease in event rate of PE was not reproducible in a more recent meta-analysis, including data from 27,000 subjects.[15] In this study, twice-daily and thrice daily dosing yielded similar event rates of DVT, PE, and major bleeding. The investigators of both large meta-analyses note that a head-to-head trial of twice-daily versus thrice daily UFH would have to enroll 150,000 subjects to show a 10% difference in VTE event rates. Despite lack of convincing evidence that thrice daily dosing is superior to twice-daily dosing, it is reasonable to dose UFH based on its half-life of 1.0 hour to 1.5 hours, which confers a duration of action of 4.0 hours to 7.5 hours.

Low-Molecular-Weight Heparin Versus Placebo

Compared with UFH, LMWH is longer acting, inhibits antithrombin with more specificity, and has increased bioavailability. Protamine sulfate neutralizes only 40-60% of its activity, making it theoretically less favorable than UFH in those at high risk for bleeding.[16] Systematic reviews of the literature demonstrate that nadroparin, tinzaparin, certoparin, dalteparin, and enoxaparin are effective in preventing VTE.[9] Although nadroparin was the first LMWH approved for VTE prophylaxis abroad, the more commonly used agents in the United States are enoxaparin and dalteparin. The MEDENOX

and PREVENT clinical trials, similarly designed, compared the efficacy of enoxaparin and dalteparin, respectively, to placebo. The MEDENOX trial randomized patients to enoxaparin, 20 mg or 40 mg, or placebo and showed that 40-mg daily dosing is most effective and decreased the incidence of asymptomatic DVT at 14 days from 13.9% to 5.5%.[17] Alikhan and colleagues[18] performed a post hoc analysis of high-risk subgroups of this trial. In patients with acute New York Heart Association class III to class IV congestive heart failure, chronic heart failure, acute or chronic respiratory failure, or age greater than 75 years, the rate of VTE decreased by 72% to 78%. Those with cancer, obesity, and acute rheumatic disease saw 50% to 59% fewer VTE events. In 2004, the PREVENT trial investigators showed an asymptomatic DVT incidence of 1.8% with dalteparin versus 3.7% with placebo at 21 days.[19] Although risk reduction was greatest in patents older than 75 years, dalteparin did not reproduce the same degree of risk reduction as enoxaparin in those with heart and respiratory failure. The rate of major bleeding was not significantly different in those who received LMWH compared with placebo (0.49% with dalteparin and 1.7% with enoxaparin). Together, the data from LMWH trials are robust and consistent; both enoxaparin and dalteparin should be considered first-line agents for VTE prophylaxis.

Unfractionated Heparin Versus Low-Molecular-Weight Heparin

It is reasonable to hypothesize that LMWHs may be more favorable for VTE prophylaxis than UFH due to their more predictable dose response. Fluctuating renal function and concern for bleeding risk, however, limit their use. The LMWHs enoxaparin, nadroparin, and certoparin have been studied in comparison to UFH. A large meta-analysis of 36 studies sought to compare the 2 classes of agents.[14] Despite limitations of the meta-analysis, including heterogeneity in medical populations and types of LMWH studied, there was a clear trend toward decreased DVT events in those receiving LMWH (relative risk [RR] 0.68; 95% CI, 0.52–0.88) whereas there was no statistically significant difference in rates of PE or major bleeding. Similar results were reported in a more recent systematic review on the use of heparins to prevent VTE in acutely ill medical patients. Again, there was a decreased risk of DVT in those receiving LMWH compared with UFH, but no difference between the 2 agents in effectiveness of preventing nonfatal and fatal PE.[9] This systematic review also found a statically significant reduction in major bleeding in the LMWH group compared with the UFH group (odds ratio [OR] 0.43; 95% CI, 0.22–0.83). Despite data that support the use of LMWH over UFH, guidelines hesitate to universally recommend it over UFH, citing that the trials have not been powered to detect a mortality benefit and any bleeding risk reduction may be negligible.[8]

Pentasaccharides

Like UFH and LMWH, pentasaccharides decrease factor Xa activity via stimulation of antithrombin III. Unlike heparins, pentasaccharides have much longer half-lives and do not cause heparin-induced thrombocytopenia (HIT). Fondaparinux was the first drug developed in its class and remains the only pentasaccharide available in the United States. Due to its long duration of action and lack of a reversal agent, it is used with some caution in the acute care setting when the bleeding risk is unknown. The use of fondaparinux compared with placebo for VTE prophylaxis in medical patients was studied by Cohen and colleagues[20] in the ARTEMIS trial. Fondaparinux reduced VTE events by 46.7% compared with placebo in subjects who were ages 60 years or older and admitted for acute respiratory failure, congestive heart failure, or inflammatory illness. Bleeding complications were rare in each group and not significantly different. Despite few data on pentasaccharides for VTE prophylaxis, it can be considered in patients with a history HIT who have a low bleeding risk.

Direct Oral Anticoagulants Versus Low-Molecular-Weight Heparin for Extended-Duration Venous Thromboembolism Prophylaxis

In recent years, several investigators have hypothesized that direct oral factor Xa inhibitors could achieve effective and safe VTE prophylaxis. These agents are of particular interest to clinicians who plan to extend VTE prophylaxis from the inpatient to the outpatient setting due to their oral route of administration, predictable pharmacokinetics, and minimal drug interactions. The EXCLAIM trial of enoxaparin for extended-duration prophylaxis laid the framework for the ADOPT, MAGELLAN, and APEX studies that tested apixaban, rivaroxaban, and betrixaban, respectively. Enoxaparin, 40 mg, administered once daily in the 10 ±4 days after hospitalization, was found to decrease VTE events from 4% in the placebo group to 2.5% in the treatment group.[21] This amounted to 6 fewer proximal DVTs per 1000 persons at an average of 38 days' follow-up, with reported episodes of major bleeding in 5 per 1000

persons.[8] Consequently, the ACCP guidelines recommend against extended-duration VTE prophylaxis. Since guideline publication in 2012, betrixaban emerged on the market as the only FDA-approved direct oral anticoagulants in hospitalized medical patients who are at high risk for thrombotic events. The evidence stems from the APEX trial that randomized 7513 patients to short-term treatment with enoxaparin for 6 days to 14 days or with betrixaban, 40 mg or 80 mg, daily for 35 days to 42 days. The results showed a decrease in composite outcome (fatal PE, nonfatal PE, and asymptomatic and symptomatic proximal DVT) in those treated with betrixaban, 80 mg, compared with enoxaparin (6.27% vs 8.39%; $P = .023$).[22] There was no significant difference in major bleeding between groups.

The ADOPT trial, which evaluated the efficacy of apixaban versus enoxaparin for VTE prophylaxis, reported that primary outcome of death, PE, and DVT occurred in 2.7% of patients on apixaban versus 3.1% of patients on enoxaparin.[23] The study was underpowered, however, and results did not reach statistical significance. It was stopped early due to increased major bleeding in the apixaban group (0.47% vs 0.19%; $P = .04$). The investigators conclude that apixaban is not superior to enoxaparin for extended prophylaxis in hospitalized medical patients at high-risk for VTE.

The MAGELLAN trial compared the safety and efficacy of rivaroxaban to enoxaparin and found that rivaroxaban, 40 mg once daily, was noninferior to enoxaparin at 10 days and superior to placebo after 35 days.[24] Like apixiban, rivaroxaban led to more major bleeding events than enoxaparin across the entire study period. Rivaroxaban for VTE prophylaxis is still under examination by the MARINER trial investigators who are currently enrolling high-risk medical patients to receive 45 days of rivaroxaban or placebo. In the coming years, the authors of this article predict that extended VTE prophylaxis in high-risk individuals will be used more readily. Further studies must evaluate efficacy and safety in subsets of acutely ill medical patients to determine which patients will benefit most from anticoagulation when they leave the hospital.

Mechanical Prophylaxis

Patients at high risk for thrombosis should be treated with pharmacologic prophylaxis. In the event that strict contraindications to anticoagulation exist, clinicians should use mechanical methods. The most readily available options are IPC devices and GCS. Mechanical prophylaxis increases venous blood flow and decreases venous pressure, consequently increasing the arteriovenous pressure gradient. Changes in flow cause stretch and shear stress on endothelial cells, leading to an increase in circulating tissue plasminogen activator, prostacyclin, and nitric oxide.[25] Although the theoretic benefits of increased fibrinolysis, antiplatelet aggregation, and vasodilation are compelling, in vivo validation in acutely ill medical patients is lacking. A majority of data are from studies in surgical subpopulations that consistently show a decrease in VTE with IPC or GCS use.[26] Translation of this work to the medical wards started in patients who presented with acute myocardial infarction.[27] Data to support modern use of mechanical prophylaxis in acutely ill medical patients are from the CLOTS trial of immobilized stroke patients. In this patient population, thigh-high GCS did not decrease rate of DVT compared with controls and had adverse outcomes of skin complications (blisters, ulcers, breaks, and necrosis) at a rate of 5.1%.[28] IPC devices were studied by the CLOTS 3 investigators and produced more favorable and statistically significant outcomes.[29] Of the 1438 patients who received IPC, VTE occurred in 8.5% compared with 12.1% of the 1438 controls leading to RR reduction of 0.69 (95% CI, 0.55–0.86).

Despite the limitations of extrapolating these data to other high-risk acutely ill medical patients, the authors of this article recommend IPC over GCS stockings when pharmacologic prophylaxis is contraindicated or interrupted.

Malignancy as a Special Population

Malignancy promotes a prothrombotic state through a host of biological mechanisms marked by release of procoagulants and inflammatory cytokines by tumor cells and decreased fibrinolytic activity.[30] The risk of VTE is compounded when chemotherapy includes an antiangiogenic agent, when tumors cause venous compression, or when management includes surgery.[31] Compared with the general population, individuals with cancer are at a 5-fold to 9-fold increased risk of VTE.[31] VTE events occur most commonly in adenomas of pancreas, lung, and gastrointestinal tract due not only to the prothrombotic mechanisms of mucinous producing tumors but also to the prevalence of these tumors.[32,33] Brain and ovarian cancers also carry high risk of VTE, but they are more rare and account for a smaller fraction of cancer-related VTE events overall. In several oncologic studies, VTE was found to be an independent risk factor for mortality.[34,35] Increased mortality associated with VTE might be related to

biologically aggressive cancers, other comorbid conditions, or the complications of VTE and its treatment.[34] The well-established risk of VTE during malignancy resulted in several studies designed to determine the safety and efficacy of VTE prophylaxis in this population.

The ACCP and National Comprehensive Cancer Network (NCCN) recommend VTE prophylaxis in patients with both presumed and confirmed active malignancy with either UFH or LMWH in absence of absolute contraindications. These guidelines support the use of prophylaxis in those with at least 1 other risk factor for VTE, such as previous venous thrombosis, immobilization, hormonal therapy, or use of angiogenesis inhibitors, or for up to 4 weeks after high-risk abdominal or pelvic surgery.[8] In the outpatient and perioperative settings, there is extensive literature evaluating the use of aspirin, warfarin, UFH, LMWH, fondaparinux, and direct oral anticoagulants for primary VTE prophylaxis over a variety of treatment durations. A Cochrane review from 2016 sought to analyze the available data, which yielded consistent evidence that LMWH reduces VTE events in ambulatory cancer patients compared with no prophylaxis (RR 0.54; 95% CI, 0.38–0.75; no heterogeneity, $Tau^2 = 0.00\%$).[36] In comparison with other active forms of prophylaxis, LMWH was found superior to warfarin and noninferior to aspirin in patients with multiple myeloma. When the ultra-LMWH, semuloparin, was compared with placebo in patients with lung, pancreatic, stomach, colon or rectum, bladder, or ovarian cancer, it was found to decrease the rate of symptomatic VTE from 3.4% to 1.2% (hazard ratio 0.36; 95% CI, 0.21–0.60; $P<.001$) without increased bleeding risk.[37] This study, along with numerous others, included subjects without regard to the list of additional risk factors noted by the ACCP and NCCN guidelines.[31] The recently published NCCN guidelines address this by suggesting consideration of primary VTE prophylaxis in subjects at high risk based on the validated Khorana RAM.[38] The guidelines cite a lack of high-quality evidence on the risk of clinically relevant bleeding as the primary factor limiting more widespread use of primary VTE prophylaxis in oncology patients.

CRITICALLY ILL MEDICAL PATIENTS

The incidence of VTE in critically ill patients without prophylaxis varies greatly, but most studies report a value of 10% to 40%.[39] Incidence rates differ due to heterogeneity of inclusion criteria and methods for detecting VTE events. Even among patients who receive adequate prophylaxis, the risk of VTE does not diminish completely. One prospective observational trial at a large academic center found that 8% of critically ill medical patients on risk-stratified prophylaxis still developed VTE.[40] Most studies that try to determine the incidence of VTE in intensive care unit (ICU) patients screen all subjects. Because not all VTE events are clinically relevant, 1 group of investigators performed a retrospective cohort study of 12,338 patients from 12 ICUs in Canada and found a shockingly low event rate of symptomatic VTE of 1% to 2%.[41] The low rate of symptomatic VTE can be attributed to the difficulty in diagnosing VTE in immobilized, ventilated, and sedated patients who cannot describe leg or chest pain or develop unilateral leg swelling as reliably as ambulatory patients.

Unfractionated Heparin or Low-Molecular-Weight Heparin Versus Placebo

In critically ill adults, UFH dosed twice a day has been compared with placebo in 2 randomized control trials. The first of the 2 studies reported a decrease in DVT from 17/59 (29%) to 8/60 (13%).[42] Similar statistics emerged from a larger trial conducted by Kapoor and colleagues,[43] who published a decrease in DVT from 122/309 (39%) to 44/401 (11%) in a cohort of medical ICU patients. Fraisse and colleagues[44] studied the efficacy and safety of nadroparin compared with placebo for the prevention of DVT in mechanically ventilated patients admitted to medical ICUs in France. Despite participation of 34 ICUs, the investigators only enrolled 223 patients of whom the primary outcome was assessed in 169 with venography. This LMWH was associated with a DVT RR reduction of 45%. On the basis of trials, such as these, and data from surgical populations, routine pharmacologic prophylaxis is recommended by the ACCP over no prophylaxis.

Unfractionated Heparin Versus Low-Molecular-Weight Heparin

When considering which type of parenteral prophylaxis to administer, the decision is most often between UFH and LMWH. A meta-analysis published in 2015 aimed to determine which of the 2 agents is superior in critically ill adults.[45] This study included 8 trials that involved trauma, surgical, and medical patients. The results showed a 10% decrease in DVT and PE in those who received LMWH versus UFH. In several of the studies included in the analysis, mechanical prophylaxis was also used and the inclusion criteria did not discriminate based on type of LMWH or dosing of UFH causing readers to question whether confounding limits application of these results. One of the most often cited studies on this topic is the PROTECT trial that compared twice-daily UFH to once-daily dalteparin in 3600 critically ill adults, of whom 76% were medical.[46] Dalteparin was considered an ideal LMWH to study due to evidence that it does not lead to bioaccumulation in renal failure as previously reported with enoxaparin.[47,48] There was no difference in the primary outcome of all VTE between the 2 groups, but there was a trend toward decreased PE in the dalteparin group. The risk of major bleeding between groups was the same at 5.5%. Since the ACCP published their guidelines in 2012, there is no new compelling evidence to push medical intensivists toward more regular use of LMWH over UFH, but there does seem to be indirect evidence from mixed population meta-analyses that favor LMWH.

Mechanical Prophylaxis

Data extrapolated from surgical literature led the ACCP to recommend IPC over no prophylaxis in critically ill nonsurgical adults. At the time of the most recent guideline publication, the authors were not aware of any clinical trials that compared mechanical prophylaxis to placebo in a critically ill medical population. There is a small body of evidence, however, that supports the use of IPC devices for this purpose. Zhang and colleagues[49] enrolled 162 critically ill medical patients into a randomized trial that compared IPC with no prophylaxis and found that the IPC group had a significantly lower rate of DVT than the control group (3.8% [3/79] versus 19.28% [16/83]; $P<.01$). This study was included in a meta-analysis published in 2016 that analyzed data from multiple trials that used IPC in either a control arm or treatment arm and showed a trend toward decreased VTE events in IPC versus no prophylaxis, but the results did not reach statistical significance.[50] Despite widespread use of IPC in medical ICUs, reproducible efficacy data are lacking.

Inferior Vena Cava Filters

Neither nonsurgical nor surgical ACCP guidelines recommend the use of inferior vena cava filters for primary VTE prophylaxis. The utility of inferior vena cava filters is addressed in a Brian P. Holly and colleagues' article, "IVC Filters: Why, Who, and for How Long?," in this issue.

SUMMARY

More than 40 years of research supports the use of VTE prophylaxis in high-risk hospitalized medical patients. The ACCP guidelines recommend heparins as first-line agents and mechanical prophylaxis as second-line agents. The risk of major bleeding with anticoagulants is less than 1% and not significantly different among recommended or approved agents.[8,9] Although data support the use of UFH, LMWH, or fondaparinux, there is a trend toward superiority of LMWH in both nonsurgical patients on the ward and in the ICU. Clinicians should be adept at identifying patients with high-risk features for VTE and start prophylaxis after considering bleeding risk and history of HIT (see **Fig. 1**). Despite efforts to improve VTE prophylaxis rates and methods, VTE events are not completely mitigated with the current guideline-directed therapy and clinicians should still suspect VTE in the appropriate context.

Modern research focuses on the duration of VTE prophylaxis and methods for monitoring heparin activity. Whereas traditional VTE prophylaxis methods are limited to the hospital setting, there is a growing body of literature to support extended-duration therapy. Optimizing use of heparins with anti–factor Xa levels or with thromboelastography is another area of interest, but results from small trials yield inconclusive evidence to date. Given the range of pharmacologic and mechanical prophylaxis options, clinicians can tailor therapy based on their preference for dosing frequency, bleeding risk, concern for HIT, cost of therapy, indication for extended therapy, and institutional availability.

REFERENCES

1. Grosse SD, Nelson RE, Nyarko KA, et al. The economic burden of incident venous thromboembolism in the United States: a review of estimated attributable healthcare costs. Thromb Res 2016; 137(Supplement C):3–10.
2. Alikhan R, Peters F, Wilmott R, et al. Fatal pulmonary embolism in hospitalised patients: a necropsy review. J Clin Pathol 2004;57(12):1254–7.
3. Baglin TP, White K, Charles A. Fatal pulmonary embolism in hospitalised medical patients. J Clin Pathol 1997;50(7):609.
4. Cohen AT, Tapson VF, Bergmann J-F, et al. Venous thromboembolism risk and prophylaxis in the acute hospital care setting (ENDORSE study): a multinational cross-sectional study. Lancet 2008;371(9610): 387–94.
5. The Joint Commission. Available at: https://www.jointcommission.org/venous_thromboembolism/. Accessed November 13, 2017.
6. Heit JA, O'Fallon W, Petterson TM, et al. Relative impact of risk factors for deep vein thrombosis and pulmonary embolism: a population-based study. Arch Intern Med 2002;162(11):1245–8.
7. Barbar S, Noventa F, Rossetto V, et al. A risk assessment model for the identification of hospitalized medical patients at risk for venous thromboembolism: the Padua Prediction Score. J Thromb Haemost 2010;8(11):2450–7.
8. Kahn SR, Lim W, Dunn AS, et al. Prevention of VTE in nonsurgical patients: antithrombotic therapy and prevention of thrombosis, 9th ed: American College of Chest Physicians evidence-based clinical practice guidelines. Chest 2012;141(2, Supplement): e195S–226.
9. Alikhan R, Forster R, Cohen AT. Heparin for the prevention of venous thromboembolism in acutely ill medical patients (excluding stroke and myocardial infarction). Cochrane Database Syst Rev 2014;(5):CD003747.
10. Greene MT, Spyropoulos AC, Chopra V, et al. Validation of risk assessment models of venous thromboembolism in hospitalized medical patients. Am J Med 2016;129(9):1001.e9-e8.
11. Kleber F-X, Witt C, Vogel G, et al. Randomized comparison of enoxaparin with unfractionated heparin for the prevention of venous thromboembolism in medical patients with heart failure or severe respiratory disease. Am Heart J 2003;145(4):614–21.
12. Gallus AS, Hirsh J, Tutle RJ, et al. Small subcutaneous doses of heparin in prevention of venous thrombosis. N Engl J Med 1973;288(11):545–51.
13. Belch JJ, Lowe GD, Ward AG, et al. Prevention of deep vein thrombosis in medical patients by low-dose heparin. Scottish Med J 1981;26(2):115–7.
14. Wein L, Wein S, Haas SJ, et al. Pharmacological venous thromboembolism prophylaxis in hospitalized medical patients: a meta-analysis of randomized controlled trials. Arch Intern Med 2007; 167(14):1476–86.
15. Phung OJ, Kahn SR, Cook DJ, et al. Dosing frequency of unfractionated heparin thromboprophylaxis: a meta-analysis. Chest 2011;140(2):374–81.
16. Schroeder M, Hogwood J, Gray E, et al. Protamine neutralisation of low molecular weight heparins and their oligosaccharide components. Anal Bioanal Chem 2011;399(2):763–71.
17. Samama MM, Cohen AT, Darmon JY, et al. A comparison of enoxaparin with placebo for the prevention of venous thromboembolism in acutely ill medical patients. Prophylaxis in medical patients with enoxaparin study group. N Engl J Med 1999; 341(11):793–800.
18. Alikhan R, Cohen AT, Combe S, et al. Prevention of venous thromboembolism in medical patients with enoxaparin: a subgroup analysis of the MEDENOX study. Blood Coagul Fibrinolysis 2003;14(4):341–6.
19. Leizorovicz A, Cohen AT, Turpie AGG, et al. Randomized, placebo-controlled trial of dalteparin for the prevention of venous thromboembolism in

19. acutely ill medical patients. Circulation 2004;110(7): 874–9.

20. Cohen AT, Davidson BL, Gallus AS, et al. Efficacy and safety of fondaparinux for the prevention of venous thromboembolism in older acute medical patients: randomised placebo controlled trial. BMJ 2006;332(7537):325–9.

21. Hull RD, Schellong SM, Tapson VF, et al. Extended-duration venous thromboembolism prophylaxis in acutely ill medical patients with recently reduced mobility: a randomized trial. Ann Intern Med 2010; 153(1):8–18.

22. Gibson CM, Halaby R, Korjian S, et al. The safety and efficacy of full- versus reduced-dose betrixaban in the acute medically ill VTE (Venous Thromboembolism) prevention with extended-duration betrixaban (APEX) trial. Am Heart J 2017;185:93–100.

23. Goldhaber SZ, Leizorovicz A, Kakkar AK, et al. Apixaban versus enoxaparin for thromboprophylaxis in medically ill patients. N Engl J Med 2011;365(23): 2167–77.

24. Cohen AT, Spiro TE, Buller HR, et al. Rivaroxaban for thromboprophylaxis in acutely ill medical patients. N Engl J Med 2013;368(6):513–23.

25. Chen AH, Frangos SG, Kilaru S, et al. Intermittent pneumatic compression devices – physiological mechanisms of action. Eur J Vasc Endovasc Surg 2001;21(5):383–92.

26. Gould MK, Garcia DA, Wren SM, et al. Prevention of VTE in nonorthopedic surgical patients: antithrombotic therapy and prevention of thrombosis, 9th ed: American College of Chest Physicians evidence-based clinical practice guidelines. Chest 2012;141(2 Suppl):e227S–277.

27. Kierkegaard A, Norgren L. Graduated compression stockings in the prevention of deep vein thrombosis in patients with acute myocardial infarction. Eur Heart J 1993;14(10):1365–8.

28. Dennis M, Sandercock PA, Reid J, et al. Effectiveness of thigh-length graduated compression stockings to reduce the risk of deep vein thrombosis after stroke (CLOTS trial 1): a multicentre, randomised controlled trial. Lancet 2009;373(9679): 1958–65.

29. Dennis M, Sandercock P, Graham C, et al. The Clots in Legs Or sTockings after Stroke (CLOTS) 3 trial: a randomised controlled trial to determine whether or not intermittent pneumatic compression reduces the risk of post-stroke deep vein thrombosis and to estimate its cost-effectiveness. Health Technol Assess 2015;19(76):1–90.

30. Falanga A, Donati MB. Pathogenesis of thrombosis in patients with malignancy. Int J Hematol 2001; 73(2):137–44.

31. Lee AY, Levine MN. Venous thromboembolism and cancer: risks and outcomes. Circulation 2003; 107(23 suppl 1):I17–21.

32. Spinal Cord Injury Thromboprophylaxis Investigators. Prevention of venous thromboembolism in the acute treatment phase after spinal cord injury: a randomized, multicenter trial comparing low-dose heparin plus intermittent pneumatic compression with enoxaparin. J Trauma 2003;54(6):1116–24 [discussion: 1125–6].

33. Petterson TM, Marks RS, Ashrani AA, et al. Risk of site-specific cancer in incident venous thromboembolism: a population-based study. Thromb Res 2015;135(3):472–8.

34. Chew HK, Wun T, Harvey D, et al. Incidence of venous thromboembolism and its effect on survival among patients with common cancers. Arch Intern Med 2006;166(4):458–64.

35. Sorensen HT, Mellemkjaer L, Olsen JH, et al. Prognosis of cancers associated with venous thromboembolism. N Engl J Med 2000;343(25):1846–50.

36. Di Nisio M, Porreca E, Candeloro M, et al. Primary prophylaxis for venous thromboembolism in ambulatory cancer patients receiving chemotherapy. Cochrane Database Syst Rev 2016;(12): CD008500.

37. Agnelli G, George DJ, Kakkar AK, et al. Semuloparin for thromboprophylaxis in patients receiving chemotherapy for cancer. N Engl J Med 2012;366(7): 601–9.

38. Khorana AA, Kuderer NM, Culakova E, et al. Development and validation of a predictive model for chemotherapy-associated thrombosis. Blood 2008; 111(10):4902–7.

39. Attia J, Ray JG, Cook DJ, et al. Deep vein thrombosis and its prevention in critically ill adults. Arch Intern Med 2001;161(10):1268–79.

40. Khouli H, Shapiro J, Pham VP, et al. Efficacy of deep venous thrombosis prophylaxis in the medical intensive care unit. J Intensive Care Med 2006;21(6): 352–8.

41. Patel R, Cook DJ, Meade MO, et al. Burden of illness in venous thromboembolism in critical care: a multicenter observational study. J Crit Care 2005;20(4): 341–7.

42. Cade JF. High risk of the critically ill for venous thromboembolism. Crit Care Med 1982;10(7): 448–50.

43. Kapoor M, Kupfer YY, Tessler S. Subcutaneous heparin prophylaxis significantly reduces the incidence of venous thromboembolic events in the critically ill. Crit Care Med 1999;27(12):A69.

44. Fraisse F, Holzapfel L, Couland JM, et al. Nadroparin in the prevention of deep vein thrombosis in acute decompensated COPD. The Association of Non-University Affiliated Intensive Care Specialist Physicians of France. Am J Respir Crit Care Med 2000; 161(4 Pt 1):1109–14.

45. Beitland S, Sandven I, Kjaervik LK, et al. Thromboprophylaxis with low molecular weight heparin

versus unfractionated heparin in intensive care patients: a systematic review with meta-analysis and trial sequential analysis. Intensive Care Med 2015; 41(7):1209–19.

46. PROTECT Investigators for the Canadian Critical Care Trials Group and the Australian and New Zealand Intensive Care Society Clinical Trials Group, Cook D, Meade M, Guyatt G, et al. Dalteparin versus unfractionated heparin in critically ill patients. N Engl J Med 2011;364(14): 1305–14.

47. Rabbat CG, Cook DJ, Crowther MA, et al. Dalteparin thromboprophylaxis for critically ill medical-surgical patients with renal insufficiency. J Crit Care 2005; 20(4):357–63.

48. Douketis J, Cook D, Meade M, et al. Prophylaxis against deep vein thrombosis in critically ill patients with severe renal insufficiency with the low-molecular-weight heparin dalteparin: an assessment of safety and pharmacodynamics: the DIRECT study. Arch Intern Med 2008;168(16):1805–12.

49. Zhang C, Zeng W, Zhou H, et al. The efficacy of intermittent pneumatic compression in the prevention of venous thromboembolism in medical critically ill patients. Zhongguo Wei Zhong Bing Ji Jiu Yi Xue 2011;23(9):563–5 [in Chinese].

50. Park J, Lee JM, Lee JS, et al. Pharmacological and mechanical thromboprophylaxis in critically Ill patients: a network meta-analysis of 12 trials. J Korean Med Sci 2016;31(11):1828–37.

Diagnosis of Deep Venous Thrombosis and Pulmonary Embolism
New Imaging Tools and Modalities

Farbod Nicholas Rahaghi, MD, PhD[a],*,
Jasleen Kaur Minhas, MD[b], Gustavo A. Heresi, MD, MS[c]

KEYWORDS

- Pulmonary embolism • Imaging • Computed tomography • MRI • Ultrasound

KEY POINTS

- Imaging has a key role in establishing the diagnosis of DVT and PE, particularly as integrated into diagnostic algorithms.
- Ultrasound remains the gold standard for diagnosis of DVT though CT and MRI based imaging have a role in situations where ultrasound has limitations.
- CT angiography and ventillation perfusion imaging have largely replaced pulmonary angiography as the modality of choice in assessing acute pulmonary embolus.
- MRI, nuclear imaging and dual energy CT are currently being clinically evaluated as tools for diagnosis, subtyping and prognostication in pulmonary embolism.

INTRODUCTION

Untreated venous thromboembolism carries the potential for serious complications and mortality. At the same time, there is also significant risk associated with treatment with anticoagulation and thrombolysis. This leads to a need for sensitivity in diagnosis, certainty in the decision not to treat, as well as relative urgency in making the diagnosis and initiation of treatment. Thus, there is significant impetus to develop and refine tools for detection and management of venous thrombus, both in the extremities and the lungs. Although the importance of these clinical decisions necessitates a comprehensive clinical approach to diagnosis, imaging has long played a pivotal role in detecting the presence and extent of thromboembolic disease. Although many great imaging tools already exist, furthering the application of imaging in thromboembolism remains an area of intense research and development.

Within the realm of imaging, there has been a steady progression towards using noninvasive methods to guide initial diagnosis, with invasive imaging used in complex cases or as part of an interventional strategy. Research has historically focused on the detection of clot, which then inputs into the clinical decision making pathways. However, as the number of tools and options for treatment increase, there is growing interest in using imaging for better quantification and classification

Funding Sources: F.N. Rahaghi: 1K23HL136905 (NIH), G.A. Heresi: K23HL125697 (NIH).
Disclosures: F.N. Rahaghi and J.K. Minhas have nothing to disclose; G.A. Heresi has received Advisory Board and Speaking fees from Bayer Healthcare.
[a] Pulmonary and Critical Care Medicine, Brigham and Women's Hospital, Harvard Medical School, 15 Francis Street, Boston MA 02115, USA; [b] Department of Medicine, North Shore Medical Center, 81 Highland Avenue, Salem MA 10970, USA; [c] Department of Pulmonary and Critical Care Medicine, Respiratory Institute, Cleveland Clinic, Mail Code A90, 9500 Euclid Avenue, Cleveland, OH 44195, USA
* Corresponding author.
E-mail address: frahaghi@bwh.harvard.edu

Clin Chest Med 39 (2018) 493–504
https://doi.org/10.1016/j.ccm.2018.04.003

of thromboembolic disease to improve prognostication and to guide intervention.

In this section, we review the role of imaging in the diagnosis and management of deep venous thrombosis (DVT) and pulmonary embolism (PE), highlighting the current state of the art modalities as well as areas in which current research is uncovering promising tools that may find their way to clinical use in the near future.

IMAGING IN THE DETECTION AND MANAGEMENT OF DEEP VENOUS THROMBOSIS

Contrast venography is an invasive procedure in which venous opacification is evaluated in real time. Although the gold standard for the detection of DVT, this method is rarely practiced outside of expert centers, where it is often used in the context of intervention.[1,2] This is in large part due to the myriad of noninvasive imaging techniques that are now widely available, and in particular, the use of ultrasound examination in the diagnosis of DVT.

Methods using ultrasound examination to evaluate venous thrombosis were developed in the 1960s[3] and were perfected in the following decades. The measurement of venous blood flow as well as venous compressibility[4,5] were also developed. The evaluation of venous compressibility in combination with color and Spectral Doppler assessment of flow and phase is now the recommended approach for detection of a venous clot[2,6] (**Fig. 1**). This is largely due to the availability and ease of deployment in a variety of clinical settings.[6] Although the incidence of upper extremity DVT is much lower than the lower extremity, its presence leads to a significant risk of PE and associated morbidity.[7,8] Imaging approaches similar to the lower extremity can be used for the detection of clot in the upper extremities. However, restrictions imposed by the clavicle significantly limit ultrasound-based techniques.[2,9]

Other imaging modalities have been investigated for clot detection and have shown promising results, although none have replaced ultrasound-based methods in routine clinical settings. As an analogue of direct venography, computed tomography (CT)-based venography (involving direct injection of contrast into the veins) has been shown to have great sensitivity in detection of DVT[10] while reducing contrast load by as much as 80% compared with conventional venography. Additionally, venography using contrast injected in a distal site, for example, in the context of a CT angiography of the chest, have also been investigated.[11] This approach is proposed given the common risk factors between PE and DVT as well as the observation that many individuals with no evidence of PE on CT angiography are noted to have DVT.[11] This approach to CT angiography also improves the ability to detect proximal clots in the pelvis.[12] Subsequent studies of these combined approaches have shown limited usefulness with additional radiation (but not contrast exposure given the need for both angiography

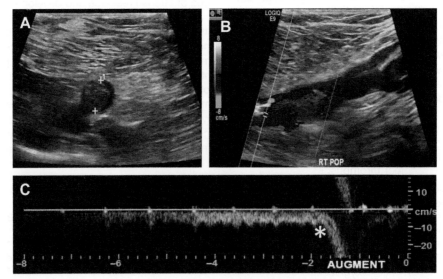

Fig. 1. Ultrasound evidence of deep venous thrombosis at the bifurcation of the right popliteal vein. (*A*) Demonstration of partially occlusive thrombus in the right popliteal vein and accompanying color flow Doppler imaging (*B*) showing decreased flow in the right popliteal vein. Spectral waveforms measuring the velocity of flow demonstrate an increase in velocity during an augmentation (marked by the *yellow star*) (*C*), consistent with the presence of residual flow.

and venography. Thus, despite initially promising results, the routine use of this combination remains controversial.[13,14]

Many promising studies have been performed to assess the usefulness of MRI venography as a tool for detection of DVT. Those with contrast have had a good sensitivity, but carry risks associated with contrast loads.[15,16] Noncontrast studies have limited the ability to visualize subacute and chronic clot.[17] Metaanalyses of these studies[18,19] have not yielded sufficient evidence for replacement of ultrasound approaches by MRI as standard of care.

Although the dominance of ultrasound-based techniques has made this the most commonly used tool for detection of DVT, alternative imaging modalities have an evolving role in clot detection in cases where ultrasound examination has limitations, as well as for defining the chronicity and composition of clot. Although ultrasound imaging is widely available, patient body habitus can provide a significant limitation in the use of ultrasound techniques.[2,19] Additionally, ultrasound-based techniques are not reliable in cases of suspected proximal DVT.[20] In these cases, magnetic resonance venography as well as CT approaches can provide an alternative method to diagnose and define the extent of thrombus.

Determination of the age of thrombus is clinically relevant to identify cause and to establish efficacy of treatment. Ultrasound abnormalities can persist in 50% of patients a year out from the initial diagnosis of DVT,[21] leading to a diagnostic dilemma of identifying recurrent clots, particularly in the same anatomic location in at-risk patients.[22] MRI offers the opportunity to differentiate between old and new thrombi.[22] Modifications including black-blood thrombus imaging[23,24] have shown promise in dating clot chronicity. Sonographic elasticity imaging uses ultrasound-based techniques to assess the stiffness of a clot and, thus, distinguish fresh from subacute/chronic clot.[25,26] Photoacoustic imaging, combined with ultrasound imaging, may also be helpful with defining the extent and age of clot.[27] Molecular imaging, which involves using specific targeted molecules to enhance and detect thrombus, has led to a number of proposed approaches to examine clot chronicity.[28] As an example, (99m)Tc-recombinant tissue plasminogen activator has been used to determine the age of clot, given the differential activity of (99m)Tc-recombinant tissue plasminogen activator in old versus new thrombus.[29] Similarly, PET with fludeoxyglucose ^{18}F-FDG-PET scanning has shown that FDG activity of clot decreases with time and thus can be used in assessing the age of clots of size detectable by ^{18}F-FDG-PET.[30] Methods of fluorescence-based

molecular imaging have also been developed to quantify fibrin deposition.[31] Differentiating between bland and tumor thrombus is also a clinically important question because of the fundamentally different approaches to treatment. In this context, PET imaging for classification based on the activity of the thrombus has shown promise for assessing clot tumor burden.[28,32–35]

PULMONARY EMBOLISM

Untreated PE can have potentially fatal consequences. The clinical diagnosis of PE currently relies on a framework where the clinical suspicion of the presence of clot is altered by tests, usually imaging, leading to a final clinical diagnosis. This process also yields further prognostic information, including the degree of right ventricular strain and clot burden that, in addition to the patient's hemodynamic status, guides further intervention. Selective pulmonary angiography, the gold standard for the detection of pulmonary emboli (**Fig. 2**), has largely been replaced by CT angiography and nuclear ventilation-perfusion scans (V/Q scans) embedded within this clinical decision-making flow (**Fig. 3**).

Despite this, limitations exist in the detection of clot using imaging alone. In the case of CT angiography, there remains uncertainty around findings of isolated subsegmental PE.[36] Additionally, there is significant concern about contrast-induced nephropathy.[37] In the case of the V/Q scan, the degradation of the clinical usefulness of the test in the context of preexisting or coevolving lung disease presents a limitation.[38] This is further complicated by the significant presence of renal disease for CT angiography and lung disease for V/Q scans in the most at-risk populations for PE. Thus, in addition to improving these techniques, there remains significant interest in developing additional modalities for detection of clot.

Diagnostic Algorithm and the Use of Imaging Modalities

For patients with symptoms concerning for PE, the use of probability criteria such as the Wells or Geneva Score is the initial step in determining likelihood of disease. Application of both traditional and modified versions of these scores has been validated and is well-established.[39] The Pulmonary Embolism Rule-out Criteria (PERC) can be used subsequently in individuals with a low risk score. Further workup may be deferred in those with a negative PERC[39] (Appendix 1).

A low-risk probability criteria with a positive PERC warrants further testing with a D-dimer. Enzyme-linked immunosorbent based D-dimer assays have a sensitivity of greater than 95%.

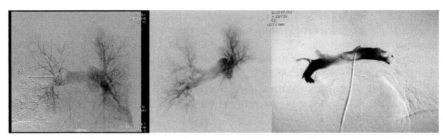

Fig. 2. Three examples of pulmonary angiography in acute pulmonary embolus. An area of lucency can be seen (example: *blue arrow*), where a clot is blocking the flow, leading to decreased opacification of the pulmonary vascular tree on the right compared with the left. Complete occlusion of flow is noted on the middle panel with minimal opacification of the lower lobes on the left. Bilateral pulmonary emboli on the rightmost panel demonstrating cutoffs and minimal flow beyond the central pulmonary artery.

D-Dimer levels normally increase with age and adjusting the upper limit of normal (age multiplied by 10 in patients ≥50 years of age) for interpretation improves the sensitivity and specificity in this population.[39] A negative D-dimer test combined with low probability criteria on the Wells or Geneva criteria negates the need for further testing.[39]

A moderate or high risk on probability criteria or positive D-dimer assay warrants a further workup for PE. CT angiography (**Fig. 4**) continues to be the mainstay for the diagnosis of acute PE owing to its high specificity. The combination of CT angiography with clinical probability criteria further increases predictive values, as demonstrated by the PIOPED II study.[40–42] Thus, a negative CT in a non–high-risk patient is adequate to rule out PE. Additionally, once a diagnosis of PE has been established, the CT finding of an increased right ventricle:left ventricle diameter ratio may further aid in risk stratification and management.[43–45]

A V/Q scan may be of use in patients with a high risk on probability criteria but potentially falsely negative CT angiography. It may also be a preferential initial diagnostic study in conditions where CT angiography is contraindicated, such renal failure or contrast allergy.[43–45]

Computed Tomography Angiography for Diagnosis and Prognostication

CT angiography has largely replaced the use of pulmonary angiography and nuclear studies in the detection of PE. Although initially the low resolution of CT scanning led to concerns about poor detection of smaller emboli,[46] the advent of multidetector CT (MDCT) scanning leading to higher resolution has improved detection of smaller clot.[47] The PIOPED II study has been largely used to define the role of CT angiography in the context of a decision-making algorithm.[48] The study showed a high specificity of CT angiography for the detection of PE (96%), but also raised concerns about sensitivity (83%), particularly for the detection of small subsegmental PE.[36] It also noted the limited sensitivity of CT angiography in the context of high clinical suspicion and

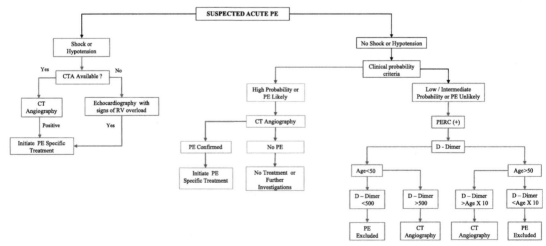

Fig. 3. Suspect acute algorithm for pulmonary embolism. CT, computed tomography; CTA, computed tomography angiography; PE, pulmonary embolism; PERC, Pulmonary Embolism Rule-out Criteria; RV, right ventricular.

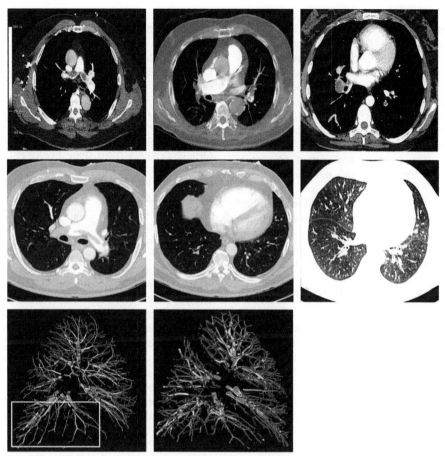

Fig. 4. Examples of computed tomography findings in acute pulmonary embolism (PE). From top left: example of a saddle PE, example of a lobar PE, and example of a doughnut sign (partial arterial obstruction). Second row: Example of a saddle embolus, with corresponding right ventricular dilation and heterogeneous perfusion of the lung. Third row: Vascular reconstruction of the subject from the second row demonstrating areas with decreased detection of vessels corresponding to the areas of decreased perfusion as compared with a normal subject (*right*).

recommended further investigations if CT angiography was negative in this population. Many centers in PIOPED II used 4-slice MDCT; currently, 64-slice MDCT are increasingly common with 256- and 512-slice MDCT becoming available.[49] Thus, further studies are needed to clarify the impact of improving scanner technology on detection of a small PE.

The risk of contrast-induced nephropathy has been a major barrier to use of CT angiography because many patients at risk for PE either have chronic kidney disease or are suffering from acute kidney injury in the context of hemodynamic compromise.[37,50–52] Although it is generally believed that this risk is significant, it has not been well-quantified, and recent studies suggest that it may be overestimated.[53–55] These discrepancies arise from lack of randomized controls, differing definitions of clinically relevant acute kidney injury, and fluctuations in creatinine in such

populations,[56] as well as changes in the nature and dosing of contrast currently administered as compared with the initial studies.[53]

CT angiography has also been explored as a means for prognostication. Recently, prognostication models have been developed leveraging CT imaging to detect evidence of right ventricular strain. Although most CT angiograms are non-electrocardiogram gated, which leads to an imprecise size estimation of the ventricles, initial studies suggest that cardiac size obtained from non–electrocardiogram-gated scans still contain prognostic information.[57] The most commonly studied and validated marker has been the ratio of the diameter of the right ventricle to the left ventricle, which is used to detect right ventricular strain as a precursor to impending right ventricular failure. This measure has shown validity in predicting progression to right ventricular failure,[43–45] in particular when combined with other clinical information.[58] The detection and calculation of this ratio has recently been automated requiring no human operator input[59] and is becoming increasingly a part of the prognostic information used for triaging patients with the potential for deterioration. However, its lack of specificity requires additional studies such as echocardiography for critical decision making.[60]

Subjective and objective quantification of the location and burden of clot has also been explored.[61] The location and extent of clot is known to be associated with evidence of heart dysfunction.[62,63] Quantity of clot can be integrated into models to predict right ventricular dysfunction,[64] including those assessing maximal clot size.[65] Although these methods are promising, further studies to build consensus on the best method of measuring clot burden are ongoing.

Assessing Regional Perfusion Using Nuclear Imaging

Evaluation of lung perfusion defects using nuclear imaging, combined with concurrent imaging of ventilation defects, continues to be a key approach to the evaluation of PE.[66] The PIOPED I study established the usefulness of the V/Q scan in the detection of PE and, in particular, the diagnostic value of a normal V/Q study.[67,68] Significant research has led to improvement of interpretation of V/Q scans and the data from PIOPED I study and the subsequent PIOPED II study have led to the modifications of PIOPED II guidelines for image interpretation.[40–42]

Single photon emission computed tomography (SPECT) imaging uses tomographic techniques to create 3-dimensional (3D) reconstructions like CT scans, but instead uses gamma rays emitted from injected tracers. Unlike traditional V/Q scans, which are based on multiple planes, this method creates true 3D images. The use of 3D reconstruction information has been shown to improve diagnostic accuracy over planar reconstructions,[69–71] particularly when used in conjunction with CT.[72] However, large multi-center studies are currently lacking to define the role of SPECT and CT-SPECT in detection of PE.[73,74]

The Role of MRI in Pulmonary Embolism

Non–contrast-enhanced and contrast-enhanced MRI techniques have been leveraged for many years in detecting PE[75–77] with similar findings to CT scans, including luminal filling defects and vascular "cutoff" (**Fig. 5**). However, the nature of numerous tissue–air transitions and significant artifacts limit the use of traditional MRI in detection of small pulmonary emboli,[78] leading to concerns about sensitivity in detection.[79,80] The usefulness of gadolinium-enhanced MRI in clot detection was evaluated systematically in the PIOPED III study, which demonstrated great specificity (99%) but low sensitivity (78%), and further highlighted the variations between centers in terms of the adequacy of the imaging acquired.[81]

Thus, the use of traditional MRI techniques as a general initial approach for detection of PE is not currently recommended.[82,83] However, single-center experiences suggest that, with appropriate tools, training, and a program-focused approach, MRI can be used for this purpose.[84]

In an effort to improve clot detection using MRI, research has focused on the use of molecular markers targeted toward fibrin,[85,86] alpha2-antiplasmin,[87,88] and platelets.[78] Additionally, stepwise protocols have been proposed and assessed that take advantage of the variety of MRI protocols available to improve the speed and accuracy of clot detection using MRI.[89]

In addition to the detection of PE, MRI is also being considered for novel uses, such as noninvasive estimation of pulmonary vascular resistance[90] as well as the development of perfusion mapping,

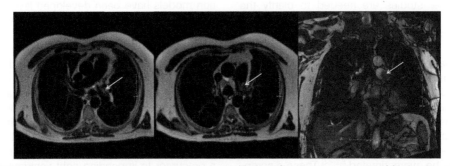

Fig. 5. MRI without intravenous contrast owing to impaired kidney function in a 65-year-old man. Scanning using axial half-Fourier acquisition single-shot turbo spin echo imaging; and axial, sagittal, and coronal true fast imaging with steady-state precession. There is a filling defect in the main left pulmonary artery extending into the ascending and descending branches (*arrows*).

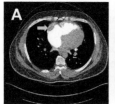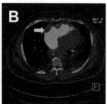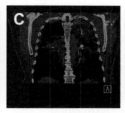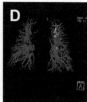

Fig. 6. Images from a dual energy computed tomography (CT) scan. (*A*) Mixed CT Image in mediastinal window setting shows occlusive thrombi in both lower lobar pulmonary arteries. Also noted is right atrial thrombus (*arrow*). (*B, C*) Axial and coronal perfused blood volume images demonstrate large wedge shaped perfusion defects in both lungs, most severe in lower lobes. (*D*) Lung vessel image shows distribution of iodine containing and non-opacified pulmonary arteries. The iodine containing pulmonary arterial branches are coded in blue, and the non-opacified arteries are coded in red. (*Courtesy of* Rahul Renapurkar, MD, Cleveland, Ohio.)

similar in concept to those obtained using nuclear studies.

Dual Energy Computed Tomography

The response of materials being penetrated by x-ray is used in CT to generate 3D representation of material density, which is the basis for CT imaging. However, when two x-rays of differing energies are present, the differential response to each energy provides the ability to infer material composition in addition to density. Although this potential has been known since the 1970s,[91] the technologic limitation of simultaneously emitting and detecting two different x-ray energies while not exposing the patient to double the dose of radiation limited the clinical deployment of this technology. Multiple solutions to this technical challenge have been developed and tested resulting in dual energy CT scans becoming clinically available in many centers. In the current implementations, the radiation dosage, use of contrast, and the patient/provider experience are not significantly different, and thus these scanners can be incorporated into routine clinical care without significant retooling of the workflow.

A common use of dual energy CT is to create quantifiable perfusion maps based on the density of iodine outside of the vasculature, which provide a more robust 3D representation of penetration of iodine into the distal tissue (**Fig. 6**).[92] This is then used to detect perfusion defects in a similar manner to MRI and SPECT approaches[93] with comparable results.[94] Multiple studies have evaluated the usefulness of dual energy CT in improving the diagnosis of PE.[95] Blood volume detected using this approach has also been shown to be related to right heart strain in patients with PE[93] and to improve the detection of pulmonary embolus, particularly in the peripheral lung.[96,97] Dual energy CT has also shown significant promise in the study of chronic thromboembolic pulmonary

hypertension,[39,98] as well as in distinguishing tumor embolism from thromboembolism.[99]

SUMMARY

Imaging continues to play a pivotal role in the diagnosis of venous thromboembolism. Advances in imaging technology continue to improve the diagnostic usefulness of imaging and increasing experience with imaging has allowed it to become integrated into clinical decision making tools. The development of new technology and processing algorithms continue to expand the role of imaging in both prognostication and subtyping of disease, which is likely to improve the usefulness of imaging in clinical treatment of venous thromboembolism.

REFERENCES

1. de Valois JC, van Schaik CC, Verzijlbergen F, et al. Contrast venography: from gold standard to 'golden backup' in clinically suspected deep vein thrombosis. Eur J Radiol 1990;11(2):131–7.
2. Karande GY, Hedgire SS, Sanchez Y, et al. Advanced imaging in acute and chronic deep vein thrombosis. Cardiovasc Diagn Ther 2016; 6(6):493–507.
3. Sigel B, Popky GL, Wagner DK, et al. Comparison of clinical and Doppler ultrasound evaluation of confirmed lower extremity venous disease. Surgery 1968;64(1):332–8.
4. Cronan JJ. History of venous ultrasound. J Ultrasound Med 2003;22(11):1143–6.
5. Raghavendra BN, Horii SC, Hilton S, et al. Deep venous thrombosis: detection by probe compression of veins. J Ultrasound Med 1986;5(2):89–95.
6. Tapson VF, Carroll BA, Davidson BL, et al. The diagnostic approach to acute venous thromboembolism. Clinical practice guideline. American Thoracic Society. Am J Respir Crit Care Med 1999;160(3):1043–66.

7. Munoz FJ, Mismetti P, Poggio R, et al. Clinical outcome of patients with upper-extremity deep vein thrombosis: results from the RIETE Registry. Chest 2008;133(1):143–8.

8. Kooij JD, van der Zant FM, van Beek EJ, et al. Pulmonary embolism in deep venous thrombosis of the upper extremity: more often in catheter-related thrombosis. Neth J Med 1997;50(6):238–42.

9. Chin EE, Zimmerman PT, Grant EG. Sonographic evaluation of upper extremity deep venous thrombosis. J Ultrasound Med 2005;24(6):829–38 [quiz: 839–40].

10. Baldt MM, Zontsich T, Stumpflen A, et al. Deep venous thrombosis of the lower extremity: efficacy of spiral CT venography compared with conventional venography in diagnosis. Radiology 1996; 200(2):423–8.

11. Cham MD, Yankelevitz DF, Shaham D, et al. Deep venous thrombosis: detection by using indirect CT venography. The pulmonary angiography-indirect CT venography cooperative group. Radiology 2000;216(3):744–51.

12. Loud PA, Katz DS, Bruce DA, et al. Deep venous thrombosis with suspected pulmonary embolism: detection with combined CT venography and pulmonary angiography. Radiology 2001;219(2): 498–502.

13. Goodman LR, Sostman HD, Stein PD, et al. CT venography: a necessary adjunct to CT pulmonary angiography or a waste of time, money, and radiation? Radiology 2009;250(2):327–30.

14. Reichert M, Henzler T, Krissak R, et al. Venous thromboembolism: additional diagnostic value and radiation dose of pelvic CT venography in patients with suspected pulmonary embolism. Eur J Radiol 2011;80(1):50–3.

15. Moody AR. Magnetic resonance direct thrombus imaging. J Thromb Haemost 2003;1(7):1403–9.

16. Arnoldussen C, Strijkers R, Lambregts D, et al. Feasibility of identifying deep vein thrombosis characteristics with contrast enhanced MR-venography. Phlebology 2014;29(1 suppl):119–24.

17. Westerbeek RE, Van Rooden CJ, Tan M, et al. Magnetic resonance direct thrombus imaging of the evolution of acute deep vein thrombosis of the leg. J Thromb Haemost 2008;6(7):1087–92.

18. Sampson FC, Goodacre SW, Thomas SM, et al. The accuracy of MRI in diagnosis of suspected deep vein thrombosis: systematic review and meta-analysis. Eur Radiol 2007;17(1):175–81.

19. Abdalla G, Fawzi Matuk R, Venugopal V, et al. The diagnostic accuracy of magnetic resonance venography in the detection of deep venous thrombosis: a systematic review and meta-analysis. Clin Radiol 2015;70(8):858–71.

20. Davidson BL, Elliott CG, Lensing AW. Low accuracy of color Doppler ultrasound in the detection of proximal leg vein thrombosis in asymptomatic high-risk patients. The RD Heparin Arthroplasty Group. Ann Intern Med 1992;117(9):735–8.

21. Piovella F, Crippa L, Barone M, et al. Normalization rates of compression ultrasonography in patients with a first episode of deep vein thrombosis of the lower limbs: association with recurrence and new thrombosis. Haematologica 2002;87(5):515–22.

22. Huisman MV, Klok FA. Current challenges in diagnostic imaging of venous thromboembolism. Hematology Am Soc Hematol Educ Program 2015;2015:202–9.

23. Xie G, Chen H, He X, et al. Black-blood thrombus imaging (BTI): a contrast-free cardiovascular magnetic resonance approach for the diagnosis of non-acute deep vein thrombosis. J Cardiovasc Magn Reson 2017;19(1):4.

24. Treitl KM, Treitl M, Kooijman-Kurfuerst H, et al. Three-dimensional black-blood T1-weighted turbo spin-echo techniques for the diagnosis of deep vein thrombosis in comparison with contrast-enhanced magnetic resonance imaging: a pilot study. Invest Radiol 2015;50(6):401–8.

25. Lubinski MA, Emelianov SY, O'Donnell M. Speckle tracking methods for ultrasonic elasticity imaging using short-time correlation. IEEE Trans Ultrason Ferroelectr Freq Control 1999; 46(1):82–96.

26. Rubin JM, Xie H, Kim K, et al. Sonographic elasticity imaging of acute and chronic deep venous thrombosis in humans. J Ultrasound Med 2006; 25(9):1179–86.

27. Karpiouk AB, Aglyamov SR, Mallidi S, et al. Combined ultrasound and photoacoustic imaging to detect and stage deep vein thrombosis: phantom and ex vivo studies. J Biomed Opt 2008;13(5): 054061.

28. Houshmand S, Salavati A, Hess S, et al. The role of molecular imaging in diagnosis of deep vein thrombosis. Am J Nucl Med Mol Imaging 2014; 4(5):406–25.

29. Brighton T, Janssen J, Butler SP. Aging of acute deep vein thrombosis measured by radiolabeled 99mTc-rt-PA. J Nucl Med 2007;48(6):873–8.

30. Rondina MT, Lam UT, Pendleton RC, et al. (18) F-FDG PET in the evaluation of acuity of deep vein thrombosis. Clin Nucl Med 2012;37(12): 1139–45.

31. Hara T, Bhayana B, Thompson B, et al. Molecular imaging of fibrin deposition in deep vein thrombosis using fibrin-targeted near-infrared fluorescence. JACC Cardiovasc Imaging 2012;5(6): 607–15.

32. Sharma P, Kumar R, Jeph S, et al. 18F-FDG PET-CT in the diagnosis of tumor thrombus: can it be differentiated from benign thrombus? Nucl Med Commun 2011;32(9):782–8.

33. Sharma P, Kumar R, Singh H, et al. Imaging thrombus in cancer patients with FDG PET-CT. Jpn J Radiol 2012;30(2):95–104.

34. Erhamamci S, Reyhan M, Nursal GN, et al. Incidental diagnosis of tumor thrombosis on FDG PET/CT imaging. Rev Esp Med Nucl Imagen Mol 2015;34(5):287–94.

35. Davidson T, Goitein O, Avigdor A, et al. 18F- FDG-PET/CT for the diagnosis of tumor thrombosis. Isr Med Assoc J 2009;11(2):69–73.

36. Carrier M, Righini M, Wells PS, et al. Subsegmental pulmonary embolism diagnosed by computed tomography: incidence and clinical implications. A systematic review and meta-analysis of the management outcome studies. J Thromb Haemost 2010;8(8):1716–22.

37. Kooiman J, Klok FA, Mos IC, et al. Incidence and predictors of contrast-induced nephropathy following CT-angiography for clinically suspected acute pulmonary embolism. J Thromb Haemost 2010;8(2):409–11.

38. Hayes SA, Soff GA, Zabor EC, et al. Clinical consequences of an indeterminate CT pulmonary angiogram in cancer patients. Clin Imaging 2014;38(5):637–40.

39. Hoey ET, Mirsadraee S, Pepke-Zaba J, et al. Dual-energy CT angiography for assessment of regional pulmonary perfusion in patients with chronic thromboembolic pulmonary hypertension: initial experience. AJR Am J Roentgenol 2011;196(3):524–32.

40. Yazdani M, Lau CT, Lempel JK, et al. Historical evolution of imaging techniques for the evaluation of pulmonary embolism. Radiographics 2015;35(4):1245–62.

41. Sostman HD, Miniati M, Gottschalk A, et al. Sensitivity and specificity of perfusion scintigraphy combined with chest radiography for acute pulmonary embolism in PIOPED II. J Nucl Med 2008;49(11):1741–8.

42. Sostman HD, Stein PD, Gottschalk A, et al. Acute pulmonary embolism: sensitivity and specificity of ventilation-perfusion scintigraphy in PIOPED II study. Radiology 2008;246(3):941–6.

43. Lu MT, Cai T, Ersoy H, et al. Interval increase in right-left ventricular diameter ratios at CT as a predictor of 30-day mortality after acute pulmonary embolism: initial experience. Radiology 2008;246(1):281–7.

44. Kumamaru KK, Hunsaker AR, Wake N, et al. The variability in prognostic values of right ventricular-to-left ventricular diameter ratios derived from different measurement methods on computed tomography pulmonary angiography: a patient outcome study. J Thorac Imaging 2012;27(5):331–6.

45. Jia D, Zhou XM, Hou G. Estimation of right ventricular dysfunction by computed tomography pulmonary angiography: a valuable adjunct for evaluating the severity of acute pulmonary embolism. J Thromb Thrombolysis 2017;43(2):271–8.

46. Rathbun SW, Raskob GE, Whitsett TL. Sensitivity and specificity of helical computed tomography in the diagnosis of pulmonary embolism: a systematic review. Ann Intern Med 2000;132(3):227–32.

47. Goodman LR. Small pulmonary emboli: what do we know? Radiology 2005;234(3):654–8.

48. Stein PD, Fowler SE, Goodman LR, et al. Multidetector computed tomography for acute pulmonary embolism. N Engl J Med 2006;354(22):2317–27.

49. Douma RA, Hofstee HM, Schaefer-Prokop C, et al. Comparison of 4- and 64-slice CT scanning in the diagnosis of pulmonary embolism. Thromb Haemost 2010;103(1):242–6.

50. Schrader R. Contrast material-induced renal failure: an overview. J Interv Cardiol 2005;18(6):417–23.

51. Mitchell AM, Kline JA, Jones AE, et al. Major adverse events one year after acute kidney injury after contrast-enhanced computed tomography. Ann Emerg Med 2015;66(3):267–74.e4.

52. Mitchell AM, Jones AE, Tumlin JA, et al. Incidence of contrast-induced nephropathy after contrast-enhanced computed tomography in the outpatient setting. Clin J Am Soc Nephrol 2010;5(1):4–9.

53. Hinson JS, Ehmann MR, Fine DM, et al. Risk of acute kidney injury after intravenous contrast media administration. Ann Emerg Med 2017;69(5):577–86.e4.

54. McDonald RJ, McDonald JS, Bida JP, et al. Intravenous contrast material-induced nephropathy: causal or coincident phenomenon? Radiology 2013;267(1):106–18.

55. McDonald JS, McDonald RJ, Carter RE, et al. Risk of intravenous contrast material-mediated acute kidney injury: a propensity score-matched study stratified by baseline-estimated glomerular filtration rate. Radiology 2014;271(1):65–73.

56. Sinert R, Brandler E, Subramanian RA, et al. Does the current definition of contrast-induced acute kidney injury reflect a true clinical entity? Acad Emerg Med 2012;19(11):1261–7.

57. Gutte H, Mortensen J, Mork ML, et al. Non-ECG-gated CT pulmonary angiography and the prediction of right ventricular dysfunction in patients suspected of pulmonary embolism. Clin Physiol Funct Imaging 2017;37(6):575–81.

58. Kumamaru KK, George E, Ghosh N, et al. Normal ventricular diameter ratio on CT provides adequate assessment for critical right ventricular strain among patients with acute pulmonary embolism. Int J Cardiovasc Imaging 2016;32(7):1153–61.

59. Kumamaru KK, George E, Aghayev A, et al. Implementation and performance of automated software for computing right-to-left ventricular diameter ratio from computed tomography pulmonary angiography images. J Comput Assist Tomogr 2016;40(3):387–92.

60. Dudzinski DM, Hariharan P, Parry BA, et al. Assessment of right ventricular strain by computed tomography versus echocardiography in acute pulmonary embolism. Acad Emerg Med 2017; 24(3):337–43.

61. Qanadli SD, El Hajjam M, Vieillard-Baron A, et al. New CT index to quantify arterial obstruction in pulmonary embolism: comparison with angiographic index and echocardiography. AJR Am J Roentgenol 2001;176(6):1415–20.

62. Aviram G, Soikher E, Bendet A, et al. Automatic assessment of cardiac load due to acute pulmonary embolism: saddle vs. central and peripheral emboli distribution. Heart Lung 2016;45(3): 261–9.

63. Gouin B, Blondon M, Jimenez D, et al. Clinical prognosis of nonmassive central and noncentral pulmonary embolism: a registry-based cohort study. Chest 2017;151(4):829–37.

64. El-Menyar A, Nabir S, Ahmed N, et al. Diagnostic implications of computed tomography pulmonary angiography in patients with pulmonary embolism. Ann Thorac Med 2016;11(4):269–76.

65. Hariharan P, Dudzinski DM, Rosovsky R, et al. Relation among clot burden, right-sided heart strain, and adverse events after acute pulmonary embolism. Am J Cardiol 2016;118(10): 1568–73.

66. Metter D, Tulchinsky M, Freeman LM. Current status of ventilation-perfusion scintigraphy for suspected pulmonary embolism. AJR Am J Roentgenol 2017;208(3):489–94.

67. PIOPED Investigators. Value of the ventilation/perfusion scan in acute pulmonary embolism. Results of the prospective investigation of pulmonary embolism diagnosis (PIOPED). JAMA 1990; 263(20):2753–9.

68. Worsley DF, Alavi A. Comprehensive analysis of the results of the PIOPED Study. Prospective investigation of pulmonary embolism diagnosis study. J Nucl Med 1995;36(12):2380–7.

69. Reinartz P, Wildberger JE, Schaefer W, et al. Tomographic imaging in the diagnosis of pulmonary embolism: a comparison between V/Q lung scintigraphy in SPECT technique and multislice spiral CT. J Nucl Med 2004;45(9):1501–8.

70. Bajc M, Olsson B, Palmer J, et al. Ventilation/Perfusion SPECT for diagnostics of pulmonary embolism in clinical practice. J Intern Med 2008;264(4):379–87.

71. Reinartz P, Kaiser HJ, Wildberger JE, et al. SPECT imaging in the diagnosis of pulmonary embolism: automated detection of match and mismatch defects by means of image-processing techniques. J Nucl Med 2006;47(6):968–73.

72. Gutte H, Mortensen J, Jensen CV, et al. Detection of pulmonary embolism with combined ventilation-perfusion SPECT and low-dose CT: head-to-head comparison with multidetector CT angiography. J Nucl Med 2009;50(12):1987–92.

73. Non-contrast 4DCT to detect pulmonary thromboembolic events. Available at: https://ClinicalTrials.gov/show/NCT03183063. Accessed August 7, 2017.

74. Comparison of 3 diagnostic strategies of PE: planar V/Q scan, CTPA, and V/Q SPECT. Available at: https://ClinicalTrials.gov/show/NCT02983760. Accessed August 7, 2017.

75. Ohno Y, Yoshikawa T, Kishida Y, et al. Unenhanced and contrast-enhanced MR angiography and perfusion imaging for suspected pulmonary thromboembolism. AJR Am J Roentgenol 2017;208(3):517–30.

76. Hatabu H, Gefter WB, Kressel HY, et al. Pulmonary vasculature: high-resolution MR imaging. Work in progress. Radiology 1989;171(2):391–5.

77. Kluge A, Luboldt W, Bachmann G. Acute pulmonary embolism to the subsegmental level: diagnostic accuracy of three MRI techniques compared with 16-MDCT. AJR Am J Roentgenol 2006;187(1):W7–14.

78. Heidt T, Ehrismann S, Hovener JB, et al. Molecular imaging of activated platelets allows the detection of pulmonary embolism with magnetic resonance imaging. Sci Rep 2016;6:25044.

79. Li J, Feng L, Li J, et al. Diagnostic accuracy of magnetic resonance angiography for acute pulmonary embolism - a systematic review and meta-analysis. Vasa 2016;45(2):149–54.

80. Revel MP, Sanchez O, Couchon S, et al. Diagnostic accuracy of magnetic resonance imaging for an acute pulmonary embolism: results of the 'IRM-EP' study. J Thromb Haemost 2012;10(5):743–50.

81. Stein PD, Chenevert TL, Fowler SE, et al. Gadolinium-enhanced magnetic resonance angiography for pulmonary embolism: a multicenter prospective study (PIOPED III). Ann Intern Med 2010;152(7): 434–43. W142–433.

82. Jaff MR, McMurtry MS, Archer SL, et al. Management of massive and submassive pulmonary embolism, iliofemoral deep vein thrombosis, and chronic thromboembolic pulmonary hypertension: a scientific statement from the American Heart Association. Circulation 2011;123(16): 1788–830.

83. Konstantinides SV, Torbicki A, Agnelli G, et al. 2014 ESC guidelines on the diagnosis and management of acute pulmonary embolism. Eur Heart J 2014; 35(43):3033–69, 3069a–k.

84. Nagle SK, Schiebler ML, Repplinger MD, et al. Contrast enhanced pulmonary magnetic resonance angiography for pulmonary embolism: building a successful program. Eur J Radiol 2016;85(3):553–63.

85. Spuentrup E, Katoh M, Wiethoff AJ, et al. Molecular magnetic resonance imaging of pulmonary emboli

with a fibrin-specific contrast agent. Am J Respir Crit Care Med 2005;172(4):494–500.

86. Vymazal J, Spuentrup E, Cardenas-Molina G, et al. Thrombus imaging with fibrin-specific gadolinium-based MR contrast agent EP-2104R: results of a phase II clinical study of feasibility. Invest Radiol 2009;44(11):697–704.

87. Miserus RJ, Herias MV, Prinzen L, et al. Molecular MRI of early thrombus formation using a bimodal alpha2-antiplasmin-based contrast agent. JACC Cardiovasc Imaging 2009;2(8):987–96.

88. Temme S, Grapentin C, Quast C, et al. Noninvasive imaging of early venous thrombosis by 19F magnetic resonance imaging with targeted perfluorocarbon nanoemulsions. Circulation 2015; 131(16):1405–14.

89. Hosch W, Schlieter M, Ley S, et al. Detection of acute pulmonary embolism: feasibility of diagnostic accuracy of MRI using a stepwise protocol. Emerg Radiol 2014;21(2):151–8.

90. Garcia-Alvarez A, Fernandez-Friera L, Garcia-Ruiz JM, et al. Noninvasive monitoring of serial changes in pulmonary vascular resistance and acute vasodilator testing using cardiac magnetic resonance. J Am Coll Cardiol 2013;62(17):1621–31.

91. Brooks RA. A quantitative theory of the Hounsfield unit and its application to dual energy scanning. J Comput Assist Tomogr 1977;1(4):487–93.

92. Ferda J, Ferdova E, Mirka H, et al. Pulmonary imaging using dual-energy CT, a role of the assessment of iodine and air distribution. Eur J Radiol 2011; 77(2):287–93.

93. Bauer RW, Frellesen C, Renker M, et al. Dual energy CT pulmonary blood volume assessment in acute pulmonary embolism - correlation with D-dimer level, right heart strain and clinical outcome. Eur Radiol 2011;21(9):1914–21.

94. Meysman M, Everaert H, Buls N, et al. Comparison of ventilation-perfusion single-photon emission computed tomography (V/Q SPECT) versus dual-energy CT perfusion and angiography (DECT) after 6 months of pulmonary embolism (PE) treatment. Eur J Radiol 2015;84(9):1816–9.

95. Lu GM, Zhao Y, Zhang LJ, et al. Dual-energy CT of the lung. AJR Am J Roentgenol 2012;199(5 Suppl): S40–53.

96. Hwang HJ, Hoffman EA, Lee CH, et al. The role of dual-energy computed tomography in the assessment of pulmonary function. Eur J Radiol 2017;86: 320–34.

97. Okada M, Kunihiro Y, Nakashima Y, et al. Added value of lung perfused blood volume images using dual-energy CT for assessment of acute pulmonary embolism. Eur J Radiol 2015;84(1):172–7.

98. Le Faivre J, Duhamel A, Khung S, et al. Impact of CT perfusion imaging on the assessment of peripheral chronic pulmonary thromboembolism: clinical experience in 62 patients. Eur Radiol 2016; 26(11):4011–20.

99. Chang S, Hur J, Im DJ, et al. Dual-energy CT-based iodine quantification for differentiating pulmonary artery sarcoma from pulmonary thromboembolism: a pilot study. Eur Radiol 2016;26(9): 3162–70.

100. Kline JA, Mitchell AM, Kabrhel C, et al. Clinical criteria to prevent unnecessary diagnostic testing in emergency department patients with suspected pulmonary embolism. J Thromb Haemost 2004; 2(8):1247–55.

101. Wells PS, Anderson DR, Rodger M, et al. Excluding pulmonary embolism at the bedside without diagnostic imaging: management of patients with suspected pulmonary embolism presenting to the emergency department by using a simple clinical model and d-dimer. Ann Intern Med 2001;135(2): 98–107.

102. Le Gal G, Righini M, Roy PM, et al. Prediction of pulmonary embolism in the emergency department: the revised Geneva score. Ann Intern Med 2006;144(3):165–71.

APPENDIX 1:

Pulmonary Embolism Rule-Out Criteria[100]	
Age $\geq$50	1 point
SaO$_2$ on room air <95%	1 point
Heart rate $\geq$100 bpm	1 point
Unilateral leg swelling	1 point
Recent surgery or trauma; that is, $\leq$4 wk ago requiring general anesthesia	1 point
Hemoptysis	1 point
Previous pulmonary embolism or deep venous thrombosis	1 point
Hormone use (oral contraceptive, hormone replacement or estrogenic hormones use in male or female patients)	1 point
Score	*Risk*
0	<2% chance of pulmonary embolism
$\geq$1	Rule cannot be used to rule out in a patient with pulmonary embolism

Wells Criteria for Pulmonary Embolism[101]		
Clinical signs of deep venous thrombosis		3 points
PE is #1 diagnosis or equally likely		3 points
Heart rate >100		1.5 points
Immobilization at least 3 d or surgery in previous 4 wk		1.5 points
Previous, objectively diagnosed pulmonary embolism or deep venous thrombosis		1.5 points
Hemoptysis		1 point
Malignancy w/treatment within 6 mo		1 point
Score	*Risk*	*Prevalence*
0–1	Low risk	1.3%
2–6	Moderate risk	16.2%
>6	High risk	37.5%

Revised Geneva Score for Pulmonary Embolism[102]		
Age >65		1 point
Surgery (under general anesthesia) or lower limb fracture in past month		2 points
Active malignant condition (solid or hematologic malignancy, currently active or cured <1 y)		2 points
Unilateral limb pain		3 points
Previous pulmonary embolism or deep venous thrombosis		3 points
Hemoptysis		2 points
Pain on limb palpation		4 points
Heart rate (bpm)		
<75		0 points
75–94		3 points
$\geq$95		5 points
Score	*Risk*	*Incidence*
0–3	Low risk	<10%
4–10	Moderate risk	10%–60%
>11	High risk	>60%

Intraluminal Arterial Filling Defects Misdiagnosed as Pulmonary Emboli: What Else Could They Be?

Anastasiia A. Rudkovskaia, MD*,
Debabrata Bandyopadhyay, MD

KEYWORDS

- Nonthrombotic pulmonary embolism • Amniotic fluid embolism • Tumor embolism
- Pulmonary artery sarcoma • Computed tomography angiography • Stenosis or obstruction
- Cement embolism • Pulmonary hypertension

KEY POINTS

- Pulmonary artery filling defects can be observed in pathologic conditions other than pulmonary embolism.
- Nonthrombotic pulmonary embolism with biological and nonbiological materials and intrinsic pulmonary artery lesions have been described among these conditions.
- Fibrosing mediastinitis and congenital absence or stenosis of pulmonary artery, pulmonary parenchymal and airway malignancies are some other rare causes of misdiagnosis.
- Correct diagnosis is based on the appropriate clinical suspicion with full scope of clinical, laboratory and radiologic data.

INTRODUCTION

The incidence of pulmonary embolism (PE) is estimated to be 112 cases per 100,000 US population. Since 1998, the incidence of PE has nearly doubled, but mortality from PE has significantly decreased in the same period.[1,2] This trend is attributed to early diagnosis and intervention. Computed tomography pulmonary angiography (CTPA) has become the investigation of choice for the imaging of pulmonary arteries in patients with suspected PE and has largely replaced the gold standard pulmonary angiography.[3] The PIOPED II trial reported a sensitivity of 83% and specificity of 96% for CTPA to detect PE.[4]

CTPA has a high diagnostic accuracy, demonstrating partial or complete intraluminal filling defects in pulmonary arteries. The filling defects characteristically show signs, such as the doughnut sign, railroad sign, or abrupt cutoff of the vessels. However, the positive predictive value of a positive CTPA is much lower (58%) in patients with a low probability of PE.[5] Therefore, caution must be used before diagnosing all filling defects as pulmonary thromboembolic disease, particularly with atypical presenting symptoms. In clinical practice, PE is more common; however, other causes of filling defects, although rare, can lead to inappropriate diagnosis and a delayed intervention. Certain filling defect patterns, such as the involvement of entire main pulmonary arteries

Disclosure Statement: No disclosures.
Pulmonary and Critical Care Medicine, Geisinger, 100 North Academy Avenue, Danville, PA 17822-1334, USA
* Corresponding author.
E-mail address: aarudkovskaia@geisinger.edu

Clin Chest Med 39 (2018) 505–513
https://doi.org/10.1016/j.ccm.2018.04.004
0272-5231/18/© 2018 Elsevier Inc. All rights reserved.

chestmed.theclinics.com

and one of its branches, delayed and heterogeneous contrast enhancement of the lesion, and globular filling defects, are more suggestive of an etiology other than PE. Hence, an accurate timely diagnosis is often challenging.[6]

The primary purpose of this article is to describe other etiopathologic processes causing intraluminal filling defects of the pulmonary arteries, which radiographically mimic PE and often misdiagnosed as PE. The filling defect can arise from embolization into the pulmonary vasculature, referred to as nonthrombotic PE (NTPE), or de novo pulmonary vascular lesions.

NONTHROMBOTIC PULMONARY EMBOLISM

NTPE refers to the obstruction of pulmonary circulation by embolization of different biologic and nonbiologic materials. NTPE is less common than thrombotic PE, which explains the low clinical suspicion and frequent misdiagnosis.[7-9]

The mechanism of NTPE is multifactorial. It involves both mechanical obstruction of the pulmonary vasculature and activation of the inflammatory and coagulation cascades as in the pulmonary tumor thrombotic microangiopathy. These events lead to stenosis or occlusion of the vessel, with development of pulmonary hypertension (PH), right heart failure, and sudden death.[8]

NTPE frequently presents with atypical signs and symptoms, making clinical diagnosis an arduous task. Symptomatology of NTPE is largely similar to thrombotic PE, for example, dyspnea, pleuritic chest pain, cough, hemoptysis, and syncope. The clinical appearance may range from being asymptomatic to sudden death. Patients may present with hemodynamic instability and acute respiratory distress syndrome (ARDS). Embolism owing to fat, amniotic fluid, and septic embolism usually have a more dramatic presentation. Patients can present with subacute to chronic dyspnea owing to development of chronic thromboembolic PH and congestive heart failure. This finding is more common with talc, cement, and tumor embolism.[10] The clinical signs are variable, and include tachycardia, tachypnea, cyanosis, low oxygen saturation, and hypotension.

A laboratory diagnosis of NTPE is nonspecific. The D-dimer test does not have diagnostic value in NTPE, unlike in PE.[11] Many patients show elevated troponin as an expression of right ventricular strain.[12] The diagnosis of NTPE is largely based on radiologic imaging. The CTPA in NTPE can follow 2 distinct patterns, macroembolic and microembolic, all based on the nature and location of the emboli. The macroembolism usually presents with visible pulmonary artery obstruction (Table 1). Owing to the hyperdense nature of some of the nonbiological materials, they can be obscured by the bright contrast material, and thus remain undetected.[13] The imaging characteristics secondary to pulmonary artery occlusion include enlargement of central pulmonary artery (Fleischner sign), pleural-based wedge-shaped opacity (Hampton sign), peripheral radiolucency owing to decreased vascularity (Westermark sign), and hemidiaphragm elevation. However, these signs are nonspecific, are often seen in any type of pulmonary occlusion.[10]

Conversely, microembolism owing to fat, talcum, amniotic fluid, septic material, and many tumors may not cause filling defects in CTPA (Fig. 1; see Table 1). They present with signs of PH, parenchymal infarction from pulmonary arterial obstruction, and pulmonary edema owing to venous obstruction.[13] The radiologic manifestation of microembolic event also depends on the site of occlusion. An occluded subsegmental pulmonary artery at centrilobular region can cause a tree-in-bud appearance like mucoid impaction or peribronchiolar inflammation.[10] The spectrum of radiographic manifestations owing to microembolism also include bilateral infiltrates consistent with ARDS, multiple pulmonary cavities seen in septic emboli, ground glass opacities, and parenchymal consolidation as a result of chemical pneumonitis.[13]

The pulmonary-specific management measures are supportive, and include adequate oxygenation, ventilatory support, hemodynamic resuscitation with fluid, and vasopressors.

Table 1
Most common causes of NTPE

Macroembolic NTPE	Microembolic NTPE
Hydatid embolism	Fat embolism
Glue embolism	Amniotic fluid
Gas embolism	embolism
Catheter embolism	Septic embolism
Pacemaker lead embolism	Bone and tissue
Cement embolism	embolism
Embolism with	Talcum embolism
angiographic and	Radioactive seed
intraoperative material	embolism
Bullet embolism	Mercury embolism
Ventriculoperitoneal	Silicone embolism
shunt embolism	Trophoblastic
Tumor embolism	embolism

Some types of nonthrombotic pulmonary embolism may have both microembolic and macroembolic presentation; the table reflects the most common presentation.

Abbreviation: NTPE, nonthrombotic pulmonary embolism.

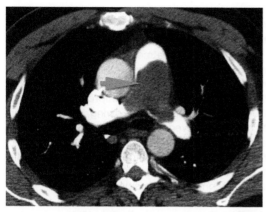

Fig. 1. Computed tomography pulmonary angiography with the *arrowhead* pointing at the filling defect of the pulmonary artery in a patient with pulmonary artery sarcoma.

Nonthrombotic Pulmonary Embolism Owing to Biological Materials

Pulmonary tumor embolism

Pulmonary tumor embolism (PTE) refers to the embolisation of pulmonary vasculature with tumor cells, which is an end-stage manifestation of many malignancies. PTE differs from hematogenous metastases because the latter tends to invade the arterial wall.[14] Common sources of PTE include gastric, hepatic, pancreatic, hepatocellular, renal cell, prostate, breast, and choriocarcinomas. Autopsy series reveal the incidence of PTE between 2.5% and 26.0%.[15]

PTE can present as (a) macroscopic emboli occluding main pulmonary arteries, (b) microscopic arteriolar emboli, (c) diffuse interstitial opacities with septal thickening owing to microvascular invasion by tumor emboli, or (d) any combination of the above.[16] Pulmonary tumor thrombotic microangiopathy is a related phenomenon, most common in advanced gastric adenocarcinoma, and caused by microscopic tumor cell emboli inducing thrombotic microangiopathy. Pathologically, pulmonary tumor thrombotic microangiopathy demonstrates fibrocellular intimal proliferation and occlusion of the affected vessels, unlike PTE.[17]

The most common clinical manifestation of PTE is subacute or chronic onset of dyspnea (60%–100% cases) and hypoxemic respiratory failure. Other symptoms, such as pleuritic chest pain, cough, hemoptysis, fatigue, and weight loss, have been reported. Eventually, patients develop PH and progressive right ventricular failure in 15% to 20% cases. Marked cardiopulmonary derangements are usually noticeable after about 60% to 80% of the arterial bed is affected.[16] On physical examination, signs of cor pulmonale are the most frequent. Crackles may be present owing to the associated lymphangitic carcinomatosis.[14]

Diagnosis is mostly confirmed after autopsy; even in patients with known malignancy, only 6% are diagnosed antemortem.[18] Tumor emboli affects small and medium size arteries, which appear beaded with tree-in-bud appearance on CT scans of the chest.[19] Filling defects of the pulmonary arteries are not characteristic of this disease. Rarely, macroscopic PTE can cause filling defect by occluding main or lobar pulmonary arteries. This type of radiologic findings is usually owing to direct invasion of the inferior vena cava and right ventricular spread by solid tumors, such as sarcoma, hepatocellular, renal cell, or choriocarcinoma.[20]

The prognosis is usually grim. Complete cure after surgical resection of the primary tumor is possible in renal cell carcinoma and choriocarcinoma.[14] Chemotherapy is generally not recommended, although favorable results are reported in breast cancer and choriocarcinoma.[21]

Fat embolism syndrome

The fat embolism syndrome refers to adipose tissue release by an identifiable injury causing obstruction of pulmonary and systemic circulation. It usually occurs 12 to 72 hours after the insult, and presents with respiratory distress (hypoxemia), neurologic sequalae (focal neurodeficit, seizures, confusion, coma), and cutaneous (petechial rash) abnormalities.[8,22] It is commonly associated with the release of fat globules from the bone marrow of fractured long bones and pelvic bones, endomedullary nailing, placement of joint prostheses, and severe trauma.[22] The incidence of fat embolism after long bone fracture is 1% to 3% and in severe trauma it is 10% to 20%.[23] Less commonly, it happens after other fatty tissue injury, such as liposuction, major burns or necrosis of steatotic liver, acute pancreatitis, and rarely with lipid-based infusions.

The exact pathogenesis of fat embolism syndrome is unknown, but several hypotheses have been proposed: (a) mechanical obstruction of the pulmonary vasculature by the fat droplets or (b) biochemical injury from release of free fatty acids causing endothelial injury, activation of inflammatory reactions and coagulation cascade leading to accumulation of neutrophils and other inflammatory cells, and intravascular fibrins.[10]

Diagnosis is mostly clinical in the appropriate setting with the triad of respiratory symptoms, unexplained cerebral manifestations, and petechial rash. The laboratory abnormalities include anemia, thrombocytopenia, coagulation abnormalities consistent with disseminated intra-vascular coagulation, a high erythrocyte sedimentation rate, hyperbilirubinemia, and renal dysfunction. CT scan demonstrates an ARDS pattern with diffuse areas of homogenous and heterogenous ground glass opacities owing to microembolic nature of the process. Rarely, fat embolism syndrome presents with macroembolism identified on the CT scans as pulmonary artery obstruction by a low-density material.[22]

Primary prevention with early mobilization, and open reduction and external fixation of fractures are important in management of fat embolism.[22] Treatment consists of supportive care, such as adequate oxygenation, mechanical ventilation, fluid resuscitation, and vasopressors. Transfusion of blood products and bronchodilators improve oxygenation and correct disseminated intravascular coagulation. The routine use of heparin, low-molecular-weight dextran, and aprotinin is not recommended.[24] The role of steroid remains controversial because the beneficial results from small studies were not replicated in large, well-designed trials.[25] The successful use of venovenous extracorporeal member oxygenation has been reported to treat this condition.[26] Fat embolism syndrome is largely self-limiting and has a good outcome. The mortality ranges between 10% and 20%.

Hydatid embolism
Hydatid cysts (echinococcosis) is a parasitic infection caused by the larval stage of the tapeworm *Eccinococcus granulosus*. Humans are infected by ingestion of eggs. The cysts develop commonly in human liver (75%) and lung (15%). It is endemic in the Middle East, Latin America, and Mediterranean countries. Rarely, the cysts reach right ventricle via portal vessels or lymphatic channels from liver or lung. Hydatid embolism develops as a consequence of (a) rupture of cysts into the right ventricle, (b) hematogenous dissemination of hepatic hydatid cysts into hepatic vein and inferior vena cava,[27] and (c) seldom, pulmonary cysts burrow into pulmonary arterial wall.[28]

Clinically, hydatid embolism presentation varies: (a) asymptomatic (most common), (b) rupture of cysts causing fatal anaphylactic reaction, (c) subacute PH leading to right heart failure and death within 1 year, or (d) chronic PH. Hemoptysis is the most common symptom, others include cough, dyspnea, and chest pain.

Serologic tests are more specific but less sensitive than imaging techniques.[29] Transesophageal echocardiography can detect Hydatid embolism in main pulmonary arteries. Chest CT and magnetic resonance angiography show pulmonary

artery occlusion by hypodense cystic structures. Magnetic resonance angiography is more sensitive in detecting hydatid cysts.[30]

Early surgical treatment with embolectomy is recommended in hydatid embolism. In disseminated cases, combined surgery and antiparasitic treatment with albendazol improves outcomes. Overall, prognosis is poor owing to progression to chronic PH even after embolectomy in the presence of distal cysts, focal inflammation, and fibrosis. Successful outcome with PH-specific therapies have been reported.[31] Lung transplantation is recommended in selected cases.[32]

Septic pulmonary embolism
Septic PE (SPE) usually presents with insidious onset of fever, pulmonary symptoms, and infiltrates. It is caused by embolization of infected thrombi, often containing bacteria, parasites, or fungi, and leading to pulmonary infarction and cavitary lesions.

The most common sources of SPE are intravenous drug abuse, an infected intravascular device or catheter, and soft tissue infections.[33] An increasing number of recent SPE cases can be attributed to increasing use of intravascular and intracardiac devices.

Patients usually present with fever, cough, dyspnea, hemoptysis, and fatigue. Extrapulmonary symptoms depend on the source of infection. In severe cases, progression to respiratory failure, empyema, septic shock, ad renal insufficiency can occur. Pulmonary crackles, audible murmur, and stigmata of infective endocarditis can be found on physical examination.

Most cases of SPE are associated with bacteremia. In 1 published series, the majority of the blood cultures grew methicillin-sensitive or -resistant *Staphylococcus aureus*.[34] Echocardiography revealed right-sided vegetation in more than one-half of the cases. A transesophageal echocardiography is superior in detecting small thrombi, prosthetic valve vegetations, and perivalvular abscesses. Chest CT findings are often nonspecific, including diffuse or focal pulmonary infiltrates, wedge-shaped opacities, and pleural effusions. Findings of multiple, scattered, and sometimes cavitating nodules in the lower lobes are more characteristic of SPE. Pulmonary nodules in SPE are characterized by the feeding vessel sign, representing a vessel leading directly to the nodule, and the halo sign, ground-glass attenuation from perilesional hemorrhagic infarction.[23] Owing to the small size of septic emboli, SPE mostly leads to segmental and subsegmental pulmonary artery occlusion and intravascular filling defects are usually not found on chest CT.[35]

Amniotic fluid embolism

Amniotic fluid embolism (AFE) is a catastrophic complication of pregnancy and early postpartum period resulting from passage of fetal and amniotic fragments into the maternal circulation through the uterine veins. It occurs as early as the second trimester of pregnancy, up to 24 hours after delivery.[36] The incidence of AFE is 7 to 8 per 100,000 births.[37] The maternal and fetal mortality remains high; 56% die within 2 hours.[38]

Mechanisms of pulmonary injury are similar to those observed in fat embolism syndrome: (a) obstruction of the pulmonary artery by amniotic debris and (b) an immunologic response to the amniotic tissue associated with intense inflammatory reaction, activation of complement system, and stimulation of coagulation cascade. Clinically, it results in anaphylactoid reactions, ARDS with respiratory failure, cardiogenic shock, disseminated intravascular coagulation, and death.

AFE is characterized by a rapidly progressive clinical course with dyspnea, hypoxia, hypotension, and at a later stage hemorrhagic shock and neurologic complications like seizures and coma. AFE can be responsible for sudden maternal death after delivery.[39]

There are no uniform diagnostic criteria for AFE. The histologic confirmation of fetal tissue in maternal circulation can be confirmed by Alcian blue or Atwood stain. Immunostaining using antibody to THK-2 is a sensitive method to detect amniotic fluid derived mucin in lung biopsy specimen.[40] Many other stains, such as cytokeratin AE1/E3 and ZnCp-1, have been used to detect components of amniotic fluid in the maternal circulation. However, fetal tissue is detected in only 50% of maternal circulation with AFE.[37]

High clinical suspicion and prompt diagnosis is paramount. Delivery within 5 minutes of maternal cardiac arrest improves outcome. Treatment is directed toward maintaining adequate oxygenation, hemodynamic support, and correction of the coagulopathy.[8] Successful use of inhaled nitric oxide, cardiopulmonary bypass, intraaortic balloon pump counterpulsation, and extracorporeal member oxygenation has been reported.[41,42]

Trophoblastic embolism

Gestational trophoblastic neoplasia refers to the abnormal proliferation of trophoblastic tissue of placenta. This neoplastic growth arises from fetal tissue. Two benign variants (partial or complete hydatiform mole) and 3 malignant variants (invasive mole, choriocarcinoma, and trophoblastic tumor) have been described. Lung metastases may occur after gestation, during hysterectomy or evacuation of moles and as side effects of chemotherapy for choriocarcinoma.

Pulmonary emboli largely are a coincidental finding. Most patients present with vaginal bleeding. Preeclampsia is a common association. Self-limited respiratory distress lasting for 1 to 3 days can occur during the manipulation of molar tissue. Cardiopulmonary compromise like elevated pulmonary artery pressure, wedge pressure, pulmonary vascular resistance, and a decrease in cardiac output are rare. Different CT chest appearances with military, nodular, or snowstorm opacities have been reported, along with pleural effusion. Signs of embolic occlusion of pulmonary arteries have also been described.[43]

Acute treatment involves diuresis and ventilatory support. Gestational trophoblastic neoplasia is treated with multiagent regimens owing to the increased risk of drug resistance to a single agent. Chemotherapy-resistant malignancies are usually treated with surgical resection such as embolectomy.[44] The prognosis is usually good. Source control often resolves the pulmonary complications.

Nonthrombotic Pulmonary Embolism Owing to Nonbiological Materials

Cement pulmonary artery embolism

Cement pulmonary artery embolism (CPAE) is described in association with vertebroplasty and kyphoplasty owing to embolization of polymethyl-methacrylate (cement). The incidence of CPAE is 4% to 23%. Interestingly, CPAE does not occur when it is used in putty consistency in hip or knee replacements. The occurrence of CPAE is independent of the volume of injected cement; a high focal pressure may aid its entry into the venous system.

Most CPAE is asymptomatic, but persistent PH and fatal outcome are reported.[45] Chest CT demonstrates radiopaque bandlike intraluminal filling defect. Different medical and surgical therapeutic interventions have been suggested. In mild cases, anticoagulation is continued for 3 to 6 months to prevent thrombus formation. Surgical embolectomy has been performed in hemodynamic instability.[46]

Air embolism

Air embolism is frequently iatrogenic and occurs as a complication of procedures, such as central venous catheter insertions, transthoracic needle biopsy, or radiofrequency ablations. The noniatrogenic causes include diving, aviation, and trauma. The risk of death is related to the amount of air and speed of delivery.[23] It can rarely cause PH, right ventricular failure, and arterial embolism through a patent foramen ovale.

Treatment is directed toward the maintenance of circulation and preventing further air embolization. Once suspected, a right lateral decubitus position is recommended. A CT scan is done in this position to make a diagnosis after visualization of air in the pulmonary arteries. Hyperbaric oxygen reduces bubble size and improves oxygenation.

Iodinated oil and glue embolism

Pulmonary artery embolism with cyanoacrylate and glutaraldehyde has been reported after surgical procedures for embolization of brain arteriovenous malformations and fundal varices, after chemoembolization for hepatocellular carcinoma and vertebroplasty. On chest CT, it presents as radiopaque material coursing the pulmonary vessels.[47–49]

Talc embolism

Talc embolism owing to magnesium trisilicate is seen in intravenous drug users. It is an insoluble component of many oral narcotics, which are crushed and then injected. These particulates cause vascular obstruction, thrombosis, inflammation, and giant cell reaction. This syndrome gives rise to a vessel wall tree-in-bud appearance on CT chest in addition to widespread pulmonary nodules. PH may also develop.

Silicone embolism

Polydimethylsiloxane (liquid silicone) is used for cosmetic purposes in breast implants and subcutaneous injections in gluteal and vaginal regions. In some, the inert material enters the venous system and pulmonary artery, causing embolism and pneumonitis. Dyspnea, hemoptysis, alveolar hemorrhage, hypoxia, petechiae, and an altered sensorium are commonly observed. A 25% mortality has been reported. A multitude of rare causes of embolism with a variety of substances have been reported. They are listed in **Table 1**.

Intrinsic Pulmonary Lesions Causing Pulmonary Artery Filling Defect

Primary pulmonary artery sarcoma

Primary pulmonary artery sarcoma (PPAS) is a rare tumor arising from the mesenchymal cells. The true incidence is unknown owing to the frequent misdiagnosis as PE and chronic thromboembolic PH. Different histologic types of PPAS have been reported in the literature: leiomyosarcoma, spindle cell sarcoma, fibrous histiocytoma, undifferentiated, angiosarcoma, myofibroblastic sarcoma, chondrosarcoma, osteosarcoma, and so on.[6]

Most commonly, patients present with dyspnea and shortness of breath. Other symptoms, such as cough, chest pain, fever, fatigue, weight loss, and syncope owing to PH, have been reported.[6] Hemoptysis occurs in cases of bronchial infiltration by PPAS. Patients usually present with clinical signs of PH in chronic cases. Atypical features, such as a lack of predisposing risk factors for thromboembolism and failure of anticoagulation, should raise suspicion for PPAS.[50]

Characteristic radiologic findings have been described in the literature. In contrast with the classic PE, the filling defects in CTPA tend to be more central, unilateral, and lobular (see **Fig. 1**). Additionally, filling defects in PPAS tend to form acute angles with the pulmonary artery wall, and areas of hemorrhage with necrosis and ossification may be observed within the mass.[51] CTPA might not be sufficient for the diagnosis and additional imaging with gadolinium-enhanced MRI, fluorodeoxyglucose, or PET is often required.[52] Other radiologic features are hilar mass, metastatic lesions, unilateral pulmonary artery enlargement, decreased pulmonary vascular markings, peripheral pulmonary opacities, pleural effusions, and hemidiaphragm elevation.

Even with appropriate diagnosis, the overall prognosis is dismal; up to 50% of the patients have lung metastasis by the time of diagnosis.[53] Therapeutic options are limited. Complete surgical resection, if feasible, improves survival. Early diagnosis and combination treatment with surgical resection and chemotherapy show the most favorable outcomes and survival benefits.[6]

Takayasu arteritis

Takayasu arteritis is a large vessel arteritis with primary involvement of aorta and its branches, commonly found in young females. Recent studies describe pulmonary arterial involvement between 14% and 86%.[54,55] Rare cases of isolated pulmonary artery involvement have been reported.[56]

Pulmonary arteritis is often asymptomatic or associated with nonspecific symptoms of dyspnea, hemoptysis, chest pain, and signs of PH. Associated systemic symptoms such as fever, weight loss, and arthralgia are often present. The presence of systemic hypertension, arterial bruits, diminished pulses, and renal involvement in a young female should raise suspicion for Takayasu arteritis.

Anemia and an elevated erythrocyte sedimentation rate are characteristic of Takayasu arteritis.[56] CTPA demonstrates occlusion of segmental or subsegmental pulmonary arteries, rarely lobar or main pulmonary artery. CTPA has a high diagnostic accuracy, clearly depicts wall thickening and enhancement, and mural calcium deposition.[57] Nonetheless, it is often misdiagnosed as chronic thromboembolic disease. The presence of systemic manifestations and evidence of bronchial artery collaterals such as rib notching distinguishes this condition.

Other Etiologies

Unusual pulmonary artery filling defects have been described in the presence of systemic to pulmonary arterial shunts and in the setting of chronic lung diseases.[58] Other rarely described cases of pulmonary artery filling defects include congenital absence or stenosis of pulmonary artery and fibrosing mediastinitis, which mimics PE.

SUMMARY

Radiologic findings of pulmonary artery filling defects can be observed in a spectrum of pathologic processes other than PE. Additionally, the relative rarity of these conditions in general clinical practice may lead to a reduced awareness and consequent misdiagnosis and inappropriate intervention. Hence, a high index of suspicion in the appropriate clinical background is paramount to allow a prompt and precise diagnosis. The diagnosis is largely based on the unique clinical features, laboratory findings and additional radiologic clues inferring a pathology other than PE.

REFERENCES

1. Wiener RS, Schwartz LM, Woloshin S. Time trends in pulmonary embolism in the United States: evidence of overdiagnosis. Arch Intern Med 2011; 171(9):831–7.
2. Sogaard KK, Schmidt M, Pedersen L, et al. 30-year mortality after venous thromboembolism: a population-based cohort study. Circulation 2014; 130(10):829–36.
3. Henschke CI, Mateescu I, Yankelevitz DF. Changing practice patterns in the workup of pulmonary embolism. Chest 1995;107(4):940–5.
4. Stein PD, Fowler SE, Goodman LR, et al. Multidetector computed tomography for acute pulmonary embolism. N Engl J Med 2006;354(22):2317–27.
5. Konstantinides SV, Torbicki A, Agnelli G, et al. 2014 ESC guidelines on the diagnosis and management of acute pulmonary embolism. Eur Heart J 2014; 35(43):3033–69, 3069a–k.
6. Bandyopadhyay D, Panchabhai TS, Bajaj NS, et al. Primary pulmonary artery sarcoma: a close associate of pulmonary embolism-20-year observational analysis. J Thorac Dis 2016;8(9): 2592–601.
7. Rossi SE, Goodman PC, Franquet T. Nonthrombotic pulmonary emboli. AJR Am J Roentgenol 2000; 174(6):1499–508.
8. Jorens PG, Van Marck E, Snoeckx A, et al. Nonthrombotic pulmonary embolism. Eur Respir J 2009;34(2):452–74.
9. Khashper A, Discepola F, Kosiuk J, et al. Nonthrombotic pulmonary embolism. AJR Am J Roentgenol 2012;198(2):W152–9.
10. Unal E, Balci S, Atceken Z, et al. Nonthrombotic pulmonary artery embolism: imaging findings and review of the literature. AJR Am J Roentgenol 2017; 208(3):505–16.
11. Huang HK, Huang CH, Wu CC, et al. An unusual cause of acute pulmonary embolism. Int J Cardiol 2011;149(2):e88–9.
12. Montagnana M, Cervellin G, Franchini M, et al. Pathophysiology, clinics and diagnostics of nonthrombotic pulmonary embolism. J Thromb Thrombolysis 2011;31(4):436–44.
13. Bach AG, Restrepo CS, Abbas J, et al. Imaging of nonthrombotic pulmonary embolism: biological materials, nonbiological materials, and foreign bodies. Eur J Radiol 2013;82(3):e120–41.
14. Chan CK, Hutcheon MA, Hyland RH, et al. Pulmonary tumor embolism: a critical review of clinical, imaging, and hemodynamic features. J Thorac Imaging 1987;2(4):4–14.
15. Veinot JP, Ford SE, Price RG. Subacute cor pulmonale due to tumor embolization. Arch Pathol Lab Med 1992;116(2):131–4.
16. Roberts KE, Hamele-Bena D, Saqi A, et al. Pulmonary tumor embolism: a review of the literature. Am J Med 2003;115(3):228–32.
17. Rudkovskaia AA, Lo YC, Brady V, et al. A 49-year-old man with subacute respiratory failure and interstitial lung opacities. Am J Case Rep 2017;18:941–4.
18. Brock SJ, Fuller C, Iveson TJ. Pulmonary tumour emboli: a difficult ante-mortem diagnosis. Clin Oncol (R Coll Radiol) 2000;12(1):56–7.
19. Rossi SE, Franquet T, Volpacchio M, et al. Tree-in-bud pattern at thin-section CT of the lungs: radiologic-pathologic overview. Radiographics 2005;25(3):789–801.
20. Winterbauer RH, Elfenbein IB, Ball WC Jr. Incidence and clinical significance of tumor embolization to the lungs. Am J Med 1968;45(2):271–90.
21. Schriner RW, Ryu JH, Edwards WD. Microscopic pulmonary tumor embolism causing subacute cor pulmonale: a difficult antemortem diagnosis. Mayo Clin Proc 1991;66(2):143–8.
22. Parisi DM, Koval K, Egol K. Fat embolism syndrome. Am J Orthop (Belle Mead NJ) 2002;31(9): 507–12.
23. Pena E, Dennie C, Franquet T, et al. Nonthrombotic pulmonary embolism: a radiological perspective. Semin Ultrasound CT MR 2012;33(6):522–34.

24. Mellor A, Soni N. Fat embolism. Anaesthesia 2001; 56(2):145–54.

25. Schonfeld SA, Ploysongsang Y, DiLisio R, et al. Fat embolism prophylaxis with corticosteroids. A prospective study in high-risk patients. Ann Intern Med 1983;99(4):438–43.

26. Webb DP, McKamie WA, Pietsch JB. Resuscitation of fat embolism syndrome with extracorporeal membrane oxygenation. J Extra Corpor Technol 2004; 36(4):368–70.

27. Pedrosa I, Saiz A, Arrazola J, et al. Hydatid disease: radiologic and pathologic features and complications. Radiographics 2000;20(3):795–817.

28. Kiresi DA, Karabacakoglu A, Odev K, et al. Uncommon locations of hydatid cysts. Acta Radiol 2003; 44(6):622–36.

29. Babba H, Messedi A, Masmoudi S, et al. Diagnosis of human hydatidosis: comparison between imagery and six serologic techniques. Am J Trop Med Hyg 1994;50(1):64–8.

30. Salem R, Zrig A, Joober S, et al. Pulmonary embolism in echinococcosis: two case reports and literature review. Ann Trop Med Parasitol 2011;105(1):85–9.

31. Bulman W, Coyle CM, Brentjens TE, et al. Severe pulmonary hypertension due to chronic echinococcal pulmonary emboli treated with targeted pulmonary vascular therapy and hepatic resection. Chest 2007;132(4):1356–8.

32. Franquet T, Plaza V, Llauger J, et al. Hydatid pulmonary embolism from a ruptured mediastinal cyst: high-resolution computed tomography, angiographic, and pathologic findings. J Thorac Imaging 1999;14(2):138–41.

33. Cook RJ, Ashton RW, Aughenbaugh GL, et al. Septic pulmonary embolism: presenting features and clinical course of 14 patients. Chest 2005;128(1):162–6.

34. Ye R, Zhao L, Wang C, et al. Clinical characteristics of septic pulmonary embolism in adults: a systematic review. Respir Med 2014;108(1):1–8.

35. Huang RM, Naidich DP, Lubat E, et al. Septic pulmonary emboli: CT-radiographic correlation. AJR Am J Roentgenol 1989;153(1):41–5.

36. Clark SL. New concepts of amniotic fluid embolism: a review. Obstet Gynecol Surv 1990;45(6):360–8.

37. Balinger KJ, Chu Lam MT, Hon HH, et al. Amniotic fluid embolism: despite progress, challenges remain. Curr Opin Obstet Gynecol 2015;27(6): 398–405.

38. Kramer MS, Rouleau J, Baskett TF, et al, Maternal Health Study Group of the Canadian Perinatal Surveillance System. Amniotic-fluid embolism and medical induction of labour: a retrospective, population-based cohort study. Lancet 2006; 368(9545):1444–8.

39. Sinicina I, Pankratz H, Bise K, et al. Forensic aspects of post-mortem histological detection of amniotic fluid embolism. Int J Legal Med 2010;124(1):55–62.

40. Kobayashi H, Ooi H, Hayakawa H, et al. Histological diagnosis of amniotic fluid embolism by monoclonal antibody TKH-2 that recognizes NeuAc alpha 2-6GalNAc epitope. Hum Pathol 1997;28(4):428–33.

41. Hsieh YY, Chang CC, Li PC, et al. Successful application of extracorporeal membrane oxygenation and intra-aortic balloon counterpulsation as lifesaving therapy for a patient with amniotic fluid embolism. Am J Obstet Gynecol 2000;183(2):496–7.

42. Stanten RD, Iverson LI, Daugharty TM, et al. Amniotic fluid embolism causing catastrophic pulmonary vasoconstriction: diagnosis by transesophageal echocardiogram and treatment by cardiopulmonary bypass. Obstet Gynecol 2003;102(3):496–8.

43. Gamer EI, Garrett A, Goldstein DP, et al. Significance of chest computed tomography findings in the evaluation and treatment of persistent gestational trophoblastic neoplasia. J Reprod Med 2004; 49(6):411–4.

44. El-Helw LM, Hancock BW. Treatment of metastatic gestational trophoblastic neoplasia. Lancet Oncol 2007;8(8):715–24.

45. Krueger A, Bliemel C, Zettl R, et al. Management of pulmonary cement embolism after percutaneous vertebroplasty and kyphoplasty: a systematic review of the literature. Eur Spine J 2009;18(9):1257–65.

46. Lee SH, Kim WH, Ko JK. Multiple pulmonary cement embolism after percutaneous vertebroplasty. QJM 2013;106(9):877–8.

47. Pelz DM, Lownie SP, Fox AJ, et al. Symptomatic pulmonary complications from liquid acrylate embolization of brain arteriovenous malformations. AJNR Am J Neuroradiol 1995;16(1):19–26.

48. Weng MT, Chen CH. Education and imaging. Hepatobiliary and pancreatic: pulmonary emboli after transcatheter arterial chemoembolization for hepatocellular carcinoma. J Gastroenterol Hepatol 2010; 25(8):1466.

49. Kim DJ, Willinsky RA, Krings T, et al. Intracranial dural arteriovenous shunts: transarterial glue embolization–experience in 115 consecutive patients. Radiology 2011;258(2):554–61.

50. Delany SG, Doyle TC, Bunton RW, et al. Pulmonary artery sarcoma mimicking pulmonary embolism. Chest 1993;103(5):1631–3.

51. Gutierrez A, Sauler M, Mitchell JM, et al. Unresolved pulmonary embolism leading to a diagnosis of pulmonary artery sarcoma. Heart Lung 2014;43(6):574–6.

52. Lee EJ, Moon SH, Choi JY, et al. Usefulness of fluorodeoxyglucose positron emission tomography in malignancy of pulmonary artery mimicking pulmonary embolism. ANZ J Surg 2013;83(5):342–7.

53. Blackmon SH, Reardon MJ. Pulmonary artery sarcoma. Methodist Debakey Cardiovasc J 2010;6(3): 38–43.

54. Sharma S, Kamalakar T, Rajani M, et al. The incidence and patterns of pulmonary artery

involvement in Takayasu's arteritis. Clin Radiol 1990;42(3):177–81.

55. Yamato M, Lecky JW, Hiramatsu K, et al. Takayasu arteritis: radiographic and angiographic findings in 59 patients. Radiology 1986;161(2):329–34.

56. Kerr KM, Auger WR, Fedullo PF, et al. Large vessel pulmonary arteritis mimicking chronic thromboembolic disease. Am J Respir Crit Care Med 1995; 152(1):367–73.

57. Castaner E, Gallardo X, Rimola J, et al. Congenital and acquired pulmonary artery anomalies in the adult: radiologic overview. Radiographics 2006; 26(2):349–71.

58. Ansari-Gilani K, Gilkeson RC, Hsiao EM, et al. Unusual pulmonary arterial filling defect caused by systemic to pulmonary shunt in the setting of chronic lung disease demonstrated by dynamic 4D CTA. J Radiol Case Rep 2015;9(11):17–23.

Venous Thromboembolism in Special Populations
Preexisting Cardiopulmonary Disease, Cirrhosis, End-Stage Renal Disease, and Asplenia

Quyen Nguyen, MD, Belinda N. Rivera-Lebron, MD, MS, FCCP*

KEYWORDS

- Pulmonary embolism • Venous thromboembolism • Cardiopulmonary disease • Cirrhosis
- Renal failure • Asplenia • Splenectomy

KEY POINTS

- Preexisting cardiopulmonary disease, such as atrial fibrillation, heart failure, and chronic obstructive pulmonary disease, is associated with worse prognosis in venous thromboembolic disease.
- Chronic liver disease patients have substantially increased risk of venous thromboembolism (VTE), and the risk for deep vein thrombosis is higher than for PE.
- Patients with renal disease have increased risk for VTE, suffer worse outcomes, and have limitations to anticoagulation due to bleeding and drug clearance.
- Asplenia, in particular splenectomy for hematologic disease, is associated with increased risk for VTE.

INTRODUCTION

Venous thromboembolism (VTE) includes deep vein thrombosis (DVT) and pulmonary embolism (PE). There are approximately 900,000 cases of VTE per year in the United States, of which 150 to 250,000 are PE-related hospitalizations and 60 to 100,000 PE-related deaths, making it the third most common cause of cardiovascular death.[1]

VTE is associated with inherited (factor V Leiden, prothrombin mutation, antithrombin deficiency, protein C and S deficiency, and so forth) and acquired risk factors (immobilization, trauma, major surgery, malignancy, pregnancy, congestive heart failure, chronic obstructive pulmonary disease, nephrotic syndrome, liver disease, and so forth). Some of these risk factors, along with other clinical assessments, are included in the Wells rule and Geneva scores, to classify patients into pretest probability of PE diagnosis.[2–4]

Acute PE spans a wide spectrum of clinical outcomes mainly based on the right ventricle capacity to tolerate strain. The PE score index (PESI) is a validated clinical prediction rule that classifies patients with increasing risk of mortality and/or other adverse medical outcomes.[5,6] Heart failure (HF) and chronic lung disease are both included in the PESI calculation (**Table 1**).

Disclosure Statement: B. Rivera-Lebron has participated in advisory boards for Bayer Pharmaceutics and Gilead Sciences and serves as site principal investigator for a clinical trial sponsored by Actelion Pharmaceuticals. Q. Nguyen has nothing to disclose.
Division of Pulmonary, Allergy and Critical Care Medicine, University of Pittsburgh, UPMC Montefiore, 3459 Fifth Avenue, Pittsburgh, PA 15213, USA
* Corresponding author. Division of Pulmonary, Allergy and Critical Care Medicine, University of Pittsburgh, UPMC Montefiore, Room S652.1, 3459 Fifth Avenue, Pittsburgh, PA 15213.
E-mail address: riveralebronbn@upmc.edu

Clin Chest Med 39 (2018) 515–524
https://doi.org/10.1016/j.ccm.2018.04.006
0272-5231/18/

Table 1
Summary of characteristics of venous thromboembolism in special population

Special Population	Examples of Specific Conditions	Effect on Venous Thromboembolism Risk or Incidence	Effect on Venous Thromboembolism Outcomes	Therapeutic Considerations
Cardiopulmonary disease	AF	PE is a risk factor for AF.[14] May Increase VTE risk[18–20]	Higher mortality[17]	No specific recommendation
	Heart failure	N/A	Worse prognosis[5,6] Higher mortality[21]	
	AE-COPD	Increased VTE risk[28–31]	Worse prognosis[5,6]	
Cirrhosis		Increased VTE risk[41–44]	Increased length of stay and hospitalization cost[41]	LMWH is preferred over VKA[35]
Renal disease		Increased VTE risk[51–53]	Worse outcomes[47,48] Increased bleeding complications[48,57–60]	VKA is preferred anticoagulant[35] LMWH may increase bleeding.[63] DOACs not indicated in CrCl <30 mL/min or dialysis[67–70]
Asplenia	Surgical splenectomy Trauma Hematologic Thalassemia Hemolytic Anemia Sickle cell disease	Increased VTE risk[71,73–77]	Higher PE mortality[75]	Do not withhold thromboprophylaxis for patients undergoing splenectomy.[78]

Abbreviations: AE-COPD, acute exacerbation of chronic obstructive pulmonary disease; AF, atrial fibrillation; CrCl, creatinine clearance; DOAC, direct oral anticoagulant; LMWH, low molecular weight heparin; PE, pulmonary embolism; VKA, vitamin K antagonist; VTE, venous thromboembolism.

The goal of this review is to discuss the intrinsic details of patients with preexisting cardiopulmonary diseases, cirrhosis, renal dysfunction, and asplenia. Presence of these conditions not only increases the risk of VTE but also carries worse outcomes. The complexity of the use and choice of anticoagulation in these special populations are also reviewed.

CARDIOPULMONARY DISEASE
Cardiovascular Disease

Preexisting cardiovascular disease is common in VTE patients. Clinical characteristics of 1023 patients presenting with PE between 2000 and 2007 showed that 44% of patients had cardiovascular disease, including ischemic heart disease, stroke, heart failure, peripheral vascular disease, valvular heart disease (with or without prosthetic valve), and/or atrial fibrillation/flutter (AF).[7] These patients with underlying cardiovascular disease at baseline had a 2.2-fold (95% CI, 1.75–2.72; *P*<.0001) increased risk of death during long-term follow-up compared with those without baseline cardiovascular disease when presenting with acute PE.[7] In a Taiwanese population-based retrospective study, an increased risk of major adverse cardiovascular events (adjusted hazard ratio [HR] 1.86, 95% CI, 1.65–2.09; *P*<.0001) in patients with VTE, including acute coronary syndrome and stroke, was observed.[8] This risk increased with age and was up to 15-fold higher (95% CI, 8.14–28.95; *P*<.0001) in patients over 75 years old. Also comorbidities, such as diabetes mellitus, hypertension, and stroke, increased the risk of major adverse cardiovascular events, but hyperlipidemia reduced the risks of cardiovascular events.[8]

Atrial Fibrillation

AF is the most common sustained chronic cardiac arrhythmia, with a lifetime prevalence of up to

25%.[9,10] AF causes atrial stasis with increased risk of systemic thrombus formation and embolization that may result in ischemic stroke.[11]

PE and AF have common risk factors, such as age, obesity, heart failure, myocardial infarction, and hypertension.[12] AF may be both the causal factor and the consequence of VTE. Abnormal hemostasis, including increased fibrin and platelet activation, can occur in AF, and it may promote thrombi development, such as DVT and/or isolated PE.[13] On the other hand, paroxysmal AF can occur as a consequence of sudden increase in right atrial pressure and right ventricle strain.[14]

PE is a risk factor for AF.[14] The prevalence of AF in patients with PE ranges from 15% to 20%.[15,16] In a cohort of 391 hospitalized PE patients, those with paroxysmal AF had higher pulmonary artery systolic pressure by echocardiogram compared with those with permanent AF or sinus rhythm(56 versus 48 versus 47, respectively; $P = .001$).[17] In-hospital mortality was higher in permanent AF compared with paroxysmal and sinus rhythm (25% vs 6.5% vs 5%; $P<.001$).[17] Moreover, patients with AF have a higher all-cause mortality at 1 month (35% vs 17%; $P = .001$; OR 3.16; 95% CI, 1.61–6.21) and 6 months after discharge (46% vs 17%; $P<.001$; OR 4.67; 95% CI, 2.37–9.21).[15] Therefore, occurrence of AF may be an indicator of PE severity.[17]

Although less studied, AF may be a risk factor for PE.[18–20] The risk of VTE was substantially increased during the first 6 months after diagnosis of AF during a 16-year population-based cohort study (HR 8.44; 95% CI, 5.61–12.69) and the risk remained increased throughout the study period (HR 1.43; 95% CI, 1.43–1.99).[20] Furthermore, AF exhibited higher risk estimates for PE than for DVT, particularly in the period more than 6 months after AF diagnosis.[20] These findings support the theory that isolated PE in AF may originate from right intra-atrial thrombi.

Heart Failure

Congestive HF carries a worse prognosis in patients with PE. HF is included in the PESI calculation as a predictor of mortality.[5,6] In a study of 87 patients with HF and PE, those with PE had higher 6-month overall and cardiovascular mortality, 34% and 29% versus 13% and 12%, respectively ($P = .02$ and $P = .02$).[21] Moreover, PE in patients with HF was an independent risk factor for mortality at 6 months (HR = 2.7; 95% CI, 1.1–24.4; $P = .04$).[21]

HF with preserved ejection fraction or diastolic dysfunction is responsible for more than half of the cases of HF.[22] In a retrospective study of 205 patients of hemodynamically stable PE, presence of diastolic dysfunction on echocardiogram carried a nonsignificant increased in-hospital mortality (HR 2.7; 95% CI, 0.6–12.4).[23] Further studies with a larger population is needed to determine the implications of diastolic dysfunction in PE.

Chronic Obstructive Pulmonary Disease

Chronic obstructive pulmonary disease (COPD) is currently the third leading cause of mortality and morbidity worldwide.[24] Acute exacerbations (AE) of COPD are primarily caused by respiratory infections, but in up to 30% of cases, no clear cause is identified.[25,26]

COPD is a recognized negative prognostic factor for VTE and it has been integrated in the prognostic scores, such as PESI.[5,6] Diagnosing PE in AE-COPD is challenging, however, because presenting symptoms are often similar. Undiagnosed PE was found in an autopsy study in up to 30% of COPD patients.[27]

The prevalence of DVT and PE in AE-COPD is 12%[28] and 16% to 25%, respectively.[28–31] This prevalence might be explained by increased markers of systemic inflammation that contribute to thrombosis, such as C-reactive protein, fibrinogen, and tumor necrosis factor α.[31] Additionally, the use of glucocorticoids to treat AE-COPD increases the risk of VTE.[31,32]

Some studies showed that the presence of pleuritic chest pain was reported more frequently in AE-COPD with PE than in AE-COPD without PE,[33,34] and some did not show a difference.[29,31] On the other hand, symptoms suggestive of respiratory tract infection were reported less frequent in AE-COPD with PE.[29,31] Two-thirds of the PE were found in main pulmonary arteries and segmental arteries, which have a clear indication for anticoagulation; and one-third were isolated subsegmental arteries.[31] The new 2016 antithrombotic VTE guidelines from the American College of Chest Physicians (ACCP) recommend that in patients with subsegmental PE and no proximal DVT with low risk of recurrent VTE, clinical surveillance is preferred over anticoagulation.[35] These guidelines, however, do not specify if presence of COPD is considered an increased risk of VTE recurrence.

In the Registro Informatizado de la Enfermedad TromboEmbólica (RIETE), a multicenter prospective registry of VTE patients, a lower use of thrombolytics and inferior vena cava filter was seen in COPD compared with non-COPD patients.[36] Presence of PE in COPD carried an increased overall mortality, minor bleeding, and PE recurrence at 7 and 90 days.[36,37] COPD patients had a statistically insignificant 1.3-fold increase risk of death during long-term follow-up compared with those without lung disease when presenting with acute PE (odds ratio [OR] 1.3; 95% CI, 0.98–1.73; $P = .07$).[7]

CIRRHOSIS

There are approximately 3.9 million patients with cirrhosis in the United States.[38] One of the most common complications of liver disease is bleeding due to endogenous coagulation disorder. Cirrhotic patients are often referred to as "auto-anticoagulated" due to defective coagulation factor synthesis, resulting in prolonged conventional coagulation tests, such as prothrombin time. This underlying coagulopathy has led to the assumption that these patients may be at lower risk for developing thrombosis.

It has been demonstrated, however, that patients with liver cirrhosis are also hypercoagulable by having decreased antithrombin III, protein C, and protein S activities.[39,40] These may lead to thrombotic complications, such as portal vein thrombosis, nonsplanchnic venous thrombosis, and VTE as well as portopulmonary hypertension.

Prevalence and Outcomes of Venous Thromboembolism in Cirrhosis

The prevalence of VTE in cirrhosis ranges from 0.5% to 6.3%.[41–43] Patients with chronic liver disease have increased risk of VTE, varying from an adjusted relative risk (RR) of 1.74 (95% CI, 1.54–1.95) for liver cirrhosis to an RR of 1.87 (95% CI, 1.73 to 2.03) for noncirrhotic liver disease and an RR of 1.75 (95% CI, 1.56 −1.97) in those with cirrhosis and hepatocellular carcinoma.[44] Patients with liver disease and VTE were more commonly seen in alcoholic, nonalcoholic steatohepatitis, or cryptogenic cirrhosis.[42] In 1 study, VTE in cirrhosis was not associated with greater in-hospital mortality but with increased length of stay and hospitalization cost.[41]

Lower serum albumin was found more frequently in cirrhotics with VTE than in those without VTE.[42] Elevated international normalized ratio (INR) was found in all patients with liver cirrhosis, independent of the presence of VTE.[42] In a retrospective cohort that followed patients with chronic liver disease, there was no significant difference in the incidence of VTE between INR quartiles,[43] suggesting that an elevated INR in the setting of liver disease does not appear protective against developing a VTE.

Anticoagulation in Cirrhosis

The most recent antithrombotic therapy for VTE guidelines from the ACCP recommend low-molecular-weight heparin (LMWH) as the preferred anticoagulation in patients with liver disease and coagulopathy.[35] LMWHs are preferred over vitamin K antagonists (VKAs) given difficulty in relying on INR to monitor VKA dosing. Most recently, there has been increased usage of direct-acting oral anticoagulants (DOACs) for treatment of VTE. Unfortunately, patients with cirrhosis were excluded from DOACs pivotal trials due to presence of liver disease. Emerging retrospective data show that DOACs have similar efficacy and safety compared with VKAs.[45] The precise role and use of DOACs in this population, however, remain unclear and require further investigation.[46]

RENAL DISEASE

VTE in patients with renal disease, which includes chronic kidney disease (CKD) and end-stage renal disease (ESRD), is common and is associated with high mortality and complication rates.[47,48] In clinical practice, impaired renal function poses certain challenges for diagnosis, prevention, and treatment of VTE. Thus, managing VTE in patients with renal disease requires specific considerations.

Venous Thromboembolism Risk in Renal Disease

The clinical spectrum of thrombosis in renal disease comprises DVT and PE, hemodialysis vascular access–related thrombosis, and arterial thrombosis (related to atherosclerosis: acute coronary syndrome, stroke, and peripheral vascular disease). There has been much interest in establishing whether renal insufficiency itself poses increased risk for spontaneous VTE.

In renal disease, platelet dysfunction, compounded by uremia, has been well recognized as producing a bleeding tendency. Biological support, however, for a prothrombotic state in renal disease also exists due to derangements in endothelial and coagulation factors, specifically elevated procoagulant factors plasminogen activator inhibitor type 1; elevated tissue factor; D-dimer; C-reactive protein; fibrinogen; factors VII, VIII, and IX–XII and von Willebrand factor; and decreased anticoagulant factors antithrombin and protein C.[49,50] Although factors VII, VIII, IX, and XI; fibrinogen; and D-dimer have been associated with VTE in the general population, a link between these hemostatic derangements and increased VTE incidence in renal disease has not specifically been established.

Current epidemiologic evidence supports renal dysfunction as a risk factor for VTE. Early autopsy studies had previously suggested that VTE was uncommon in ESRD.[50] A subsequent study, however, showed a higher age-adjusted overall incidence of PE in dialysis patients compared with the general population.[51] In the Longitudinal Investigation of Thromboembolism Etiology study, patients with moderate to severe CKD had a 2.09 RR (95% CI, 1.47–2.96) of VTE compared with those with normal kidney function, after adjustment for age, gender, race, center, and cardiovascular risk factors.[52] The Atherosclerosis Risk in Communities study showed adjusted HRs of VTE for normal, mildly impaired, and moderate-to-severe renal function to be 1.0, 1.26, and 1.6, respectively ($P = 0.04$).[53] Taken together, the biological and epidemiologic data identify patients with renal dysfunction as a group at high risk for VTE.

Presentation and Diagnosis of Venous Thromboembolism in Renal Disease

Renal dysfunction itself can confound the recognition and diagnosis of VTE, which may delay management for a population already at increased risk for VTE and its serious complications. The presentation of VTE in patients with renal disease may differ from the general population. Daneschvar and colleagues[54] showed that among patients with DVT, those with CKD more often presented with upper extremity DVT and less often with typical DVT symptoms. Clinicians should also be aware that patients with hemodialysis-dependent ESRD are uniquely at risk for vascular access thrombosis and subsequent embolic phenomena, including PE.[55]

The use of radiologic contrast in CT angiography for the diagnosis of PE must be carefully considered in patients with preexisting renal insufficiency due to the risk of renal failure from contrast-induced nephropathy. Also, clinical algorithms recommend CT angiography for intermediate/high pretest probability of PE based on D-dimer levels, which may be already elevated in renal disease. The sensitivity of D-dimer less than 500 µg/L to rule out PE in patients with renal disease is high, whereas the specificity is low and decreases further with declining renal function.[56] Thus, some investigators argue that PE clinical risk assessment scores using D-dimer cutoffs for those with normal renal function may be overexposing those with renal disease to the risk of contrast-induced nephropathy. At present, guidelines do not endorse adjusting D-dimer cutoffs based on reduced renal function. Further investigation into alternate strategies to diagnose PE in patients with renal disease will likely benefit these patients.

Outcomes of Venous Thromboembolism in Renal Disease

Acute PE is associated with high mortality, and renal impairment seems to worsen PE outcomes. In the RIETE, patients with moderate and severe renal impairment had a higher incidence of fatal PE (OR 2.7; 95% CI, 1.6–4.4, and OR 7.2; 95% CI, 1.9–11, respectively) compared with those with normal kidney function. Those with renal disease were more likely to be older and have underlying lung disease and heart failure.[48] A nationwide US database similarly showed that compared with those with normal renal function, patients with CKD and ESRD who were hospitalized for PE had higher adjusted in-hospital mortality (for CKD, OR 1.57; 95% CI, 1.27–1.93, and for ESRD, OR 1.92; 95% CI, 1.17–3.15) and longer median length of stay (1 day for CKD and 2 days for ESRD; $P<.001$). ESRD and CKD patients also had higher rates of mechanical ventilation requirement and cardiac arrest. Patients with renal impairment were older, more likely to have cardiopulmonary comorbidities, and present with severe PE. Thus, the investigators surmised that diminished cardiopulmonary reserve due to comorbidities in patients with CKD and ESRD likely led to increased severity of PE and mortality.[47]

Patients hospitalized with VTE and renal disease also have increased bleeding complications.[48,57–60] Monreal and colleagues[48] showed renal insufficiency to independently predict fatal bleeding in patients with acute VTE. In those with severe renal dysfunction, the 5.4% incidence of major bleeding and 1.2% incidence of fatal bleeding did not exceed the 6.6% incidence of fatal PE. Nonetheless, bleeding complications demand additional management and resources and significantly augment the morbidity faced by this patient group.

Anticoagulation in Renal Disease

Pharmacologic therapy for VTE in patients with renal disease is challenging due to their bleeding diathesis and altered drug kinetics. Thrombolysis improves mortality in acute hemodynamically unstable PE but carries an increased risk of bleeding, which may be further enhanced with worsening renal function. Patel and colleagues[61] recently examined the safety of thrombolysis for PE in patients with CKD using propensity score matching and found that CKD did not independently increase in-hospital mortality or hemorrhage. As such, renal dysfunction and dialysis dependence are not considered contraindications to receiving thrombolytics for VTE.

Heparin infusion is the mainstay for the treatment of VTE. The use of LMWHs are increasingly favored over unfractionated heparin due to multiple advantages, including a more predictable anticoagulant effect and higher therapeutic efficacy.[62] It is unclear that patients with renal disease reap the same therapeutic benefits of LMWHs, which must also be balanced with the risks associated with diminished renal clearance. Because LMWHs are renally cleared, their elimination half-life is significantly increased in patients with renal dysfunction. Accordingly, the use of LMWH in patients with renal dysfunction has been shown to increase bleeding.[63] Nonetheless, a lower mortality in patients with severe renal impairment (but not moderate impairment) and PE treated with LMWH compared with unfractionated heparin was reported, with similar bleeding rates.[64]

For decades, VKAs were the only available oral anticoagulant. Patients with renal disease on VKAs spend less time within therapeutic range and more time with supratherapeutic levels leading to increased bleeding.[65] CKD patients, therefore, require more frequent laboratory monitoring and dosing adjustments than those with normal renal function.[65] For the prevention of recurrent VTE and VTE-related death in renal disease, DOACs have been shown to have similar efficacy and bleeding outcomes as VKAs, including within CKD subgroups (creatinine clearance 30–60 mL/min).[66–70] Patients with severe renal impairment (creatinine clearance <30 mL/min) and on dialysis were excluded from trials evaluating the use of DOAC in VTE.[67–70] As such, there is no evidence to support use of DOACs in patients with severe renal dysfunction and on dialysis.

ASPLENIA

Asplenic and hyposplenic states may be congenital, functional (as in the case of hematologic and certain immunologic disorders), or acquired after splenectomy. Trauma is the overall most common indication for surgical splenectomy. The most common medical indication for splenectomy is hematologic disorders, such as autoimmune hemolytic anemia, thalassemia, immune thrombocytopenic purpura, and non-Hodgkin lymphoma.[71] The risk of thrombotic complications after splenectomy is well recognized and may be influenced by both the asplenic state and the underlying hematologic disorder for which splenectomy was performed.[71]

Venous Thromboembolism Risk in Asplenic States

Portal venous thrombosis incidence is increased after splenectomy and can be ascribed to local surgical factors rather than the asplenic state itself.[71] Portal venous thrombosis incidence is increased with the laparoscopic versus open approach.[72] With respect to VTE outside the portal system, increased PE-related death has been described in splenectomized patients compared with those who underwent other surgery (35.6% vs 9.7%; P<.001) in a large autopsy study of more than 37,000 patients.[73] In another large retrospective study of more than 375,000 patients in the Nationwide Inpatient Sample who underwent abdominal surgery, splenectomy conferred the highest risk for VTE (OR 2.69; 95% CI, 2.03–3.56).[74] Among more than 8000 cancer-free US veterans who underwent splenectomy and were followed for up to 27 years, the incidence of VTE was increased (DVT RR 2.18; 95% CI, 1.99–2.4; PE RR 2.24; 95% CI, 1.97–2.55), with a 4.5-fold increased risk of death from PE.[75]

Patients with thalassemia and splenectomy have a well-documented increased risk for VTE. In 89 patients with β-thalassemia who were followed for 10 years, 29% developed VTE; all but 1 had undergone splenectomy. In a study of 8860 patients with thalassemia intermedia (TI) and thalassemia major (TM), the overall incidence of VTE was 1.65%, with TI patients 4.38 times (P<.001) more likely than TM patients to develop VTE; 94% of TI patients with VTE had undergone splenectomy.[76] High VTE incidence postsplenectomy has also been reported to occur in sickle cell disease (autosplenectomy), hereditary spherocytosis, and hereditary stomatocytosis.[71,77]

Postsplenectomy thrombocytosis occurs in 3% to 13% of patients[77,78] although its contribution to VTE is controversial. Among patients who underwent splenectomy for sideroblastic anemia, hemolytic anemia, hemoglobinopathies, or thalassemia, 10% developed VTE in association with thrombocytosis.[79] Patients with congenital asplenia syndrome and associated heart defects were found to have higher platelet count than those with similar heart defects without asplenia as well as a higher incidence of VTE (28% vs 10%; P = .030).[80] In contrast, in a study of 318 splenectomized patients, Boxer and colleagues[81] did not find a statistically significant increase in VTE incidence among those with thrombocytosis compared to those with normal platelet counts.

Mechanisms of Hypercoagulability in Asplenia

The pathogenesis of hypercoagulability after splenectomy involves an intersection of the loss of protection from thrombosis provided by the spleen and the prothrombotic nature of underlying hematologic disorders. Proposed mechanisms for a prothrombotic state after splenectomy include increased platelet activation, altered red blood cell (RBC)-endothelium interactions, altered lipid profiles, and thrombocytosis.[71,78] A major function of the spleen is to filter damaged or senescent RBCs, which contribute to hypercoagulability when they persist in the circulation. Damaged RBCs, which are increased in hemolysis,[82,83] express phosphatidylserines, which typically target them for removal in the spleen. Cappellini and colleagues[77,84] showed that these phosphatidylserine-expressing RBCs can replace activated platelets as sources of anionic phospholipids in the conversion of prothrombin to thrombin, thereby directly contributing to thrombosis. During hemolysis and apoptosis, RBCs release microvesicular remnants called cell-derived microparticles, which are also highly procoagulant. Cell-derived microparticle levels are shown to be elevated after splenectomy for several hematologic disorders.[85–87] The link between postsplenectomy thrombocytosis and hypercoagulability is postulated to arise from increased platelet activation and aggregation, compounded by elevated interleukin 6, tumor necrosis factor, and C-reactive protein.[78]

Venous Thromboembolism Prophylaxis in Asplenia

Currently the ACCP does not specify different thromboprophylaxis guidelines for those undergoing splenectomy versus other abdominal surgeries or for those with postsplenectomy thrombocytosis.[35] Nonetheless, concerns about bleeding after splenectomy sometimes delay decisions to initiate postoperative thromboprophylaxis,[78] potentially placing a vulnerable population at risk for serious thrombotic events. Based on the preceding discussion of VTE risk after splenectomy, clinicians are advised to carefully consider VTE prophylaxis, particularly where the indication for splenectomy is malignancy or a hematologic disorder.

SUMMARY

VTE carries high morbidity and mortality, particularly when it occurs in patients with certain underlying diseases. Preexisting cardiopulmonary disease, cirrhosis, renal dysfunction, and asplenic states are common in the real world and are associated with increased risk for VTE. Current guidelines, however, do not feature whether VTE in patients with these preexisting conditions should be managed differently. The enhanced thrombotic risk intrinsic to these disease states should be recognized when facing decisions about thromboprophylaxis in these groups. When patients with these diseases develop VTE, the outcomes are more serious and costly. Long-term management of VTE in these groups, in particular those with renal and hepatic dysfunction, is challenging due to altered drug metabolism. Further studies are warranted to improve risk assessment and management of VTE in these special populations.

REFERENCES

1. Blood clots: a serious but preventable medical condition. 2016. Available at: http://www.cdc.gov/ncbddd/dvt/documents/blood-clots-fact-sheet.pdf. Accessed May 6, 2016.
2. Wells PS, Anderson DR, Rodger M, et al. Derivation of a simple clinical model to categorize patients probability of pulmonary embolism: increasing the models utility with the SimpliRED D-dimer. Thromb Haemost 2000;83(3):416–20.
3. Aujesky D, Fine MJ. Does guideline adherence for empiric antibiotic therapy reduce mortality in community-acquired pneumonia? Am J Respir Crit Care Med 2005;172(6):655–6.
4. Le Gal G, Righini M, Roy PM, et al. Prediction of pulmonary embolism in the emergency department: the revised Geneva score. Ann Intern Med 2006;144(3):165–71.
5. Jimenez D, Aujesky D, Moores L, et al. Simplification of the pulmonary embolism severity index for prognostication in patients with acute symptomatic pulmonary embolism. Arch Intern Med 2010;170(15):1383–9.
6. Aujesky D, Obrosky DS, Stone RA, et al. Derivation and validation of a prognostic model for pulmonary embolism. Am J Respir Crit Care Med 2005;172(8):1041–6.
7. Ng AC, Chung T, Yong AS, et al. Long-term cardiovascular and noncardiovascular mortality of 1023 patients with confirmed acute pulmonary embolism. Circ Cardiovasc Qual Outcomes 2011;4(1):122–8.
8. Chang WT, Chang CL, Ho CH, et al. Long-term effects of unprovoked venous thromboembolism on mortality and major cardiovascular events. J Am Heart Assoc 2017;6(5) [pii:e005466].
9. Lloyd-Jones DM, Wang TJ, Leip EP, et al. Lifetime risk for development of atrial fibrillation: the Framingham Heart Study. Circulation 2004;110(9):1042–6.
10. Heeringa J, van der Kuip DA, Hofman A, et al. Prevalence, incidence and lifetime risk of atrial fibrillation: the Rotterdam study. Eur Heart J 2006;27(8):949–53.
11. Vadmann H, Nielsen PB, Hjortshoj SP, et al. Atrial flutter and thromboembolic risk: a systematic review. Heart 2015;101(18):1446–55.
12. Konstantinides SV, Torbicki A, Agnelli G, et al. 2014 ESC guidelines on the diagnosis and management

of acute pulmonary embolism. Eur Heart J 2014; 35(43):3033–69, 3069a-k.

13. Watson T, Shantsila E, Lip GY. Mechanisms of thrombogenesis in atrial fibrillation: Virchow's triad revisited. Lancet 2009;373(9658):155–66.

14. Fuster V, Ryden LE, Cannom DS, et al. ACC/AHA/ESC 2006 guidelines for the management of patients with atrial fibrillation: a report of the American College of Cardiology/American Heart Association Task Force on Practice Guidelines and the European Society of Cardiology Committee for Practice Guidelines (writing committee to revise the 2001 guidelines for the management of patients with atrial fibrillation): developed in collaboration with the European Heart Rhythm Association and the Heart Rhythm Society. Circulation 2006;114(7):e257–354.

15. Barra SN, Paiva LV, Providencia R, et al. Atrial fibrillation in acute pulmonary embolism: prognostic considerations. Emerg Med J 2014;31(4):308–12.

16. Koracevic G, Atanaskovic V. Is atrial fibrillation a prognosticator in acute pulmonary thromboembolism? Med Princ Pract 2010;19(2):166.

17. Krajewska A, Ptaszynska-Kopczynska K, Kiluk I, et al. Paroxysmal atrial fibrillation in the course of acute pulmonary embolism: clinical significance and impact on prognosis. Biomed Res Int 2017; 2017:5049802.

18. Flegel KM. When atrial fibrillation occurs with pulmonary embolism, is it the chicken or the egg? CMAJ 1999;160(8):1181–2.

19. Piszko P, Lewczuk J, Lenartowska L, et al. Pulmonary thromboembolism in 102 consecutive patients with chronic atrial fibrillation. Diagnostic value of echocardiography. Kardiol Pol 2007;65(3):246–51 [discussion: 252–3].

20. Enga KF, Rye-Holmboe I, Hald EM, et al. Atrial fibrillation and future risk of venous thromboembolism: the Tromso study. J Thromb Haemost 2015;13(1): 10–6.

21. Gromadzinski L, Targonski R, Januszko-Giergielewicz B, et al. The influence of acute pulmonary embolism on early and delayed prognosis for patients with chronic heart failure. Cardiol J 2012; 19(6):625–31.

22. Hogg K, Swedberg K, McMurray J. Heart failure with preserved left ventricular systolic function; epidemiology, clinical characteristics, and prognosis. J Am Coll Cardiol 2004;43(3):317–27.

23. Cho JH, Kaw R, Chhabra J, et al. Prognostic implications of diastolic dysfunction in patients with acute pulmonary embolism. BMC Res Notes 2014;7:610.

24. Murray CJ, Lopez AD. Measuring the global burden of disease. N Engl J Med 2013;369(5):448–57.

25. Sapey E, Stockley RA. COPD exacerbations. 2: aetiology. Thorax 2006;61(3):250–8.

26. Connors AF Jr, Dawson NV, Thomas C, et al. Outcomes following acute exacerbation of severe chronic obstructive lung disease. The SUPPORT investigators (Study to Understand Prognoses and Preferences for Outcomes and Risks of Treatments). Am J Respir Crit Care Med 1996;154(4 Pt 1):959–67.

27. Neuhaus A, Bentz RR, Weg JG. Pulmonary embolism in respiratory failure. Chest 1978;73(4):460–5.

28. Rizkallah J, Man SFP, Sin DD. Prevalence of pulmonary embolism in acute exacerbations of COPD: a systematic review and metaanalysis. Chest 2009; 135(3):786–93.

29. Tillie-Leblond I, Marquette CH, Perez T, et al. Pulmonary embolism in patients with unexplained exacerbation of chronic obstructive pulmonary disease: prevalence and risk factors. Ann Intern Med 2006; 144(6):390–6.

30. Shapira-Rootman M, Beckerman M, Soimu U, et al. The prevalence of pulmonary embolism among patients suffering from acute exacerbations of chronic obstructive pulmonary disease. Emerg Radiol 2015; 22(3):257–60.

31. Aleva FE, Voets L, Simons SO, et al. Prevalence and localization of pulmonary embolism in unexplained acute exacerbations of COPD: a systematic review and meta-analysis. Chest 2017;151(3):544–54.

32. Johannesdottir SA, Horvath-Puho E, Dekkers OM, et al. Use of glucocorticoids and risk of venous thromboembolism: a nationwide population-based case-control study. JAMA Intern Med 2013;173(9):743–52.

33. Gunen H, Gulbas G, In E, et al. Venous thromboemboli and exacerbations of COPD. Eur Respir J 2010; 35(6):1243–8.

34. Akpinar EE, Hosgun D, Akpinar S, et al. Incidence of pulmonary embolism during COPD exacerbation. J Bras Pneumol 2014;40(1):38–45.

35. Kearon C, Akl EA, Ornelas J, et al. Antithrombotic therapy for VTE disease: CHEST guideline and expert panel report. Chest 2016;149(2):315–52.

36. Bertoletti L, Quenet S, Mismetti P, et al. Clinical presentation and outcome of venous thromboembolism in COPD. Eur Respir J 2012;39(4):862–8.

37. Bertoletti L, Quenet S, Laporte S, et al. Pulmonary embolism and 3-month outcomes in 4036 patients with venous thromboembolism and chronic obstructive pulmonary disease: data from the RIETE registry. Respir Res 2013;14:75.

38. Center for Disease Control and Prevention. Chronic liver disease and cirrhosis. 2016. Available at: https://www.cdc.gov/nchs/fastats/liver-disease.htm. Accessed November 6, 2017.

39. Castelino DJ, Salem HH. Natural anticoagulants and the liver. J Gastroenterol Hepatol 1997;12(1): 77–83.

40. Raya-Sanchez JM, Gonzalez-Reimers E, Rodriguez-Martin JM, et al. Coagulation inhibitors in alcoholic liver cirrhosis. Alcohol 1998;15(1):19–23.

41. Ali M, Ananthakrishnan AN, McGinley EL, et al. Deep vein thrombosis and pulmonary embolism in

hospitalized patients with cirrhosis: a nationwide analysis. Dig Dis Sci 2011;56(7):2152–9.

42. Northup PG, McMahon MM, Ruhl AP, et al. Coagulopathy does not fully protect hospitalized cirrhosis patients from peripheral venous thromboembolism. Am J Gastroenterol 2006;101(7):1524–8 [quiz:1680].

43. Dabbagh O, Oza A, Prakash S, et al. Coagulopathy does not protect against venous thromboembolism in hospitalized patients with chronic liver disease. Chest 2010;137(5):1145–9.

44. Sogaard KK, Horvath-Puho E, Gronbaek H, et al. Risk of venous thromboembolism in patients with liver disease: a nationwide population-based case-control study. Am J Gastroenterol 2009; 104(1):96–101.

45. Intagliata NM, Henry ZH, Maitland H, et al. Direct oral anticoagulants in cirrhosis patients pose similar risks of bleeding when compared to traditional anticoagulation. Dig Dis Sci 2016;61(6):1721–7.

46. Raschi E, Bianchin M, De Ponti R, et al. Emerging therapeutic uses of direct-acting oral anticoagulants: an evidence-based perspective. Pharmacol Res 2017;120:206–18.

47. Kumar G, Sakhuja A, Taneja A, et al. Pulmonary embolism in patients with CKD and ESRD. Clin J Am Soc Nephrol 2012;7(10):1584–90.

48. Monreal M, Falga C, Valle R, et al. Venous thromboembolism in patients with renal insufficiency: findings from the RIETE registry. Am J Med 2006; 119(12):1073–9.

49. Casserly LF, Dember LM. Thrombosis in end-stage renal disease. Semin Dial 2003;16(3):245–56.

50. Wattanakit K, Cushman M. Chronic kidney disease and venous thromboembolism: epidemiology and mechanisms. Curr Opin Pulm Med 2009;15(5): 408–12.

51. Tveit DP, Hypolite IO, Hshieh P, et al. Chronic dialysis patients have high risk for pulmonary embolism. Am J Kidney Dis 2002;39(5):1011–7.

52. Wattanakit K, Cushman M, Stehman-Breen C, et al. Chronic kidney disease increases risk for venous thromboembolism. J Am Soc Nephrol 2008;19(1): 135–40.

53. Folsom AR, Lutsey PL, Astor BC, et al. Chronic kidney disease and venous thromboembolism: a prospective study. Nephrol Dial Transplant 2010; 25(10):3296–301.

54. Daneschvar HL, Seddighzadeh A, Piazza G, et al. Deep vein thrombosis in patients with chronic kidney disease. Thromb Haemost 2008;99(6):1035–9.

55. Konigsbrugge O, Lorenz M, Auinger M, et al. Venous thromboembolism and vascular access thrombosis in patients with end-stage renal disease on maintenance hemodialysis: cross-sectional results of the Vienna InVestigation of AtriaL fibrillation and thromboembolism in patients on hemoDIalysis (VIVALDI). Thromb Res 2017;158:59–64.

56. Lindner G, Funk GC, Pfortmueller CA, et al. D-dimer to rule out pulmonary embolism in renal insufficiency. Am J Med 2014;127(4):343–7.

57. Gerlach AT, Pickworth KK, Seth SK, et al. Enoxaparin and bleeding complications: a review in patients with and without renal insufficiency. Pharmacotherapy 2000;20(7):771–5.

58. Spinler SA, Inverso SM, Cohen M, et al. Safety and efficacy of unfractionated heparin versus enoxaparin in patients who are obese and patients with severe renal impairment: analysis from the ESSENCE and TIMI 11B studies. Am Heart J 2003;146(1):33–41.

59. Thorevska N, Amoateng-Adjepong Y, Sabahi R, et al. Anticoagulation in hospitalized patients with renal insufficiency: a comparison of bleeding rates with unfractionated heparin vs enoxaparin. Chest 2004;125(3):856–63.

60. Farooq V, Hegarty J, Chandrasekar T, et al. Serious adverse incidents with the usage of low molecular weight heparins in patients with chronic kidney disease. Am J Kidney Dis 2004;43(3):531–7.

61. Patel B, Sablani N, Shah M, et al. Evaluating safety of thrombolysis in chronic kidney disease patients presenting with pulmonary embolism using propensity score matching. J Thromb Thrombolysis 2017; 44(3):324–9.

62. Hetzel GR, Sucker C. The heparins: all a nephrologist should know. Nephrol Dial Transplant 2005; 20(10):2036–42.

63. Lim W, Dentali F, Eikelboom JW, et al. Meta-analysis: low-molecular-weight heparin and bleeding in patients with severe renal insufficiency. Ann Intern Med 2006;144(9):673–84.

64. Trujillo-Santos J, Schellong S, Falga C, et al. Low-molecular-weight or unfractionated heparin in venous thromboembolism: the influence of renal function. Am J Med 2013;126(5):425–34.e1.

65. Sciascia S, Radin M, Schreiber K, et al. Chronic kidney disease and anticoagulation: from vitamin K antagonists and heparins to direct oral anticoagulant agents. Intern Emerg Med 2017;12(8):1101–8.

66. Harel Z, Sood MM, Perl J. Comparison of novel oral anticoagulants versus vitamin K antagonists in patients with chronic kidney disease. Curr Opin Nephrol Hypertens 2015;24(2):183–92.

67. Schulman S, Kearon C, Kakkar AK, et al. Dabigatran versus warfarin in the treatment of acute venous thromboembolism. N Engl J Med 2009;361(24): 2342–52.

68. Investigators E, Bauersachs R, Berkowitz SD, et al. Oral rivaroxaban for symptomatic venous thromboembolism. N Engl J Med 2010;363(26):2499–510.

69. Agnelli G, Buller HR, Cohen A, et al. Oral apixaban for the treatment of acute venous thromboembolism. N Engl J Med 2013;369(9):799–808.

70. Hokusai VTEI, Buller HR, Decousus H, et al. Edoxaban versus warfarin for the treatment of symptomatic

venous thromboembolism. N Engl J Med 2013; 369(15):1406–15.

71. Crary SE, Buchanan GR. Vascular complications after splenectomy for hematologic disorders. Blood 2009;114(14):2861–8.

72. Ikeda M, Sekimoto M, Takiguchi S, et al. High incidence of thrombosis of the portal venous system after laparoscopic splenectomy: a prospective study with contrast-enhanced CT scan. Ann Surg 2005; 241(2):208–16.

73. Pimpl W, Dapunt O, Kaindl H, et al. Incidence of septic and thromboembolic-related deaths after splenectomy in adults. Br J Surg 1989;76(5): 517–21.

74. Mukherjee D, Lidor AO, Chu KM, et al. Postoperative venous thromboembolism rates vary significantly after different types of major abdominal operations. J Gastrointest Surg 2008;12(11):2015–22.

75. Kristinsson SY, Gridley G, Hoover RN, et al. Long-term risks after splenectomy among 8,149 cancer-free American veterans: a cohort study with up to 27 years follow-up. Haematologica 2014; 99(2):392–8.

76. Taher A, Isma'eel H, Mehio G, et al. Prevalence of thromboembolic events among 8,860 patients with thalassaemia major and intermedia in the Mediterranean area and Iran. Thromb Haemost 2006;96(4): 488–91.

77. Cappellini MD, Grespi E, Cassinerio E, et al. Coagulation and splenectomy: an overview. Ann N Y Acad Sci 2005;1054:317–24.

78. Ha LP, Arrendondo M. Fatal venous thromboembolism after splenectomy: pathogenesis and management. J Am Osteopath Assoc 2012;112(5): 291–300.

79. Hirsh J, Dacie JV. Persistent post-splenectomy thrombocytosis and thrombo-embolism: a consequence of continuing anaemia. Br J Haematol 1966;12(1):44–53.

80. Yamamura K, Joo K, Ohga S, et al. Thrombocytosis in asplenia syndrome with congenital heart disease: a previously unrecognized risk factor for thromboembolism. Int J Cardiol 2013;167(5):2259–63.

81. Boxer MA, Braun J, Ellman L. Thromboembolic risk of postsplenectomy thrombocytosis. Arch Surg 1978;113(7):808–9.

82. Ataga KI, Cappellini MD, Rachmilewitz EA. Beta-thalassaemia and sickle cell anaemia as paradigms of hypercoagulability. Br J Haematol 2007;139(1):3–13.

83. Borenstain-Ben Yashar V, Barenholz Y, Hy-Am E, et al. Phosphatidylserine in the outer leaflet of red blood cells from beta-thalassemia patients may explain the chronic hypercoagulable state and thrombotic episodes. Am J Hematol 1993;44(1):63–5.

84. Cappellini MD. Coagulation in the pathophysiology of hemolytic anemias. Hematology Am Soc Hematol Educ Program 2007;74–8.

85. Fontana V, Jy W, Ahn ER, et al. Increased procoagulant cell-derived microparticles (C-MP) in splenectomized patients with ITP. Thromb Res 2008; 122(5):599–603.

86. Westerman M, Pizzey A, Hirschman J, et al. Microvesicles in haemoglobinopathies offer insights into mechanisms of hypercoagulability, haemolysis and the effects of therapy. Br J Haematol 2008;142(1): 126–35.

87. Habib A, Kunzelmann C, Shamseddeen W, et al. Elevated levels of circulating procoagulant microparticles in patients with beta-thalassemia intermedia. Haematologica 2008;93(6):941–2.

Pregnancy and Pulmonary Embolism

Christopher Deeb Dado, MD[a], Andrew Tobias Levinson, MD, MPH[b], Ghada Bourjeily, MD[c],*

KEYWORDS

- Pulmonary embolism • Venous thromboembolism • Pregnancy • Heparin • Multidetector CT
- Ventilation perfusion scan

KEY POINTS

- Venous thromboembolism (VTE) is responsible for 3% of all maternal deaths worldwide and 15% in the United States.
- The increased risk of VTE in pregnancy peaks immediately postpartum and may continue up to 12 weeks postpartum.
- The increased risk is attributed to the Virchow triad, inherited thrombophilias, as well as other common risk factors.
- The algorithm for diagnosing VTE differs during and immediately after pregnancy due to physiologic factors and fear of teratogenicity.
- Low molecular weight heparin and unfractionated heparin are medications of choice, as warfarin is teratogenic and novel oral anticoagulants have increased rates of bleeding and congenital anomalies.

INTRODUCTION

Venous thromboembolism (VTE) is responsible for 3% of all maternal deaths worldwide according to data from the World Health Organization.[1] Data from the developed world suggest that death rates from VTE are significantly higher, as VTE remains one of the leading causes of maternal deaths.[1,2] Recent analysis of maternal mortality in the United States showed that VTE accounted for 15% of all maternal deaths between 2003 and 2011.[3] Substandard care occurred in more than half of all deaths[4] from pulmonary embolism (PE) in the confidential enquiry into maternal deaths in the United Kingdom, highlighting the importance of understanding and overcoming challenges in the care of this condition in pregnancy. A clinician who does not treat pregnant women on a regular basis may not routinely consider many of the pregnancy-specific risk factors for VTE. Pretest probability is also quite complicated in pregnancy, as pretest probability rules have not been validated in this population, compelling the clinician to rely more heavily on imaging tests. Diagnostic procedures are also fraught with concerns about diagnostic accuracy in this population, as well as concerns for fetal safety, teratogenicity, and oncogenicity. Treatment strategies are complex, and providers need to balance efficacy while considering fetal safety, teratogenicity, pharmacodynamics, the unexpected nature of labor and delivery, and the subsequent need to weigh the risk of anticoagulation with the risk of clot

Funding: G. Bourjeily is funded by NICHD R01HL-130702 and R01HD-078515.
Conflicts of Interest: All authors have no conflicts of interest to report.
[a] Pulmonary and Critical Care Fellowship, Rhode Island Hospital, Warren Alpert Medical School of Brown University, 593 Eddy Street, Providence, RI 02903, USA; [b] Department of Medicine, The Miriam Hospital, Warren Alpert Medical School of Brown University, 164 Summit Avenue, Providence, RI 02904, USA; [c] Department of Medicine, The Miriam Hospital, Warren Alpert Medical School of Brown University, 146 West River Street, Suite 11C, Providence, RI 02904, USA
* Corresponding author.
E-mail address: ghada_bourjeily@brown.edu

chestmed.theclinics.com

recurrence perinatally. In this review, we examine the pregnancy-specific nuances in the risk assessment pretest probability, diagnostic evaluation, and therapeutic considerations.

Epidemiology

The risk of peripartum VTE is increased, with the postpartum period conferring a higher day-to-day risk than the antepartum period. The risk of VTE is estimated at 5 to 12 per 100,000 pregnancies antepartum compared with age-matched nonpregnant women, translating into a 0.1% absolute risk.[5,6] Although the absolute risk of VTE is lower in the postpartum period compared with the antepartum period, estimated at 0.05%,[7,8] the day-to-day risk is significantly higher when considering the significantly shorter postpartum period. The risk for VTE is highest in the first 6 weeks postpartum. Although previous data had suggested that the epidemiologic risk[9,10] and the biochemical hematological changes[11,12] that occur in pregnancy return to baseline at 6 weeks postpartum, recent claims data have shown a twofold increase in the risk of venous thrombosis (odds ratio [OR] 2.2, 95% confidence interval [CI] 1.4–3.3) from 7 to 12 weeks postpartum compared with the same time period a year later.[13]

Pathophysiology of Thromboembolic Disease in Pregnancy

Venous stasis, vascular injury, and hypercoagulable state (Virchow triad) are all responsible for the increased risk of VTE in pregnancy. Inherited thrombophilias and other risk factors also contribute to the development of VTE in pregnancy.

Venous stasis

In pregnancy, through progesterone-induced veno-dilation,[14] renal vasodilation occurs simultaneously with systemic vasodilation and leads to 30% to 50% increase in renal blood flow and glomerular filtration rate (GFR). This rise in GFR increases distal sodium delivery, allowing for escape from the sodium-retaining effect of aldosterone. The volume expansion secondary to aldosterone increases the atrial natriuretic peptide, which in turn inhibits sodium reabsorption in the distal tubules leading to an increase in systemic volume and Na retention.[15] The increase in total body blood volume leads to an increase in blood volume in the lower extremities, from 94.7 ± 27.3 mL in nonpregnant individuals to 110.1 ± 30.2 mL in pregnancy. There is also an increase in the diameter of the common femoral vein from 10.14 ± 1.24 mm to 12.72 ± 2.27 mm, as well as proportional increases in the saphenous and popliteal vein diameters.[16] This rise in venous blood volume and pressure, along with resulting distension of the vessels, leads to stasis and increased lower extremity edema. However, it has been proposed that, unlike VTE in the general population, VTE in pregnancy may start in the pelvis[17] rather than the lower extremities, as the percentage of isolated pelvic deep venous thrombosis is significantly higher in pregnancy.[18] As the right common iliac artery crosses over the left common iliac vein, a pulsatile compression of the left-sided venous system ensues. This compression is implicated in the increase in left-sided DVTs in pregnant women, with an occurrence of 90% on the left side compared with 55% of the time in nonpregnant individuals.[19,20]

Vascular dysfunction and injury

In normal pregnancy there are circulating cytokines and growth factors that may contribute to the breakdown of the endothelial monolayer. This can lead to vascular dysfunction and injury by degrading or removing cell junctional proteins.[21] Endothelial injury also can occur during normal labor, as well as during surgical delivery.[22] In addition, the increase in blood volume and diameter of vessels causes sheer stress on the vessels, potentially leading to vascular damage.[21]

Hypercoagulable state

During pregnancy, the blood becomes hypercoagulable with increases in procoagulation factors V, VII, VIII, IX, X, and XII and von Willebrand factor. Factor VII increases up to 10-fold, whereas fibrinogen rises 2-fold.[23] Von Willebrand and factor VIII are elevated in late gestation and factor XI tends to decrease during pregnancy. There is also a decrease in anticoagulant activity with a decrease in protein S with gestational age, whereas protein C activity remains unchanged.[23] Fibrinolysis is reduced in pregnancy as a result of an enhanced activity of plasminogen activator inhibitor type I and II and a decreased activity of tissue plasminogen activator.[24]

Inherited thrombophilias

Up to 40% of women who develop VTE while pregnant are found to have an inherited thrombophilia.[19] In addition, a reported OR of 51.8 (95% CI 38.7–69.2) for thrombophilia was described in women with VTE in a study of the National Inpatient Sample evaluating risk factors for VTE.[25] Inherited thrombophilias associated with increased risk of VTE in pregnancy include factor V Leiden, Prothrombin G20210 A mutation, antithrombin deficiency, protein C deficiency, and protein S deficiency.[26] Estimates of reported thrombophilias vary in the literature and are based on populations studied.[27–29] Heterozygous factor V Leiden is associated with an absolute risk of up to 3% and has been observed in up to 40% of VTE cases occurring during pregnancy. Homozygous factor V Leiden is not as common, but carries a significantly higher absolute risk, reported to be up to 14%, whereas the absolute risk of VTE among women with protein C or protein S deficiency has been reported to be up to 6%. Prothrombin G20210 A mutation has a prevalence of 3% and has been reported in up to 17% of VTE cases in pregnancy. Antithrombin deficiency has a prevalence of up to 0.6% with a 25-fold increased risk for VTE. Protein C deficiency has a prevalence of 0.2% to 0.3% with a risk for VTE of 2% to 7%, whereas protein S deficiency has a prevalence of less than 0.1% with a risk for VTE of 6% to 7%.[30]

Other risk factors

Additional risk factors for VTE in pregnancy include the same risk factors for VTE in the general nonpregnant population, as well as risk factors that are specific to pregnancy itself. Nonpregnancy-related risk factors[29] include age older than 35, obesity, varicose veins, paraplegia, sickle cell disease, and heart disease, along with other medical comorbidities such as nephrotic syndrome, systemic lupus erythematosus, and inflammatory bowel disease. Prior VTE carries an OR for subsequent VTE of 24.8 (95% CI 17.1–36).[25] Some risk factors are specific for the antepartum period, whereas others are specific for the postpartum period.

Risk factors associated with antepartum VTE include immobility, assisted reproductive technique, smoking, obesity, and antepartum hemorrhage.[29] Risk factors for postpartum VTE include immobility, placenta abruption, preeclampsia, growth restriction, Cesarean delivery,[31] postpartum infection, postpartum hemorrhage, and obesity.[29] More recently, a UK-based registry has developed a postpartum VTE risk prediction model. This model was then validated in a Sweden-based registry and showed that the most predictive risk factors included varicose veins, stillbirth, preeclampsia, postpartum infection, emergency Cesarean delivery, and medical comorbidities. Of note, this model did not assess thrombophilia or past VTE.[8] In addition, some risk factors have a synergistic effect in pregnancy. For instance, strict antepartum immobilization for at least a week in women with an elevated body mass index at the first prenatal visit is associated with a 62-fold risk for antepartum VTE and a 40-fold risk for postpartum VTE.[32]

DIAGNOSIS

Signs and symptoms of VTE in pregnancy are similar to those in nonpregnant individuals. These include shortness of breath, tachycardia, leg pain or swelling, pelvic discomfort, and chest pain. Shortness of breath is the most common presenting symptom (34.7%), followed by tachycardia (30.4%), leg pain or weakness (9.6%), and chest pain (13%).[33] In addition to history and physical examination findings, multiple laboratory and imaging tests are used in the general population to help guide and diagnose VTE in pregnancy. These tests include D-dimer, brain natriuretic peptide (BNP), troponin, chest radiographs (CXR), multidetector computed tomography with pulmonary angiogram (CTPa), compression Doppler ultrasonography (CUS), and ventilation perfusion scan (V/Q scan).

Clinical Pretest Probability Rules

In the general population, pretest probability tools are used to determine likelihood of PE. These tests can then further guide the diagnostic approach toward imaging or D-dimer testing. Pretest probability rules have not been validated in pregnancy, and although some studies have suggested good correlation between rules, such as the modified Wells score and the diagnosis of PE, these rules have not been validated to date. The existing rules do not consider pregnancy and pregnancy-specific risk factors, and include some factors that may not be relevant or applicable to the pregnant population. Although sensitivity and negative predictive value appear to be excellent in retrospective cohorts using the Wells' criteria in peripartum women, these studies are limited by their retrospective design, the lack of combining the tool with D-dimer testing in their diagnostic approach, and the small number of patients.[34,35]

Diagnostic and Prognostic Laboratory Testing

D-dimer is a fibrin degradation product that is detected in the blood following blood clot degradation. D-dimer levels increase in pregnancy with the highest levels in the third trimester in one study.[36] Levels return to baseline approximately 6 weeks postpartum.[37] In general, normal D-dimer levels in pregnancy are less than 0.95 μg/mL in the first trimester, less than 1.29 μg/mL in the second trimester, and less than 1.7 μg/mL during the third trimester.[36] Sensitivity of D-dimers has varied in different retrospective studies from 73% to 100%.[38] However, D-dimers remain nonvalidated in prospective diagnostic cohort studies in pregnancy and cannot safely exclude the diagnosis of PE.[39]

BNP is commonly used to identify patients with PE that are at high risk of clinical deterioration. In a longitudinal sample, BNP levels were similar across 3 trimesters and postpartum; however, perinatal levels were approximately twice as high as those of nonpregnant controls.[40] These findings were demonstrated with other studies.[41] In patients with preexisting heart disease, BNP levels increase throughout pregnancy and the postpartum period.[42] A BNP level of less than 100 pg/mL was shown in one study to have a negative predictive value of 100% for identifying decompensation of heart disease[42]; however, the study did not examine right heart strain as it relates to BNP. The utility of using BNP to risk stratify women with PE needs to be evaluated further.

Troponin I (TnI) is another marker commonly used in the risk stratification of patients with PEs. The use of TnI in risk stratifying pregnant women with PE has not been studied and requires validation.[43]

Imaging

Although the use of ionizing radiation is best minimized in pregnancy due to the potential risk of teratogenicity and oncogenicity, this small risk needs to be weighed against the risk of missing a PE, which could have deleterious effects on both the mother and the fetus. A false-positive diagnosis is associated with unnecessary risk of therapeutic anticoagulation during the index pregnancy, which complicates labor and delivery, unneeded prophylactic anticoagulation in future pregnancies, and slimmer contraceptive options. Imaging used to diagnose a PE in pregnancy includes CUS, CXR, V/Q scans, and CTPa.

The biggest concerns regarding exposure of the fetus to radiation are teratogenicity and oncogenicity. The minimum dose of radiation associated with an increased risk of teratogenicity in humans is yet to be firmly established. Animal studies in mice and rats have shown that a minimum exposure to radiation at levels of 0.05 to 0.25 Gy is needed to cause teratogenicity. Current guidelines suggest an exposure greater than 0.1 Gy at any time during gestation as the threshold beyond which congenital abnormalities are possible.[24] To place this information into context, performing one CXR, a V/Q scan, and a CT of the chest exposes the fetus to significantly less than 0.01 Gy.[44] Despite the relative safety of these studies in terms of teratogenicity, the clinician should work with the radiology team and their institution's physicists to take necessary steps to minimize the dose of radiation with every imaging study that exposes to ionizing radiation. These steps may include modifying imaging protocols,[45] performing ventilation scans only if perfusion scans are abnormal, frequent voiding to avoid pooling of radioactive material in the bladder, and the use of abdominal and breast shielding.

Imaging Diagnostic Approach

In 2011, the American Thoracic Society (ATS) published guidelines regarding diagnostic testing for PE in pregnancy that were based on low-quality, and very low quality, evidence,[46] and, hence, not universally adopted.[47] The recommendations from this document are quite different from the current standard of care in the nonpregnant population for many reasons that extend beyond the risk of teratogenicity. Technical limitations with enhanced studies in pregnancy constitute a major challenge[48] due to the significant increase in plasma volume, heart rate, and cardiac output potentially diluting contrast and reducing vascular enhancement. These limitations depend on injection protocol as well as dose of contrast medium used, and may be minimized with protocol modifications.[45,49] Breast radiation dose is significantly higher in CT studies compared with V/Q scans[50] and could potentially translate into a higher risk of developing breast cancer during a woman's lifetime, especially in younger women.[51,52] However, breast shields, which are now being used for imaging of any body part in women, can reduce the amount of breast radiation without significantly affecting resolution of chest studies.[53] Lastly, the use of iodine-containing contrast media, which are known to cross the placenta, is another concern with CT imaging, given the potential to interfere with thyroid function at birth. However, a study of nearly 350 newborns born to women exposed to iodinated contrast during pregnancy showed no significant effect on neonatal thyroid function.[54]

The ATS/Society of Thoracic Radiology (STR) guidelines recommend CUS as the first imaging for pregnant women with lower extremity symptoms. CUS is noninvasive and has no radiation exposure. In the nonpregnant population, the number needed to test to avoid further diagnostic workup is 11.[55] In a randomized diagnostic noninferiority trial comparing CT/D-dimer approach with a CUS/CT/D-dimer approach, DVT was diagnosed by CUS in 9% of patients suspected of PE who were randomized to this approach.[55] These statistics may be even lower in pregnancy, with the number needed to test being significantly higher, as isolated pelvic DVTs are more common[17] and the ability of this test to detect pelvic DVTs suboptimal.[43] In addition, this diagnostic modality may not be an adequate first-line test in critically ill patients with hemodynamic instability, and chest imaging may be a better approach (**Fig. 1**). However, in symptomatic patients, if the CUS reveals evidence of a lower extremity VTE, no further imaging is required and treatment for VTE can be initiated.

If the patient does not have any lower extremity symptoms or the CUS is negative for any signs of VTE, then a CXR should be the first imaging test.[46] The approximate dose of radiation the fetus is exposed to with a maternal CXR is 0.000001 Gy. If the CXR is abnormal and explains the clinical picture and the clinician is no longer concerned

for VTE, it is reasonable to withhold additional imaging and treat the underlying condition diagnosed by CXR. However, if a clinical suspicion for VTE remains despite an abnormal CXR, a CTPa should be obtained. On the other hand, if the CXR is normal, V/Q scan is an appropriate next imaging study.

The approximate amount of radiation exposure for the fetus in a V/Q scan is 0.00028 to 0.00051. This is slightly higher but comparable to the amount of radiation exposure of a CTPa. As noted in the 2011 ATS/STR guidelines,[46] most evidence in the literature is based on retrospective studies, hence limiting the ability to ascertain the diagnostic capabilities of various approaches. Both

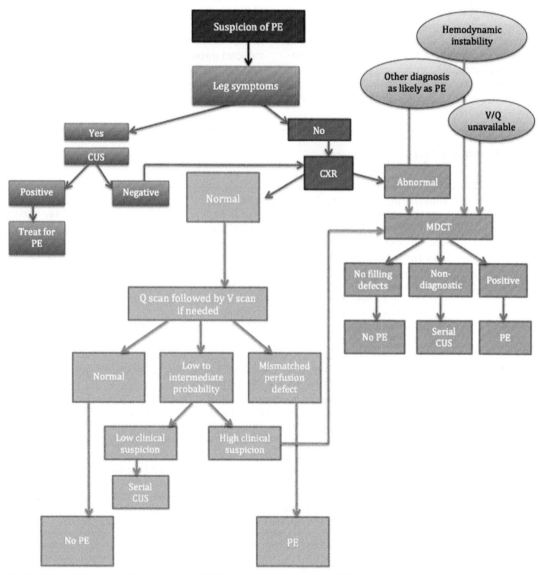

Fig. 1. Diagnostic approach to suspected PE in pregnancy. MDCT, multidetector computed tomography.

V/Q scans and CTPa appear to safely exclude PE based on these studies; however, as the incidence of PE in pregnant patients suspected of PE is quite low (close to 3%),[56–58] larger studies are needed to confirm diagnostic accuracy of these imaging approaches. Based on retrospective data, women with a normal CXR are more likely to achieve a diagnosis when evaluated using a V/Q scan as opposed to a CTPa.[59] The rate of nondiagnostic test for PE in a pregnant patient with a normal CXR is 30% for CTPa versus 5.6% when using a V/Q scan.[59] However, the rate of nondiagnostic CTPa studies decreases from 30.0% to 16.4% when initial CXR is abnormal, and the rate of nondiagnostic test in V/Q scan increases from 5.6% to 40.0%.[59]

Though the previously suggested approach (see **Fig. 1**) is feasible and reasonable when the patient is being evaluated in a hospital setting, deciding on the next available diagnostic study following a CXR may prove to be a logistical challenge in patients being evaluated in an outpatient setting. In most cases, we opt for referring a patient for CTPa. In addition, given the better availability of CT imaging compared with nuclear studies, especially after hours, and that CT may offer an alternative diagnosis when PE is not present in a population with low incidence of PE among suspected patients, many, including the authors, prefer starting with a multidetector CT. Imaging with CT may also be advantageous in patients with severe hypoxemia or hemodynamic instability.

TREATMENT

In hemodynamically stable patients, acute treatment consists of anticoagulants as the first-line treatment. Low molecular weight heparin (LMWH) and unfractionated heparin (UFH) can both be used safely in pregnancy, as they do not cross the placental barrier (**Table 1**). However, LMWH is the anticoagulant of choice for antenatal VTE due to its better bioavailability,[60] low risk of bleeding,[61–63] and low rates of heparin-induced thrombocytopenia[61] and osteopenia.[64,65] The standard dose of enoxaparin is 1 mg/kg subcutaneous injection every 12 hours given insufficient data on once-daily dosing in pregnancy.

Table 1
Safety of anticoagulant use in pregnancy

Anticoagulant	Safety and Use in Pregnancy
LMWH	Enoxaparin, Daltaparin; dose 1 mg/kg BID; does not cross the placenta, blood thinner of choice in pregnancy; may need to adjust dose with increasing weight/may need to monitor anti-Xa levels (goal 0.5–1.1 U/mL).
UFH	May be used in place of LMWH in setting of renal dysfunction, high-risk PE, or during delivery, as it has a short half-life; IV drip or injections; need to monitor anti-Xa levels as volume of distribution and weight changes during pregnancy.
NOAC/DOAC	Clinical trials for DOACs/NOACs excluded pregnant women. Association with congenital anomalies, bleeding, implantation failure in animal studies. Slight increase in risk in human reports. Registry available: http://www.surveygizmo.com/s3/2394649/international-registry-of-pregnancy-during-NOAC-use-inclusion.
VKA	Warfarin crosses the placenta and has potential of teratogenicity; 3.7%–6.4% risk of congenital abnormalities. Also risk of fetal hemorrhage after organogenesis. Should not be used for treatment of VTE in pregnancy.
Synthetic heparins	Fondaparinux is not thought to increase risk of congenital malformations. Small amounts cross the placenta and 10% detected in neonates' blood with measurable effect on neonatal anti-Xa levels. This effect was not enough to lead to a full antithrombotic effect; hence clinical significance of placental transfer is unknown.
Thrombin inhibitors	Lepirudin is not expected to increase the risk of congenital anomalies. Human case reports and animal studies do not show evidence of malformation. Lepirudin does cross the rat placenta. Argatroban use in animal studies was performed at doses lower than human doses. Rare case reports do not show evidence of congenital anomalies; safety cannot be ascertained. Argatroban has been used in cases of HIT and heparin allergy.

Abbreviations: BID, twice daily; HIT, heparin-induced thrombocytopenia; IV, intravenous; LMWH, low molecular weight heparins; NOAC/DOAC, novel/direct anticoagulants; PE, pulmonary embolism; UFH, unfractionated heparins; VKA, vitamin K antagonists; VTE, venous thromboembolism.
Data from Refs.[28,93,94]

Dosing and monitoring of LMWH remains open to debate.[29,66] Plasma volume changes significantly in pregnancy and weight is a dynamic entity in pregnancy, and thus volume of distribution of drugs, including heparins, differs significantly. Although recent guidelines do not recommend monitoring,[29] we perform anti-Xa monitoring weekly for 2 to 3 weeks at initiation, and then once per trimester. Anti-Xa levels 4 hours after injection with goal anti-Xa level of 0.5 to 1.1 units/mL are generally used,[66] although those levels have not been linked to better clinical outcomes or lower risk of recurrence.

UFH is still used in pregnancy in areas of the world where LMWH is not available. It is also preferred in cases of renal dysfunction and is used intravenously[66] in patients with high burden of thrombosis possibly requiring thrombolysis, or around labor and delivery or an anticipated procedure, as it has a short half-life and is readily reversible. Because of changes in volume of distribution and bioavailability of this drug during pregnancy and the poor reliability of activated partial thromboplastin time levels, dosing should be monitored with heparin levels.[61,67]

The duration of treatment for VTE in pregnancy is not well studied, therefore recommendations for nonpregnant patients are followed.[68] Given that the postpartum patients are high risk for recurrent VTE, it is recommended that therapy be extended for at least 6 weeks postpartum.[69]

Warfarin, an oral vitamin K agonist (VKA), is not used in pregnancy, as it crosses the placenta and can be teratogenic. The risk of congenital abnormalities with VKAs is 3.7% to 6.4%.[66] Given that LMWH and UFH are similarly efficacious but safer in pregnancy, the use of VKAs in pregnancy cannot be justified.[70] In the postpartum period, coumadin has been detected in breast milk in tiny amounts (**Table 2**) but is generally considered safe to use while breast feeding.[71] Postpartum patients on therapeutic anticoagulation may need to be bridged from LMWH or UFH to warfarin so as not to significantly increase their risk of recurrent VTE.[72] The risk of recurrence needs to be weighed against the risk of bleeding following an intervention and timing of the bridging carefully considered, especially in the case of a surgical delivery.

The direct oral anticoagulants (DOACs) are newer non–vitamin K oral anticoagulants (NOACS) that directly inhibit clotting factors. Their use has become widespread in the nonpregnant population. The largest clinical trials for DOACs excluded pregnant women. DOACs cross the placenta,[73,74] and animal studies have shown an elevated risk of anomalies, hemorrhage, and embryopathies (reprotox.org). Case reports and cohorts of pregnant women exposed to DOACs in pregnancy show an elevated risk of congenital anomalies and increased maternal bleeding.[75] Hence, DOACs should be avoided throughout pregnancy or in women trying to conceive until there are better data and better understanding of their risks.[76,77] Nonpregnant women receiving DOACs need to have proper contraceptive counseling, because use of contraceptives is complicated by history of VTE.

Table 2
Anticoagulant use and lactation

Anticoagulant	Safety and Use in Lactation
LMWH	Enoxaparin, Dalteparin; small amount excreted in breast milk but combination of low concentration and poor bioavailability when taken orally makes any clinically meaningful effect on infant unlikely.
UFH	High molecular weight, unlikely to transfer. Safe in lactation.
NOAC/DOAC	Clinical trials for DOACs/NOACs excluded pregnant women; animal studies show excretion into breast milk; contraindicated in breastfeeding women.
VKA	Detected in breast milk in small amounts but considered safe in lactation. May bridge from UFH or LMWH to VKA in postpartum patient.
Synthetic heparins	Fondaparinux transfers to breast; however, such transfer is inconsistent.
Thrombin inhibitors	One case report showed no transfer of Hirudin into breast milk; data are missing otherwise. Lepirudin is unlikely to transfer to human milk given its structure; oral bioavailability is low. Data on Argatroban use during lactation are lacking.

Abbreviations: LMWH, low molecular weight heparins; NOAC/DOAC, novel/direct anticoagulants; UFH, unfractionated heparins; VKA, vitamin K antagonists.
Data from Refs.[28,93,95]

Pregnant women who are hemodynamically unstable or severely hypoxemic should be treated with thrombolysis if there are no contraindications. Data on managing pregnant patients in shock from VTE with other interventions besides systemic anticoagulation are limited to case reports. There are case reports of the administration of thrombolytics to pregnant patients with no resulting complications to the mother or the newborn,[78] and tissue plasminogen activator (t-PA) appears to be the best thrombolytic agent. In one case series, however, the fetal fatality rate in the setting of thrombolytics was 8%.[79] The overall risk of thrombolytic administration in pregnancy for decompensating patients is similar to nonpregnant patients[80,81] and is best described in the management of acute stroke.[82] The main risk of thrombolysis is maternal bleeding, which has been reported to occur in 8% of patients treated, with no reported cases of intracranial hemorrhage reported.[81] Although reported cases of fetal death may be related to thrombolytics, it is as likely that they may be related to a hemodynamically unstable PE. Although catheter-based thrombolytic administration may have lower complication risk, as lower medication dosages are used than systemic lysis, there are currently no data to support its use in pregnancy.[83]

Other salvage therapies have been described in pregnant patients with hemodynamically unstable PE, which theoretically may have less bleeding risk than systemic thrombolytics and include extracorporeal membrane oxygenation (ECMO) and surgical thrombectomy. One recent case series described 2 cases of veno-arterial extracorporeal life support as an alternative to thrombolysis to restore hemodynamic stability in pregnant patients with massive PE.[84] As ECMO is used in severe life-threatening conditions, it is hard to withhold this therapy from pregnant patients because of safety concerns; however, a decision to use such therapy should be weighed against efficacy, safety, and availability of other options. Surgical thrombectomy is another alternative to systemic thrombolysis and also may be considered when thrombolytic therapy has failed. Limited data suggested that although maternal survival may be high after surgical thrombectomy, fetal death rates can be elevated. In one case series, of eight cases reviewed there were no maternal deaths; however, 3 fetal deaths (37.5%) and 4 preterm deliveries (50.0%) were described.[80] Temporary intravenous filters have also been successfully used in pregnancy in cases in which anticoagulation is contraindicated or to manage the risk of clot recurrence around

Table 3
Management of anticoagulation around labor and delivery

Gestational Age at Time of VTE	Management Plan
<2 wk before labor	• Treat with intravenous heparin or place an IVC filter (preferably retrievable) and consider induction. • Restart anticoagulation with LMWH or UFH postpartum and plan for removal of IVC filter.
2–4 wk before labor	• Treat initially with LMWH but consider switching to IV heparin at approximately 38 wk of gestation in consultation with the obstetric team for a planned induction. • IV heparin stopped 6 h before anticipated delivery.
More than 1 mo before labor	• Depending on patient's risk for fast labor (such as number of prior pregnancies and gestational age at delivery in prior pregnancies, cervical examination), may continue LMWH until planned induction or consider switching from LMWH to UFH at term and follow with anti-Xa levels.
Recommendations for all women on anticoagulation during pregnancy	• Patients should be instructed to stop heparin injections at the first sign of labor. • Therapeutic LMWH should be discontinued at least 24 h before regional anesthesia or planned delivery. • LMWH should not be restarted for 4 h after the use of regional anesthesia or after the epidural catheter has been removed. • The epidural catheter should not be removed within 12 h of the most recent injection of LMWH.

Abbreviations: IV, intravenous; IVC, inferior vena cava filter; LMWH, low molecular weight heparin; UFH, unfractionated heparin; VTE, venous thromboembolism.
  Data from Refs.[44,80,89]

labor and delivery when clot occurs at term. Given the impact of pregnancy on inferior vena cava (IVC) anatomy, filters are usually placed suprarenally. A recent systematic review, which included 124 pregnancies with IVC filters placed, found no fatal PEs in women with IVC filters placed along with no recorded fetal morbidity or mortality.[85] There is, however, concern for more complicated retrieval of the filter in pregnancy, possibly due to angulation and distortion of the filter by the gravid uterus.[86]

Peripartum Anticoagulation

Management of VTE during the peripartum period can be challenging. Several clinical questions need to be addressed, including the duration of an anticoagulation window and whether an IVC filter is an option in high-risk patients. The biggest challenge for anticoagulation during the peripartum period is balancing the risk of postpartum hemorrhage with the risk of clot recurrence and the need for neuraxial analgesia.

Depending on the gestational age at which VTE has occurred (**Table 3**), several management options (eg, intravenous heparin, withholding anticoagulation, placement of IVC filter) are available,[87] but may vary based on institutional preferences.

PREVENTION

Pharmacologic thromboprophylaxis is usually initiated when the absolute risk of VTE exceeds a

Table 4
Summary of recommendations for prevention recurrent VTE

Source of Recommendation/Level of Evidence		Antepartum	Postpartum
• Single prior VTE • Transient risk (NH) • No thrombophilia	ACCP (Grade 1C)[28] ACOG[96] RCOG (C)[89] Bates et al,[29] 2016	Surveillance Surveillance Individual basis Individual basis	AC prophylaxis AC prophylaxis AC prophylaxis AC prophylaxis
• Single prior VTE • Transient risk (H) • No thrombophilia	ACCP (Grade 2C)[28] ACOG[96] RCOG (C)[89] Bates et al,[29] 2016	Surveillance or AC prophylaxis AC prophylaxis AC prophylaxis Individual basis	AC prophylaxis AC prophylaxis AC prophylaxis AC prophylaxis
• Single prior VTE • Idiopathic • No thrombophilia	ACCP (Grade 1C)[28] ACOG[96] RCOG (C)[89] Bates et al,[29] 2016	AC prophylaxis or surveillance AC prophylaxis Individual basis	AC prophylaxis AC prophylaxis AC prophylaxis
• Single VTE • Thrombophilia	ACCP (Grade 1C)[28] ACOG[96] RCOG (B)[89] Bates et al,[29] 2016	AC prophylaxis or surveillance AC prophylaxis or surveillance AC prophylaxis AC prophylaxis	AC prophylaxis Surveillance or AC AC prophylaxis AC prophylaxis
• Single VTE • "Higher risk" thrombophilia	ACCP (Grade 2C)[28] ACOG[96] RCOG (C)[89] Bates et al,[29] 2016	AC prophylaxis AC prophylaxis	AC prophylaxis AC AC prophylaxis
• Multiple prior VTE, not on long-term AC	ACCP (Grade 2C)[28] ACOG[96] RCOG[89] Bates et al,[29] 2016	AC prophylaxis AC prophylaxis AC prophylaxis	AC prophylaxis AC prophylaxis AC prophylaxis
• No prior VTE • Low-risk thrombophilia	ACCP (2C)[28] ACOG[96] RCOG (D)[89] Bates et al,[29] 2016	Surveillance if − FH Surveillance or AC prophylaxis Consider AC prophylaxis Consider AC prophylaxis if + FH	Surveillance AC prophylaxis AC prophylaxis
• No prior VTE • "Higher risk" thrombophilia	ACCP (2B)[28] ACOG[96] RCOG (C/D)[89] Bates et al,[29] 2016	AC prophylaxis if + FH AC prophylaxis if + FH Consider	AC if + FH Consider if + FH AC prophylaxis if + FH

Abbreviations: −, negative; +, positive; AC, anticoagulation; ACCP, American College of Chest Physicians; ACOG, American College of Obstetricians and Gynecologists; FH, family history; H, hormonal; NH, non-hormonal; RCOG, Royal College of Obstetricians and Gynecologists; VTE, venous thromboembolism.

certain threshold and the benefit of thromboprophylaxis exceeds the risk associated with such therapy. However, risk assessment methods that estimate the risk of VTE are lacking in the perinatal population, and although it is clear that each additional risk factor increases the relative risk of VTE, the absolute risk estimate remains a challenge. This knowledge gap partly explains the discrepancies in recommendations for thromboprophylaxis by various societies.[28,88,89]

Risk stratification for VTE should be undertaken before consideration of preventive strategy; however, recommendations are mainly based on expert opinion rather than high-quality trials.[90] Possible risk factors include age older than 35, obesity, parity greater than 3, previous VTE, gross varicose veins, paraplegia, medical comorbidities, and inheritable thrombophilias.[91] One recent meta-analysis concluded that the thrombophilias associated with the highest risk in pregnancy were antithrombin deficiency, protein C deficiency, protein S deficiency, and homozygous factor V Leiden deficiency.[92] Prothrombin gene mutation has also been considered a high-risk thrombophilia.[28] Hence, guidelines have differed in their recommendations for pharmacotherapy, especially in the antepartum period (**Table 4**). Although most recommend thromboprophylaxis with LMWH for homozygous factor V Leiden or prothrombin gene mutation, recommendations for protein C, S, or antithrombin deficiency are debated.[28,88,92] Postpartum pharmacoprophylaxis is recommended for most patients with inherited thrombophilia, including those with weak thrombophilias, especially those with a family history of VTE or additional risk factors, and obviously in all women with thrombophilias associated with a high risk for VTE.[28,88] The Royal College of Obstetricians and Gynecologists also recommends thromboprophylaxis in patients with class 3 obesity and any woman with at least 2 persisting risk factors postpartum for at least 10 days.[89]

In low-risk patients, early mobilization and graduated elastic compression stockings are advised. Patients with high risk factors, including previous VTE or thrombophilic disorder, should be offered chemical prophylaxis.[92] The pharmacologic prophylaxis of choice for antenatal and postnatal thromboprophylaxis is LMWH, as it does not cross the placenta.[90] There is no evidence for the routine use of aspirin. For patients who are intolerant to heparin, fondaparinux may be used (see **Table 2**), especially in cases of heparin-induced thrombocytopenia.[22]

SUMMARY

The diagnosis and treatment of PE in pregnancy is complicated by pregnancy physiology. Much research is needed to develop pregnancy-specific pretest clinical pretest probability rules and to examine the negative predictive power of a given cutoff of D-dimers in diagnostic cohort studies. In addition, prospective research is needed to examine the positive and negative predictive value of imaging studies in confirming or excluding PE, and to determine the imaging study of choice in pregnancy from a cost-effectiveness and radiation-exposure standpoint, while examining pregnancy-specific imaging protocols. There are also numerous gaps in preventive and treatment strategies: mainly duration of therapy, appropriate dosing, adequacy of therapeutic levels in reducing recurrence, and in determination of risk assessment tools to use in prevention.

REFERENCES

1. Say L, Chou D, Gemmill A, et al. Global causes of maternal death: a WHO systematic analysis. Lancet Glob Health 2014;2:e323–33.

2. Knight M, Tuffnell D, Kenyon S, et al, editors. Saving lives, improving mothers' care—surveillance of maternal deaths in the UK 2011-13 and lessons learned to inform maternity care from the UK and Ireland confidential enquiries into maternal deaths and morbidity 2009-13. Oxford (England): National Perinatal Epidemiology Unit, University of Oxford; 2015.

3. Kuriya A, Piedimonte S, Spence AR, et al. Incidence and causes of maternal mortality in the USA. J Obstet Gynaecol Res 2016;42:661–8.

4. Cantwell R, Clutton-Brock T, Cooper G, et al. Saving mothers' lives: reviewing maternal deaths to make motherhood safer: 2006-2008. The Eighth Report of the Confidential Enquiries into Maternal Deaths in the United Kingdom. BJOG 2011;118(Suppl 1): 1–203.

5. Heit JA, Kobbervig CE, James AH, et al. Trends in the incidence of venous thromboembolism during pregnancy or postpartum: a 30-year population-based study. Ann Intern Med 2005;143:697–706.

6. Liu S, Rouleau J, Joseph KS, et al. Epidemiology of pregnancy-associated venous thromboembolism: a population-based study in Canada. J Obstet Gynaecol Can 2009;31:611–20.

7. Gherman RB, Goodwin TM, Leung B, et al. Incidence, clinical characteristics, and timing of objectively diagnosed venous thromboembolism during pregnancy. Obstet Gynecol 1999;94:730–4.

8. Sultan AA, West J, Grainge MJ, et al. Development and validation of risk prediction model for venous

thromboembolism in postpartum women: multinational cohort study. BMJ 2016;355:i6253.

9. Jacobsen AF, Skjeldestad FE, Sandset PM. Incidence and risk patterns of venous thromboembolism in pregnancy and puerperium–a register-based case-control study. Am J Obstet Gynecol 2008;198:233.e1-7.

10. Pomp ER, Lenselink AM, Rosendaal FR, et al. Pregnancy, the postpartum period and prothrombotic defects: risk of venous thrombosis in the MEGA study. J Thromb Haemost 2008;6:632–7.

11. Epiney M, Boehlen F, Boulvain M, et al. D-dimer levels during delivery and the postpartum. J Thromb Haemost 2005;3:268–71.

12. Kjellberg U, Andersson NE, Rosen S, et al. APC resistance and other haemostatic variables during pregnancy and puerperium. Thromb Haemost 1999;81:527–31.

13. Kamel H, Navi BB, Sriram N, et al. Risk of a thrombotic event after the 6-week postpartum period. N Engl J Med 2014;370:1307–15.

14. Barbagallo M, Dominguez LJ, Licata G, et al. Vascular effects of progesterone: role of cellular calcium regulation. Hypertension 2001;37:142–7.

15. Tkachenko O, Shchekochikhin D, Schrier RW. Hormones and hemodynamics in pregnancy. Int J Endocrinol Metab 2014;12:e14098.

16. Goulart VB, Cabral AC, Reis ZS, et al. Anatomical and physiological changes in the venous system of lower limbs in pregnant women and findings associated with the symptomatology. Arch Gynecol Obstet 2013;288:73–8.

17. Chan WS, Spencer FA, Ginsberg JS. Anatomic distribution of deep vein thrombosis in pregnancy. CMAJ 2010;182:657–60.

18. Goldhaber SZ, Tapson VF. A prospective registry of 5,451 patients with ultrasound-confirmed deep vein thrombosis. Am J Cardiol 2004;93:259–62.

19. Greer IA. Thrombosis in pregnancy: maternal and fetal issues. Lancet 1999;353:1258–65.

20. James AH, Tapson VF, Goldhaber SZ. Thrombosis during pregnancy and the postpartum period. Am J Obstet Gynecol 2005;193:216–9.

21. Boeldt DS, Bird IM. Vascular adaptation in pregnancy and endothelial dysfunction in preeclampsia. J Endocrinol 2017;232:R27–44.

22. Lim A, Samarage A, Lim BH. Venous thromboembolism in pregnancy. Obstet Gynaecol Reprod Med 2016;26:133–9.

23. Brenner B. Haemostatic changes in pregnancy. Thromb Res 2004;114:409–14.

24. Rosenkranz A, Hiden M, Leschnik B, et al. Calibrated automated thrombin generation in normal uncomplicated pregnancy. Thromb Haemost 2008;99:331–7.

25. James AH, Jamison MG, Brancazio LR, et al. Venous thromboembolism during pregnancy and the postpartum period: incidence, risk factors, and mortality. Am J Obstet Gynecol 2006;194:1311–5.

26. Dobbenga-Rhodes Y. Shedding light on inherited thrombophilias: the impact on pregnancy. J Perinat Neonatal Nurs 2016;30:36–44.

27. Gerhardt A, Scharf RE, Greer IA, et al. Hereditary risk factors for thrombophilia and probability of venous thromboembolism during pregnancy and the puerperium. Blood 2016;128:2343–9.

28. Bates SM, Greer IA, Middeldorp S, et al. VTE, thrombophilia, antithrombotic therapy, and pregnancy: antithrombotic therapy and prevention of thrombosis, 9th ed: American College of Chest Physicians evidence-based clinical practice guidelines. Chest 2012;141:e691S–736S.

29. Bates SM, Middeldorp S, Rodger M, et al. Guidance for the treatment and prevention of obstetric-associated venous thromboembolism. J Thromb Thrombolysis 2016;41:92–128.

30. American College of Obstetricians and Gynecologists Women's Health Care Physicians. ACOG Practice Bulletin No. 138: inherited thrombophilias in pregnancy. Obstet Gynecol 2013;122:706–17.

31. Blondon M, Casini A, Hoppe KK, et al. Risks of venous thromboembolism after cesarean sections: a meta-analysis. Chest 2016;150:572–96.

32. Jacobsen AF, Skjeldestad FE, Sandset PM. Ante- and postnatal risk factors of venous thrombosis: a hospital-based case-control study. J Thromb Haemost 2008;6:905–12.

33. Heyl PS, Sappenfield WM, Burch D, et al. Pregnancy-related deaths due to pulmonary embolism: findings from two state-based mortality reviews. Matern Child Health J 2013;17:1230–5.

34. O'Connor C, Moriarty J, Walsh J, et al. The application of a clinical risk stratification score may reduce unnecessary investigations for pulmonary embolism in pregnancy. J Matern Fetal Neonatal Med 2011;24:1461–4.

35. Cutts BA, Tran HA, Merriman E, et al. The utility of the Wells clinical prediction model and ventilation-perfusion scanning for pulmonary embolism diagnosis in pregnancy. Blood Coagul Fibrinolysis 2014;25:375–8.

36. Abbassi-Ghanavati M, Greer LG, Cunningham FG. Pregnancy and laboratory studies: a reference table for clinicians. Obstet Gynecol 2009;114:1326–31.

37. Boehlen F, Epiney M, Boulvain M, et al. Changes in D-dimer levels during pregnancy and the postpartum period: results of two studies. Rev Med Suisse 2005;1:296–8 [in French].

38. Parilla BV, Fournogerakis R, Archer A, et al. Diagnosing pulmonary embolism in pregnancy: are biomarkers and clinical predictive models useful? AJP Rep 2016;06:e160–4.

39. Bourjeily G. D-dimer use in venous thromboembolic disease in pregnancy. BJOG 2015;122:401.

40. Hameed AB, Chan K, Ghamsary M, et al. Longitudinal changes in the B-type natriuretic peptide levels in normal pregnancy and postpartum. Clin Cardiol 2009;32:E60–2.

41. Resnik JL, Hong C, Resnik R, et al. Evaluation of B-type natriuretic peptide (BNP) levels in normal and preeclamptic women. Am J Obstet Gynecol 2005;193:450–4.

42. Tanous D, Siu SC, Mason J, et al. B-type natriuretic peptide in pregnant women with heart disease. J Am Coll Cardiol 2010;56:1247–53.

43. Cutts BA, Dasgupta D, Hunt BJ. New directions in the diagnosis and treatment of pulmonary embolism in pregnancy. Am J Obstet Gynecol 2013;208:102–8.

44. Bourjeily G, Paidas M, Khalil H, et al. Pulmonary embolism in pregnancy. Lancet 2010;375:500–12.

45. Boiselle PM, Goodman LR, Litmanovich D, et al. Expert opinion: CT pulmonary angiography in pregnant patients with suspected pulmonary embolism. J Thorac Imaging 2012;27:5.

46. Leung AN, Bull TM, Jaeschke R, et al. An official American Thoracic Society/Society of Thoracic Radiology clinical practice guideline: evaluation of suspected pulmonary embolism in pregnancy. Am J Respir Crit Care Med 2011;184:1200–8.

47. Skeith L, Rodger MA. Pulmonary complications of pregnancy: venous thromboembolism. Semin Respir Crit Care Med 2017;38:135–47.

48. Gruning T, Mingo RE, Gosling MG, et al. Diagnosing venous thromboembolism in pregnancy. Br J Radiol 2016;89:20160021.

49. Schaefer-Prokop C, Prokop M. CTPA for the diagnosis of acute pulmonary embolism during pregnancy. Eur Radiol 2008;18:2705–8.

50. Astani SA, Davis LC, Harkness BA, et al. Detection of pulmonary embolism during pregnancy: comparing radiation doses of CTPA and pulmonary scintigraphy. Nucl Med Commun 2014;35:704–11.

51. Einstein AJ, Henzlova MJ, Rajagopalan S. Estimating risk of cancer associated with radiation exposure from 64-slice computed tomography coronary angiography. JAMA 2007;298:317–23.

52. Kim YK, Sung YM, Choi JH, et al. Reduced radiation exposure of the female breast during low-dose chest CT using organ-based tube current modulation and a bismuth shield: comparison of image quality and radiation dose. AJR Am J Roentgenol 2013;200:537–44.

53. Hopper KD, King SH, Lobell ME, et al. The breast: in-plane x-ray protection during diagnostic thoracic CT–shielding with bismuth radioprotective garments. Radiology 1997;205:853–8.

54. Bourjeily G, Chalhoub M, Phornphutkul C, et al. Neonatal thyroid function: effect of a single exposure to iodinated contrast medium in utero. Radiology 2010;256:744–50.

55. Righini M, Le Gal G, Aujesky D, et al. Diagnosis of pulmonary embolism by multidetector CT alone or combined with venous ultrasonography of the leg: a randomised non-inferiority trial. Lancet 2008;371:1343–52.

56. Bourjeily G, Khalil H, Raker C, et al. Outcomes of negative multidetector computed tomography with pulmonary angiography in pregnant women suspected of pulmonary embolism. Lung 2012;190:105–11.

57. Chan WS, Ray JG, Murray S, et al. Suspected pulmonary embolism in pregnancy: clinical presentation, results of lung scanning, and subsequent maternal and pediatric outcomes. Arch Intern Med 2002;162:1170–5.

58. Shahir K, Goodman LR, Tali A, et al. Pulmonary embolism in pregnancy: CT pulmonary angiography versus perfusion scanning. AJR Am J Roentgenol 2010;195:W214–20.

59. Cahill AG, Stout MJ, Macones GA, et al. Diagnosing pulmonary embolism in pregnancy using computed-tomographic angiography or ventilation-perfusion. Obstet Gynecol 2009;114:124–9.

60. Couturaud F, Julian JA, Kearon C. Low molecular weight heparin administered once versus twice daily in patients with venous thromboembolism: a meta-analysis. Thromb Haemost 2001;86:980–4.

61. Greer IA, Nelson-Piercy C. Low-molecular-weight heparins for thromboprophylaxis and treatment of venous thromboembolism in pregnancy: a systematic review of safety and efficacy. Blood 2005;106:401–7.

62. Lepercq J, Conard J, Borel-Derlon A, et al. Venous thromboembolism during pregnancy: a retrospective study of enoxaparin safety in 624 pregnancies. BJOG 2001;108:1134–40.

63. Nelson-Piercy C, Powrie R, Borg JY, et al. Tinzaparin use in pregnancy: an international, retrospective study of the safety and efficacy profile. Eur J Obstet Gynecol Reprod Biol 2011;159:293–9.

64. Pettila V, Leinonen P, Markkola A, et al. Postpartum bone mineral density in women treated for thromboprophylaxis with unfractionated heparin or LMW heparin. Thromb Haemost 2002;87:182–6.

65. Rodger MA, Kahn SR, Cranney A, et al. Long-term dalteparin in pregnancy not associated with a decrease in bone mineral density: substudy of a randomized controlled trial. J Thromb Haemost 2007;5:1600–6.

66. Bates SM. Pregnancy-associated venous thromboembolism: prevention and treatment. Semin Hematol 2011;48:271–84.

67. Chunilal SD, Young E, Johnston MA, et al. The APTT response of pregnant plasma to unfractionated heparin. Thromb Haemost 2002;87:92–7.

68. Kearon C, Akl EA, Ornelas J, et al. Antithrombotic therapy for VTE disease: CHEST guideline and expert panel report. Chest 2016;149:315–52.

69. Schulman S, Rhedin AS, Lindmarker P, et al. A comparison of six weeks with six months of oral anticoagulant therapy after a first episode of venous thromboembolism. Duration of Anticoagulation Trial Study Group. N Engl J Med 1995;332:1661–5.

70. Chan WS, Anand S, Ginsberg JS. Anticoagulation of pregnant women with mechanical heart valves: a systematic review of the literature. Arch Intern Med 2000;160:191–6.

71. De Swiet M, Lewis PJ. Excretion of anticoagulants in human milk. N Engl J Med 1977;297:1471.

72. Brandjes DP, Heijboer H, Buller HR, et al. Acenocoumarol and heparin compared with acenocoumarol alone in the initial treatment of proximal-vein thrombosis. N Engl J Med 1992;327:1485–9.

73. Bapat P, Kedar R, Lubetsky A, et al. Transfer of dabigatran and dabigatran etexilate mesylate across the dually perfused human placenta. Obstet Gynecol 2014;123:1256–61.

74. Bapat P, Pinto LS, Lubetsky A, et al. Examining the transplacental passage of apixaban using the dually perfused human placenta. J Thromb Haemost 2016;14:1436–41.

75. Beyer-Westendorf J, Michalski F, Tittl L, et al. Pregnancy outcome in patients exposed to direct oral anticoagulants—and the challenge of event reporting. Thromb Haemost 2016;116:651–8.

76. Myers B, Neal R, Myers O, et al. Unplanned pregnancy on a direct oral anticoagulant (Rivaroxaban): a warning. Obstet Med 2016;9:40–2.

77. Cohen H, Arachchillage DR, Middeldorp S, et al. Management of direct oral anticoagulants in women of childbearing potential: guidance from the SSC of the ISTH. J Thromb Haemost 2016;14:1673–6.

78. Lonjaret L, Lairez O, Galinier M, et al. Thrombolysis by recombinant tissue plasminogen activator during pregnancy: a case of massive pulmonary embolism. Am J Emerg Med 2011;29:694.e1-2.

79. Leonhardt G, Gaul C, Nietsch HH, et al. Thrombolytic therapy in pregnancy. J Thromb Thrombolysis 2006;21:271–6.

80. te Raa GD, Ribbert LS, Snijder RJ, et al. Treatment options in massive pulmonary embolism during pregnancy; a case-report and review of literature. Thromb Res 2009;124:1–5.

81. Turrentine MA, Braems G, Ramirez MM. Use of thrombolytics for the treatment of thromboembolic disease during pregnancy. Obstet Gynecol Surv 1995;50:534–41.

82. Leffert LR, Clancy CR, Bateman BT, et al. Treatment patterns and short-term outcomes in ischemic stroke in pregnancy or postpartum period. Am J Obstet Gynecol 2016;214:723.e1-11.

83. Weitz JI. Prevention and treatment of venous thromboembolism during pregnancy. Catheter Cardiovasc Interv 2009;74(Suppl 1):S22–6.

84. Bataillard A, Hebrard A, Gaide-Chevronnay L, et al. Extracorporeal life support for massive pulmonary embolism during pregnancy. Perfusion 2016;31:169–71.

85. Harris SA, Velineni R, Davies AH. Inferior vena cava filters in pregnancy: a systematic review. J Vasc Interv Radiol 2016;27:354–60.e8.

86. Gupta S, Ettles DF, Robinson GJ, et al. Inferior vena cava filter use in pregnancy: preliminary experience. BJOG 2008;115:785–8.

87. Middeldorp S. How I treat pregnancy-related venous thromboembolism. Blood 2011;118:5394–400.

88. Chan WS, Rey E, Kent NE, et al. Venous thromboembolism and antithrombotic therapy in pregnancy. J Obstet Gynaecol Can 2014;36:527–53.

89. Royal College of Obstetricians and Gynaecologists. Reducing the risk of venous thromboembolism during pregnancy and the puerperium. Green-top Guideline No. 37a. London: RCOG, 2015. Available at: https://http://www.rcog.org.uk/globalassets/documents/guidelines/gtg-37a.pdf. Accessed November 26, 2017.

90. Villani M, Ageno W, Grandone E, et al. The prevention and treatment of venous thromboembolism in pregnancy. Expert Rev Cardiovasc Ther 2017;15:397–402.

91. Skeith L, Carrier M, Robinson SE, et al. Risk of venous thromboembolism in pregnant women with essential thrombocythemia: a systematic review and meta-analysis. Blood 2017;129:934–9.

92. Croles FN, Nasserinejad K, Duvekot JJ, et al. Pregnancy, thrombophilia, and the risk of a first venous thrombosis: systematic review and Bayesian meta-analysis. BMJ 2017;359:j4452.

93. The reproductive toxicology center. Available at: http://www.reprotox.org/. Accessed September 20, 2017.

94. Mazer J, Zouein E, Bourjeily G. Treatment of pulmonary embolism in pregnancy. US Respir Dis 2012;8:30–5.

95. Hale TW. Medications and mothers' milk. Amarillo (TX): Pharmasoft Medical Pub; 2000.

96. James A. Practice bulletin no. 123: thromboembolism in pregnancy. Obstet Gynecol 2011;118:718–29.

Challenges and Changes to the Management of Pulmonary Embolism in the Emergency Department

Chris Moore, MD*, Katelyn McNamara, Rachel Liu, MD

KEYWORDS

- Pulmonary embolism • Venous thromboembolism • Emergency department • Thrombolysis
- Thrombolytics • PE response team

KEY POINTS

- Diagnosis of PE may include the use of age adjusted D-dimer and point-of-care ultrasound.
- Classification of PE is essential for prognosis and treatment and has evolved over the last decade.
- Alternative treatments such as low dose thrombolytics may be most appropriate in some patients.
- Cutting edge therapies for life threatening PEs include nitric oxide ventilation and extracorporeal membrane oxygenation.

 Video content accompanies this article at http://www.chestmed.theclinics.com.

EPIDEMIOLOGY AND DIAGNOSIS

The incidence of pulmonary embolism (PE) is slightly more than 1 per 1000 person-years, with estimates ranging as high as 900,000 PEs annually in the United States with 200,000 fatalities per year (**Box 1**).[1] Between 1 in 400 and 1 in 1500 patients presenting to US emergency departments (EDs) will be diagnosed with PE, an incidence that is highly age-related, and may increase as the population ages further.[2] With more than 140 million annual ED visits in the United States, this suggests that between 90,000 and 350,000 PEs are diagnosed annually in US EDs.[3]

In 1998 multidetector computed tomography (CT) pulmonary angiography was introduced and rapidly became the first-line test for PE.[4] CT is rapid, accurate, and essentially universally available in EDs as a diagnostic option. However, despite a near doubling of diagnostic incidence since CT replaced ventilation perfusion scanning, the age-adjusted mortality from PE has remained relatively stable, suggesting "overdiagnosis."[4]

At the same time, it is frequently posited that PE remains missed in the ED setting, and medicolegal concerns are prominent. It has been suggested that PE "should be suspected in all patients who present with worsening dyspnea, chest pain, or sustained hypotension without an alternate obvious cause."[5] However, the hallmark symptoms of PE—chest pain and shortness of breath—are among the most common presenting ED complaints. This makes ruling out a PE by objective means in all such patients neither feasible nor desirable. There are several validated clinical decision rules that can aid in deciding whether further diagnostic testing (D-dimer or CT) is needed, including the PE rule-out criteria (PERC), Wells score for PE, and the Geneva score.[2]

The PERC score defines a population in whom no testing is needed to exclude PE. Patients in

Department of Emergency Medicine, Yale University School of Medicine, 464 Congress Avenue, Suite 273, New Haven, CT 06519, USA
* Corresponding author.
E-mail address: Chris.moore@yale.edu

Clin Chest Med 39 (2018) 539–547
https://doi.org/10.1016/j.ccm.2018.04.009
0272-5231/18/© 2018 Elsevier Inc. All rights reserved.

chestmed.theclinics.com

> **Box 1**
> **Challenges and changes in ED management of PE**
>
> - Adjusted D-dimer for diagnosis
> - Classification of PE for prognosis and therapy
> - Thrombolytic therapy for intermediate-risk PE
> - Low-dose thrombolysis dosing
> - Adjunctive therapies for large PEs
>   - Nitric oxide ventilation
>   - Extracorporeal membrane oxygenation
> - Multidisciplinary PE response teams

whom PE is considered a possible diagnosis but who are "PERC negative" should not have D-dimer performed. An important concept with PERC is that it does not necessarily completely rule out all possibilities of a PE, but it defines a population in whom the likely harm of performing a D-dimer (false-positive results leading to likely unnecessary testing) outweighs the benefit based on defining a threshold level of diagnostic likelihood (~2%). It is also important not to apply the PERC rule indiscriminately—if there is no real concern for PE then it should not be used.

The Wells score for PE is the predominant scoring system and has been well validated in the ED setting.[6] It can be divided into either a two- or three-level score, with D-dimer testing used to exclude PE in low- or intermediate-risk patients. The Geneva score (including simplified and revised Geneva) is an alternate approach that is more common in Europe and has been shown in some studies to be more consistently reliable.[1] The decision about whether and which clinical prediction rule to use may be guided by the local prevalence of PE.[7] Although objective clinical prediction rules are recommended by some analyses, others have suggested that gestalt clinician pretest probability may be used and even preferred in some cases.[8,9]

Challenges and Changes: Adjusted D-dimer

D-dimer is a cornerstone of PE diagnosis. Quantitative enzyme-linked immunoassay D-dimer tests are sensitive enough to essentially rule out a PE in all but high-risk patients. Although sensitive for ruling out PE, the problem is that D-dimer is not specific and can be elevated in the absence of PE. This is the basis of the PERC score—an attempt to ensure D-dimers are not ordered indiscriminately, leading to increased CT scanning without improving diagnostic yield. D-dimer may

be elevated without PE in pregnancy, malignancy, trauma, or simply as people age. Recently several publications have supported the use of an age-adjusted D-dimer, allowing the threshold for CT angiography testing to increase with age. The most commonly used adjustment is to use age times 10 ng/mL, so while a normal threshold for abnormal is typically 500 ng/mL, an 80 year-old patient's cutoff would be 800 ng/mL. This approach is supported by the literature and expert opinion.[10] In pregnancy, D-dimer level also increases with each trimester, and a pregnancy-adjusted D-dimer along with a modified PERC rule may be considered (heart rate cutoff of 105; D-dimer threshold 50%, 100%, and 125% higher than normal cutoff by trimester).[11]

Challenges and Changes: Echocardiography and Focused Cardiac Ultrasound

Transthoracic echocardiography (TTE) can be used in both the diagnosis and prognosis of PE and can thus also influence therapy.[12] Although echo is insufficiently sensitive to completely rule out PE, the presence of findings (usually indirect evidence of right ventricular [RV] strain, occasionally actual visualized thrombus) increases the likelihood of the diagnosis and defines a subset that may benefit from more aggressive therapy.[13] When available, TTE can be performed by a certified sonographer and interpreted by a cardiologist; however, availability of cardiology echo is often limited or delayed in the ED setting.[14] The specificity of echo may be particularly helpful for "rule-in" of patients with hemodynamic instability in the ED setting.[12]

One of the more recent challenges and changes to the ED diagnosis and management of PE has been the potential incorporation of point-of-care ultrasound, or specifically focused cardiac ultrasound (FoCUS), which is an ultrasound performed by the emergency physician at the bedside.[15,16] Although echo performed by emergency physicians (EPs) has been described for at least 3 decades, evidence for FoCUS evaluation in suspected or confirmed PE has been more recent.[17] The evaluation of the right heart has consistently been included in consensus statements about FoCUS since 2010.[15,18,19] Available ultrasound technology has become higher in quality and more affordable, but the issue has always been what level of training is required to adequately perform FoCUS.[19]

The most prevalent and reliable sign of a significant PE on echo is RV strain, based on RV enlargement or hypokinesis (**Figs. 1** and **2**). RV enlargement relative to the left ventricle (LV) is

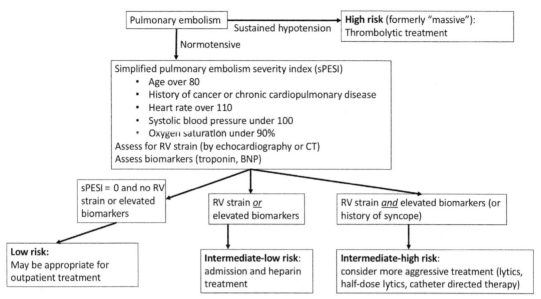

Fig. 1. This chart shows a classification scheme based on most current literature, with potential impact on therapy.

the most frequently described FoCUS measure. A normal ratio of the RV to LV is approximately 0.6:1 (measured across tips of valves in an apical view); however, a typical cutoff used for RV enlargement is an RV:LV ratio of 1:1 or greater,

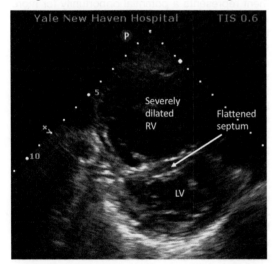

Fig. 2. This is a point-of-care FoCUS of a 37-year-old patient in cardiac arrest who came in to the ED. This is a parasternal short-axis view showing a markedly enlarged right ventricle (RV) compressing the septum into the left ventricle (LV) in a characteristic "D-shaped" pattern. Initial blood pH was 6.85 with lactate of 18 mmol/L. This patient received a total of 150 mg bolus dose tissue plasminogen activator, nitric oxide via the ventilator, and extracorporeal membrane oxygenation in the intensive care unit. Videos 1 and 2 show pre- and postthrombolysis. The patient recovered fully.

which favors specificity over sensitivity. Detection of RV enlargement by RV:LV ratio has been shown to have good interobserver agreement.[20] In a study of 146 ED patients, 30 of whom had PE, the presence of RV dilatation (1:1 or greater ratio) had a specificity of 98% for the diagnosis of PE, although sensitivity was only 50%.[21] Another study of 411 of patients by 69 different emergency providers in whom 6.2% had RV strain showed moderate agreement when comparing EPs to consultative echo.[22] In addition to aiding in diagnosis, the presence of RV strain identified by EPs in diagnosed PE has been shown on multivariate analysis to predict adverse outcomes.[23]

A potentially more objective and reliable measure of RV dysfunction secondary to PE is tricuspid annular plane systolic excursion (TAPSE). First described in the cardiology literature for more chronic diseases such as congestive heart failure and pulmonary hypertension, it has been shown to be a more reliable measure of RV dysfunction and to correlate well with other markers of acute PE severity.[20,24] A normally functioning RV contracts from base to apex and can be measured quantitatively using m-mode (motion mode), with normal movement typically being more than 16 to 20 mm, but may also be categorized qualitatively as normal or abnormal.[25] Although TAPSE also lacks sensitivity in diagnosing undifferentiated PE, a recent study showed that when PE is suspected in patients with abnormal vital signs it was sensitive for the diagnosis.

SPECTRUM OF PULMONARY EMBOLISM FOR PROGNOSIS, THERAPY, AND DISPOSITION

PE presents with a wide spectrum of severity, which is important to define for both prognosis and therapy. There is some confusion and heterogeneity regarding use of these terms and they have continued to evolve. Hemodynamic instability or hypotension at presentation is the strongest predictor of mortality and identifies patients for aggressive therapy such as thrombolysis. **Fig. 1** shows a classification scheme based on the most commonly used current stratification schema.[26–28]

Presence of hemodynamic instability has more recently been termed "high-risk" PE, previously termed "massive," and is typically defined as presence of hypotension (systolic blood pressure <90 mm Hg for at least 15 minutes not from another cause), cardiac arrest, or persistent bradycardia (<40bpm with signs and symptoms of shock).[27] Within normotensive patients there are intermediate-high and intermediate-low (formerly grouped as "submassive") and low-risk.[27,28] Although there is some variability in this area, a simplified pulmonary severity index (sPESI) score of zero has been used to define low-risk patients who may be appropriate for outpatient PE treatment. The sPESI includes age greater than 80 years, history of cancer or chronic cardiopulmonary disease, heart rate greater than 110, systolic blood pressure less than 100, or oxygen saturation less than 90%.[26] If the sPESI is greater than zero and the patients are normotensive, the presence of RV strain or elevated biomarkers (or neither) identifies intermediate-low risk (appropriate for heparin alone and admission). RV assessment may be performed using either echocardiography or CT, and elevated biomarkers typically include troponin or b-type natriuretic peptide. The presence of both RV strain and elevated biomarkers, or a history of syncope, would classify someone as having intermediate-high risk PE. Intermediate-high risk PE patients may be considered for more aggressive therapy, including full- or half-dose thrombolytics (or catheter-directed therapies). Patients presenting with hemodynamic instability from PE are estimated to have a 30-day mortality rate of ~50%, with intermediate-risk PE around 10% to 20% (perhaps lower now with improved therapy), and low-risk PE of about 1%.[27,29]

Other scoring systems include the HESTIA score and the original PE severity index (PESI).[30,31] The PESI score divides patients with diagnosed PE into 5 risk classes and was originally designed to delineate patients appropriate for outpatient treatment of PE, although it may be used to help guide patient selection for more aggressive therapy as well.[1] Both the HESTIA and PESI/sPESI scores may be used to select patients for outpatient treatment of PE, with HESTIA potentially safely identifying a larger proportion.[32] Although evidence continues to emerge, there is no consensus that there is validated data about these scoring systems for definitive treatment.[33]

THERAPY

Anticoagulation is the mainstay treatment of PE. Unfractionated heparin (UFH) can be considered a default initial treatment of PE that can be titrated and reversed if necessary, but must be administered in an inpatient setting. Low-molecular-weight heparins (LMWH) have been shown to be equivalent or better than UFH in treatment efficacy and can be administered as an outpatient.[34] Recently, novel oral anticoagulants (NOACs) that inhibit factor Xa have been approved for use in PE and may be initiated in the ED setting. Currently the NOACs approved by Food and Drug Administration (FDA) for PE treatment include apixaban (Eliquis), dabigatran (Pradaxa), rivaroxaban (Xarelto), and edoxaban (Savaysa). Outpatient treatment represents a potential opportunity for more efficient care that may also be more favorable to the patient. In patients who are at low risk (no RV strain, hypoxia, elevated biomarkers, or hemodynamic instability) and/or have low HESTIA/PESI/sPESI scores, it has been shown that they may be safely discharged from the ED on either LMWH or an NOAC with a low rate of complications.[35] It is also arguable that in some cases isolated subsegmental PEs may either be false-positive diagnoses or may be so insignificant that the harms from anticoagulation outweigh the benefits, although trials on this approach are lacking.[36]

Thrombolysis

UFH, LMWH, and NOACs have the effect of preventing new thrombus formation and allow natural processes to resolve clots but do not actively dissolve the thrombus. Thrombolytic agents (tissue plasminogen activator [tPA]) will actively dissolve clot but carries a higher risk of hemorrhage. Systemic thrombolysis is a recommended option for hemodynamically unstable (massive) PE given the high risk of death without aggressive intervention.[27] The risk of bleeding makes use of thrombolysis contraindicated for low-risk PEs. Submassive or intermediate-risk PEs represent a particular challenge in the management of PE. Systemic lysis may be of benefit, but the risk-benefit balance is slimmer and other options such as reduced dose or catheter-directed lysis may be considered.

Challenges and Changes: Thrombolysis in Intermediate-Risk Pulmonary Embolism

A 2011 review summarized the outcomes of 4 registries that reviewed thrombolysis for submassive PE, finding that data "suggest a trend towards a decrease in all-cause mortality from PE."[27] In addition to citing this mortality "trend," this review also addressed potential morbidity from submassive PEs such as pulmonary hypertension and decreased exercise tolerance. It concluded that there was also evidence to suggest decreased morbidity from thrombolytic therapy. They established with class IIb, level C evidence that "fibrinolysis may be considered for patients with submassive PE judged to have clinical evidence of adverse prognosis" but did not recommend it with "minor" RV dysfunction or "minor" myocardial necrosis (not specifically defined). In 2014 a meta-analysis in JAMA determined that "among patients with PE who were hemodynamically stable with right ventricular dysfunction, thrombolytic therapy was associated with lower rates of all-cause mortality and increased risks of major bleeding."[37] This meta-analysis included data from the ULTIMA study that used ultrasound-assisted thrombolysis and lower-dose thrombolytics, which may lower the risk of bleeding.[38]

The results of the pulmonary embolism thrombolysis (PEITHO) trial were published in 2014, representing the largest prospective evaluation of intermediate-risk PE to thrombolytic treatment, randomizing 1005 patients in a double-blind placebo controlled trial. The overall rate of "death or hemodynamic compensation" was statistically lower in the thrombolysis group (2.6%) compared with the placebo group (5.6%). A hemorrhagic stroke occurred in 2.0% of thrombolytic patients. Regarding actual patient-level decision-making, an accompanying editorial stated "data from the PEITHO trial provide valuable insight but no definitive answer."[39] A recent review of this issue in the emergency medicine literature concluded that risks and benefits be considered on a case by case basis, with incorporation of shared decision-making.[40] For a younger patient who may be more concerned about long-term morbidity and less likely to suffer an intracranial hemorrhage, lysis may be more attractive although this decision will rest on preferences and the risk tolerances of both the patient and provider. Although prior guidelines have raised the possibility of thrombolysis in intermediate-high risk patients,[27] an analysis of the PEITHO trial found no long-term difference between heparin and thrombolysis.

Thrombolytic Dosing

FDA-approved agents available for thrombolytic therapy include alteplase or recombinant tPA (brand name Activase, rt-PA) and streptokinase. The abbreviation tPA is used to encompass the class of tissue plasminogen activators, and it is recommended this abbreviation not be used when dosing medication to avoid errors.[41] Streptokinase and urokinase were used in many older trials but most EDs now have rt-PA. The FDA-approved regimen for systemic rt-PA is 100 mg infused over 2 hours. Tenecteplase (brand name TNKase, TNK) and reteplase (Retavase) are tPAs that are approved for myocardial infarction but have not been FDA-approved for PE treatment. TNK was the agent used in the PEITHO trial and has the advantage of being a single weight-based dose that ranges from 30 mg (patient weight less than 60 kg) to 50 mg (90 kg or more). It does not need an infusion, as opposed to tPA.

Challenges and Changes: Low-Dose Tissue Plasminogen Activator

In 2010 Wang and colleagues[42] published a randomized trial of 118 patients receiving full-dose tPA (100 mg over 2 hours) versus half-dose (50 mg over 2 hours). This dosing trial demonstrated similar improvements in measures of efficacy (RV dysfunction on echo and clot burden) for half-dose tPA compared with full-dose, with lower rates of significant bleeding (2% vs 10%). The MOPPET trial compared heparin alone to half-dose tPA and found improvement in symptoms without adverse events using half-dose tPA.[43] A recent meta-analysis confirmed that "low-dose" rt-PA had similar efficacy with a better safety profile.[44] Half-dose treatment thus may be more appropriate when electing to use thrombolytic for intermediate-high risk PE, although evidence is not considered definitive.[40,45]

In patients with intermediate-high risk and a subset of massive PEs (eg, low blood pressure but who are mentating and oxygenating reasonably well), a 2-hour infusion of a thrombolytic agent may be well-tolerated. However, there is a subset of ED patients who are in or near cardiac arrest from suspected or confirmed PE and who may be unlikely to survive 2 hours without more aggressive intervention. In this case, bolus dose tPA may be appropriate. At the authors' institution they have successfully used bolus dosing of tPA to resuscitate patients in near or full arrest from PE, typically using an initial bolus dose of 50 mg of rt-PA followed by infusion of the remainder, and repeated if necessary. Although this is not an FDA-approved regimen, it has been used at other institutions.[46]

Of note, the American Heart Association has recommended against thrombolysis in undifferentiated pulseless electrical activity (PEA).[27] However, they do recognize that in a patient with a high pretest probability of PE and RV dysfunction on TTE who is unstable to undergo CT scanning, aggressive therapy including thrombolysis is warranted. TTE in the ED has been described as guiding therapy in massive PE and may also help exclude other causes of hypotension.[47,48] Thus the combination of PEA with a massively dilated RV on bedside echocardiography likely merits an attempt at thrombolysis.

Another consideration in systemic thrombolysis treatment is concurrent utilization of heparin. Often these patients are started on heparin before the decision to initiate thrombolytics. The half-life of tPA is often short (~5 minutes for rt-PA) and there is a risk of rethrombosis if this medication wears off without other anticoagulants present. This needs to be balanced against the potential for increased bleeding. In the PEITHO trial, UFH was continued during the TNK infusion in both arms.[49] In another trial, the heparin dose during infusion was 10U per hour (vs regular dose of 18U/h).[43] We recommend continuing an unfractionated heparin infusion during thrombolytic infusion, possibly at reduced levels. Following thrombolytic infusion, the heparin can be adjusted to an activated partial thromboplastin level of 2.0 to 2.5 times normal.

Other Therapeutic Approaches to Large Pulmonary Embolism

In addition to systemic thrombolysis, other options for large PEs include catheter-directed thrombolysis (CDT), ultrasound-accelerated catheter-directed thrombolysis (UACDT), percutaneous mechanical thrombectomy (PMT), and surgical embolectomy. The availability of these therapeutic options vary depending on the institution and are likely only available at larger tertiary care institutions.

In PE without cardiac arrest, CDT has been shown to provide similar clinical outcomes as systemic thrombolytic therapy, while minimizing the risk of major bleeding.[50] This is achieved by the administration of thrombolytic agents locally, which allows for a much lower dose, around one-third of what would be used systemically. A 2009 meta-analysis found pooled success rates for CDT of 86.5% with major complications of 2.4%, lower than the cited risk of hemorrhagic stroke in many series of systemic thrombolysis.[51]

Another approach that is used in Europe and increasingly available in the United States is the UACDT, which delivers uniform radial ultrasound energy in addition to small continuous doses of thrombolytic. A study using the EKOS EkoSonic© UADCT system was shown to decrease the pulmonary artery pressure, lower the RV/LV ratio, and clear greater than 90% of the thrombus in more than three-quarters of patients without major bleeding complications.[52]

PMT may include clot aspiration, fragmentation, or rheolysis (high pressure saline) and may be combined with catheter-directed pharmacologic treatment. Mechanical approaches alone have a success rate of ~80% but with low rates of bleeding; inclusion of pharmacotherapy can increase success rates to 95% but increases the rate of hemorrhage.[27]

Lastly, surgical embolectomy has a history of more than 100 years and may remain an option when thrombolysis is contraindicated or fails.[53] Mortality has typically been high, although controlled trials are lacking and numbers may be skewed due to its assignation as a therapy of "last resort." Recent improvements in technique have cited improvements in outcomes, with survival approaching 90% at an experienced center using state-of-the-art techniques.[54]

Challenges and Changes: Adjunctive Therapies for Massive Pulmonary Embolism

Although mechanical obstruction by thrombus may be a primary cause of hypoxia and hemodynamic instability, pulmonary arterial vasoconstriction may play a large role. Inhaled nitric oxide (NO) ventilation can decrease pulmonary resistance and has been used as a temporary therapy to help stabilize a hemodynamically deteriorating patient pending other management options such as thrombolysis or surgical embolectomy.[55] Gas exchange and hemodynamics can improve within minutes, with as little as 1 to 2 parts per million (ppm) although optimal dosing is probably 10 to 20 ppm.[56,57] It is important that when used, NO be weaned slowly to avoid rebound pulmonary hypertension. An ongoing trial using NO in the ED setting for acute intermediate-risk PE has enrolled 78 patients to date without adverse outcomes.[58] This protocol titrated the concentration from 2 to 50 ppm and demonstrates feasibility in the ED setting.

Another option described in the literature for temporizing hypoxia and hemodynamic instability from massive PE is the use of extracorporeal membrane oxygenation (ECMO).[57,59] ECMO can be veno-venous (VV, providing no hemodynamic support) or veno-arterial (VA, providing complete cardiopulmonary bypass). Although there are no large trials, both VV and VA ECMO have been reported with survival rates of 50% to 70% and 20% to 50%, respectively.[60] The use of ECMO has increased more than 4-fold since 2006, and some centers are training ED personnel to institute ECMO.[61] Another option is a device such as the Impella RP, which is now FDA-approved for right heart failure.[62] The Impella RP is threaded through the femoral vein into the pulmonary artery, with an intake at the IVC/right atrial junction and an outlet into the pulmonary artery; it has been described as an option for massive PE.[63]

Challenges and Changes: Pulmonary Embolism Response Teams

As detailed earlier, for patients with submassive or massive PEs there are multiple options and multiple potential specialties that may be involved in patient care, including emergency medicine, pulmonary/critical care, radiology, interventional radiology, cardiology, and cardiothoracic surgery. In many cases decisions may be time critical. For high-volume centers with the capacity to do so, the creation of a multidisciplinary "pulmonary embolism response team" (PERT) has been described.[64] Over the last year the authors have implemented a PERT team at their center. Although this approach offers the potential for timely involvement of all relevant specialties, challenges include coordinating when all specialties may be available (we have only been able to staff it during daytime hours) and ensuring that involvement of "too many cooks" does not actually delay needed intervention.

SUMMARY

PE remains a common disease that is increasing in prevalence and encompasses a wide spectrum of severity and treatment options. The optimal diagnosis, prognosis, and therapy in the acute setting provide challenges that will likely continue to evolve. These include avoiding both over- and undertesting, determining appropriate prognosis and tailoring therapy to the individual situation. A multidisciplinary approach to more serious PEs is likely to provide optimal outcomes.

SUPPLEMENTARY DATA

Supplementary data related to this article can be found online at https://doi.org/10.1016/j.ccm. 2018.04.009.

REFERENCES

1. Fesmire FM, Brown MD, Espinosa JA, et al. Critical issues in the evaluation and management of adult patients presenting to the emergency department with suspected pulmonary embolism. Ann Emerg Med 2011;57:628–52.e5.

2. Kline JA, Kabrhel C. Emergency evaluation for pulmonary embolism, part 1: clinical factors that increase risk. J Emerg Med 2015;48:771–80.

3. CDC. Emergency department visits. 2017. Available at: https://www.cdc.gov/nchs/fastats/emergency-department.htm. Accessed November 28, 2017.

4. Wiener RS, Schwartz LM, Woloshin S. When a test is too good: how CT pulmonary angiograms find pulmonary emboli that do not need to be found. BMJ 2013;347:1–7.

5. Agnelli G, Becattini C. Acute pulmonary embolism. N Engl J Med 2010;363:266–74.

6. Wells PS, Anderson DR, Rodger M, et al. Excluding pulmonary embolism at the bedside without diagnostic imaging: management of patients with suspected pulmonary embolism presenting to the emergency department by using a simple clinial model and D-dimer. Ann Intern Med 2001; 135:98–107.

7. Ceriani E, Combescure C, Le Gal G, et al. Clinical prediction rules for pulmonary embolism: a systematic review and meta-analysis. J Thromb Haemost 2010;8:957–70.

8. Lucassen W, Geersing GJ, Erkens PMG, et al. Clinical decision rules for excluding pulmonary embolism: A Meta-analysis. Ann Int Med 2011;155:448–60.

9. Penaloza A, Verschuren F, Meyer G, et al. Comparison of the unstructured clinician gestalt, the wells score, and the revised Geneva score to estimate pretest probability for suspected pulmonary embolism. Ann Emerg Med 2013;62:117–24.e2.

10. Kline JA, Kabrhel C. Emergency evaluation for pulmonary embolism, part 2: diagnostic approach. J Emerg Med 2015;49:104–17.

11. ECI. Pulmonary embolism - PE - evaluation in the pregnant patient. 2017. Available at: https://www.aci.health.nsw.gov.au/networks/eci/clinical/clinical-resources/clinical-tools/respiratory/pe/pe-pregnant. Accessed July 9, 2018.

12. Fields JM, Davis J, Girson L, et al. Transthoracic echocardiography for diagnosing pulmonary embolism: a systematic review and meta-analysis. J Am Soc Echocardiogr 2017;30:714–23.e4.

13. Goldhaber SZ. Echocardiography in the management of pulmonary embolism. Ann Intern Med 2002;136:691–700.

14. Moore CL, Molina AA, Lin H. Ultrasonography in community emergency departments in the United States: access to ultrasonography performed by consultants and status of emergency physician-performed ultrasonography. Ann Emerg Med 2006; 47:147–53.

15. Labovitz AJ, Noble VE, Bierig M, et al. Focused cardiac ultrasound in the emergent setting: a

consensus statement of the American Society of Echocardiography and American College of Emergency Physicians. J Am Soc Echocardiogr 2010; 23:1225–30.

16. Moore CL, Copel JA. Point-of-care ultrasonography. N Engl J Med 2011;364:749–57.

17. Mayron R, Gaudio FE, Plummer D, et al. Echocardiography performed by emergency physicians: impact on diagnosis and therapy. Ann Emerg Med 1988;17:150–4.

18. Via G, Hussain A, Wells M, et al. International evidence-based recommendations for focused cardiac ultrasound. J Am Soc Echocardiogr 2014;27: 683.e1-e33.

19. Spencer KT, Kimura BJ, Korcarz CE, et al. Focused cardiac ultrasound: recommendations from the american society of echocardiography. J Am Soc Echocardiogr 2013;26:567–81.

20. Kopecna D, Briongos S, Castillo H, et al. Interobserver reliability of echocardiography for prognostication of normotensive patients with pulmonary embolism. Cardiovasc Ultrasound 2014;12:29.

21. Dresden S, Mitchell P, Rahimi L, et al. Right ventricular dilatation on bedside echocardiography performed by emergency physicians aids in the diagnosis of pulmonary embolism. Ann Emerg Med 2014;63:16–24.

22. Taylor RA, Moore CL. Accuracy of emergency physician-performed limited echocardiography for right ventricular strain. Am J Emerg Med 2014;32:371–4.

23. Taylor RA, Davis J, Liu R, et al. Point-of-care focused cardiac ultrasound for prediction of pulmonary embolism adverse outcomes. J Emerg Med 2013;45: 392–9.

24. Holley AB, Cheatham JG, Jackson JL, et al. Novel quantitative echocardiographic parameters in acute PE. J Thromb Thrombolysis 2009;28:506–12.

25. Daley J, Grotberg J, Pare J, et al. Emergency physician performed tricuspid annular plane systolic excursion in the evaluation of suspected pulmonary embolism. Am J Emerg Med 2017;35:106–11.

26. Jiménez D, Aujesky D, Moores L, et al. Simplification of the pulmonary embolism severity index for prognostication in patients with acute symptomatic pulmonary embolism for the RIETE investigators. Arch Intern Med 2010;170:1383–9.

27. Jaff MR, McMurtry MS, Archer SL, et al. Management of massive and submassive pulmonary embolism, iliofemoral deep vein thrombosis, and chronic thromboembolic pulmonary hypertension: a scientific statement from the American Heart Association. Circulation 2011;123:1788–830.

28. Handoko ML, de Man FS. Risk-stratification in normotensive acute pulmonary embolism. Netherlands Hear. J 2015;23:52–4.

29. Goldhaber SZ, Visani L, De Rosa M. Acute pulmonary embolism: clinical outcomes in the International Cooperative Pulmonary Embolism Registry (ICOPER). Lancet 1999;353:1386–9.

30. Aujesky D, Obrosky DS, Stone RA, et al. Derivation and validation of a prognostic model for pulmonary embolism. Am J Respir Crit Care Med 2005;172: 1041–6.

31. Zondag W, Vingerhoets LM, Durian MF, et al. Hestia criteria can safely select patients with pulmonary embolism for outpatient treatment irrespective of right ventricular function. J Thromb Haemost 2013; 11:686–92.

32. EINSTEIN–PE Investigators, Büller HR, Prins MH, Lensin AW, et al. Oral rivaroxaban for the treatment of symptomatic pulmonary embolism. N Engl J Med 2012;366:1287–97.

33. Konstantinides SV, Vicaut E, Danays T, et al. Impact of thrombolytic therapy on the long-term outcome of intermediate-risk pulmonary embolism. J Am Coll Cardiol 2017;69:1536–44.

34. Quinlan DJ, McQuillan A, Eikelboom JW. Low-molecular-weight heparin compared with intravenous unfractionated heparin for treatment of pulmonary embolism. Ann Intern Med 2004;140:175–84.

35. Roy P-M, Moumneh T, Penaloza A, et al. Outpatient management of pulmonary embolism. Thromb Res 2017;155:92–100.

36. Yoo HH, Queluz TH, El Dib R. Anticoagulant treatment for subsegmental pulmonary embolism [review]. Cochrane Database Syst Rev 2014;(4):CD010222.

37. Chatterjee S, Chakraborty A, Weinberg I, et al. Thrombolysis for pulmonary embolism and risk of all-cause mortality, major bleeding, and intracranial hemorrhage. JAMA 2014;311:2414.

38. Kucher N, Boekstegers P, Müller OJ, et al. Randomized, controlled trial of ultrasound-assisted catheter-directed thrombolysis for acute intermediate-risk pulmonary embolism. Circulation 2014;129:479–86.

39. Elliott G. Fibrinolysis of pulmonary emboli - steer closer to scylla. N Engl J Med 2014;370:1454–7.

40. Long B, Koyfman A. Current controversies in thrombolytic use in acute pulmonary embolism. J Emerg Med 2016;51:37–44.

41. Tu C-M. tPA and TNK mix-ups: clearing up the confusion. Medscape 2015.

42. Wang C, Zhai Z, Yang Y, et al. Efficacy and safety of low dose recombinant tissue-type plasminogen activator for the treatment of acute pulmonary thromboembolism: a randomized, multicenter, controlled trial. Chest 2010;137:254–62.

43. Sharifi M, Bay C, Skrocki L, et al. Moderate pulmonary embolism treated with thrombolysis (from the 'mOPETT' Trial). Am J Cardiol 2013;111:273–7.

44. Zhang Z, Zhai ZG, Liang LR, et al. Lower dosage of recombinant tissue-type plasminogen activator (rt-PA) in the treatment of acute pulmonary embolism: a systematic review and meta-analysis. Thromb Res 2014;133:357–63.

45. Wang T, Squizzato A, Dentali F, et al. The role of thrombolytic therapy in pulmonary embolism. Blood 2015;125:2191–200.

46. Prom R, Dull R, Delk B. Successful alteplase bolus administration for a presumed massive pulmonary embolism during cardiopulmonary resuscitation. Ann Pharmacother 2013;47:1730–5.

47. Kennedy Hall M, Coffey EC, Herbst M, et al. The '5Es' of emergency physician-performed focused cardiac ultrasound: a protocol for rapid identification of effusion, ejection, equality, exit, and entrance. Acad Emerg Med 2015;22:583–93.

48. Borloz MP, Frohna WJ, Phillips CA, et al. Emergency department focused bedside echocardiography in massive pulmonary embolism. J Emerg Med 2011; 41:658–60.

49. Meyer G, Vicaut E, Danays T, et al. Fibrinolysis for patients with intermediate risk pulmonary embolism. NEJM 2014;370:1402–11.

50. Kuo WT, Banerjee A, Kim PS, et al. Pulmonary embolism response to fragmentation, embolectomy, and catheter thrombolysis (PERFECT): initial results from a prospective multicenter registry. Chest 2015;148:667–73.

51. Kuo WT, Gould MK, Louie JD, et al. Catheter-directed therapy for the treatment of massive pulmonary embolism: systematic review and meta-analysis of modern techniques. J Vasc Interv Radiol 2009;20:1431–40.

52. Dumantepe M, Uyar I, Teymen B, et al. Improvements in pulmonary artery pressure and right ventricular function after ultrasound-accelerated catheter-directed thrombolysis for the treatment of pulmonary embolism. J Card Surg 2014;29:455–63.

53. He C, Von Segesser LK, Kappetein PA, et al. Acute pulmonary embolectomy. Eur J Cardiothoracic Surg 2013;43:1087–95.

54. Aklog L, Williams CS, Byrne JG, et al. Acute pulmonary embolectomy: a contemporary approach. Circulation 2002;105:1416–9.

55. Summerfield DT, Desai H, Levitov A, et al. Inhaled nitric oxide as salvage therapy in massive pulmonary embolism: a case series. Respir Care 2012; 57:444–8.

56. Szold O, Khoury W, Biderman P, et al. Inhaled nitric oxide improves pulmonary functions following massive pulmonary embolism: a report of four patients and review of the literature. Lung 2006;184:1–5.

57. Seaton A, Hodgson LE, Creagh-Brown B, et al. The use of veno-venous extracorporeal membrane oxygenation following thrombolysis for massive pulmonary embolism. J Intensive Care Soc 2017;18:342–7.

58. Kline JA, Hall CL, Jones AE, et al. Randomized trial of inhaled nitric oxide to treat acute pulmonary embolism: the iNOPE trial. Am Heart J 2017;186:100–10.

59. Cao J, Liu Y, Wang Y, et al. Salvage thrombolysis and extracorporeal membrane oxygenation for massive pulmonary embolism during the distal femur fracture surgery. Am J Emerg Med 2016;34: 1189.e3-5.

60. Weinberg A, Tapson VF, Ramzy D. Massive pulmonary embolism: extracorporeal membrane oxygenation and surgical pulmonary embolectomy. Semin Respir Crit Care Med 2017;38:066–72.

61. Mosier JM, Kelsey M, Raz Y, et al. Extracorporeal membrane oxygenation (ECMO) for critically ill adults in the emergency department: history, current applications, and future directions. Crit Care 2015; 19:431.

62. Abiomed Receives FDA PMA Approval for impella RP® for right heart failure. 2017. Available at: http://investor.abiomed.com/releasedetail.cfm?releaseid=1041176. Accessed November 28, 2017.

63. Kumar Bhatia N, Dickert NW, Samady H, et al. The use of hemodynamic support in massive pulmonary embolism. Catheter Cardiovasc Interv 2017;90: 516–20.

64. Dudzinski DM, Piazza G. Multidisciplinary pulmonary embolism response teams. Circulation 2016; 133:98–103.

The Value of Bedside Echocardiogram in the Setting of Acute and Chronic Pulmonary Embolism

David W. Lee, MD[a], Kavitha Gopalratnam, MBBS[b],
Hubert James Ford III, MD[c], Lisa J. Rose-Jones, MD[a],*

KEYWORDS

- Echocardiography • Acute pulmonary embolism • Chronic pulmonary embolism • Right ventricle
- Right heart failure • Pulmonary hypertension

KEY POINTS

- Echocardiography can be valuable in the evaluation and risk stratification of patients with acute and chronic pulmonary embolism (PE).
- Patients with acute PE who have echocardiographic evidence of right ventricular dilatation and/or right ventricular dysfunction have an increased risk of mortality.
- A minority of patients with acute PE can develop chronic thromboembolic pulmonary hypertension.
- Patients with chronic thromboembolic pulmonary hypertension often have echocardiographic evidence of elevated pulmonary arterial pressures, right ventricular hypertrophy, right ventricular dysfunction, and/or left ventricular impaired relaxation.

INTRODUCTION

Acute pulmonary embolism (PE) is associated with an estimated mortality rate of up to 11% at 2 weeks and 17% at 3 months.[1] In a large international registry of patients with acute PE, those with hemodynamic instability had an estimated 3-month mortality rate of 58%.[1] In a smaller prospective cohort, patients with normal systemic blood pressure and echocardiographic evidence of right ventricular (RV) dysfunction had an estimated 5% in-hospital mortality rate.[2] Because of the high stakes, patients with suspected acute PE require timely diagnosis and risk stratification to guide treatment. Although computed tomography pulmonary angiography remains the preferred choice of imaging for the diagnosis of PE (see Farbod N. Rahaghi and colleagues' article, "Diagnosis of DVTs and PE's – New Imaging Tools & Modalities," in this issue), bedside echocardiography (echo) guides risk stratification of patients with acute PE by providing valuable prognostic information regarding right heart structure, function, and hemodynamics. Although echo has not been associated with reduced mortality in acute hemodynamically stable PE,[3] the application of echocardiographic data to risk stratify patients with acute and chronic PE can significantly aid the clinician in determining the best therapeutic approach.

Disclosures: The authors have no financial disclosures.
[a] Division of Cardiology, University of North Carolina, 160 Dental Circle, CB #7075, Chapel Hill, NC 27599, USA;
[b] Division of Pulmonology, Yale New Haven Health, Bridgeport Hospital, 267 Grant Street, Bridgeport, CT 06610, USA; [c] Division of Pulmonary and Critical Care Medicine, University of North Carolina, 130 Mason Farm Road, CB #7020, Chapel Hill, NC 27599, USA
* Corresponding author.
E-mail address: Lisa_Rose-jones@med.unc.edu

Clin Chest Med 39 (2018) 549–560
https://doi.org/10.1016/j.ccm.2018.04.008
0272-5231/18/© 2018 Elsevier Inc. All rights reserved.

THE RIGHT VENTRICLE AND HEMODYNAMICS IN ACUTE PULMONARY EMBOLISM

There are key anatomic differences between the left ventricle (LV) and the RV.[4,5] Compared with the LV, the RV is composed of a thinner wall. The RV muscle fibers are arranged in series, creating a crescent-shaped cavity. By contrast, the LV muscle fibers are arranged in parallel, creating a concentric shaped cavity. This anatomic difference allows for the RV to have better compliance without significantly increasing pressures. Finally, the RV wall is composed of superficial circumferential muscle fibers and inner longitudinal muscle fibers. Although the circumferential fibers are responsible for inward contraction, the longitudinal fibers provide significant base-to-apex excursion. Given this unique orchestration of muscle fibers, the echocardiographic assessment of RV function can be challenging.

From a hemodynamic standpoint, both the RV and the pulmonary arterial circulation comprise a high-capacitance, low-resistance system. In acute PE, thromboembolic occlusion of the pulmonary artery (PA) leads to a sudden increase in vascular resistance, and thus RV afterload, for which the RV cannot readily compensate. When a certain threshold is reached with increased PA occlusion due to clot burden, there is decreased LV preload, which then leads to a drop in LV stroke volume and subsequent systemic hypotension. In addition, the now dilated, high-pressure RV has interventricular septal shift that encroaches on and compresses the LV. This reverse Bernheim effect further decreases LV filling and causes a further drop in LV stroke volume[6] (**Fig. 1**).

The normal PA systolic pressure (PASP) ranges between 15 and 30 mm Hg. In acute PE, depending on the severity, the PASP is typically elevated. If there is no significant gradient across the RV outflow tract, pulmonary valve, or proximal pulmonary arteries, then the PASP is equivalent to the RV systolic pressure (RVSP). The simplified Bernoulli equation using the tricuspid regurgitation (TR) jet velocity on echo can be used to estimate the RVSP.[7]

$$RVSP = 4 \times (peak\ TR\ jet\ velocity)^2 + mean\ RA\ pressure$$

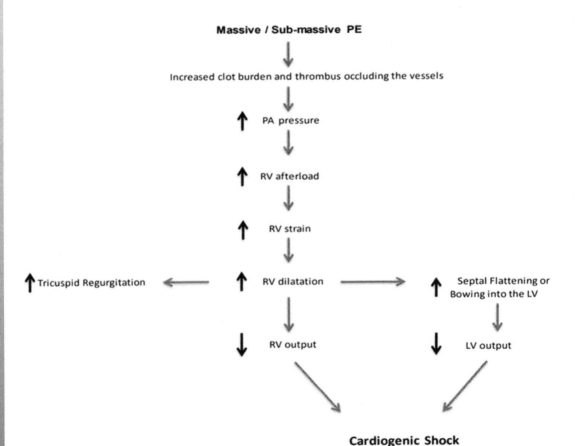

Fig. 1. Pathogenesis of RV failure leading to shock secondary to massive/submassive pulmonary embolism.

The mean right atrial (RA) pressure is approximated from the inferior vena cava (IVC) size and respiratory variation. The measurement is made as follows:

1. If the IVC diameter is less than 2.1 cm and has greater than 50% variation in the IVC size with respiration then the RA pressure is estimated to be between 0 and 5 mm Hg (mean 3 mm Hg).
2. If the IVC diameter is greater than 2.1 cm and has less than 50% variation in the IVC size with respiration then the RA pressure is estimated to be between 10 and 20 mm Hg (mean 15 mm Hg).
3. If IVC variation is between the above parameters then the RA pressure is considered to be between 5 and 10 mm Hg (mean 8 mm Hg).

Based on the American Society of Echocardiography, IVC collapsibility and IVC diameter are more accurate in predicting if RV pressure is high or low based on the cutoff values mentioned earlier and less accurate in predicting intermediate values.[7,8] Use of additional parameters such as hepatic vein Doppler tracings, RA size, and tricuspid E/e' ratio helps increase the accuracy of RA pressure measured by noninvasive methods.

IVC collapsibility and inspiratory variation is lost in RV pressure or volume overload from transmissive backup. This lack of IVC collapsibility is associated with hemodynamic changes especially in acute PE and is suggestive of RV dysfunction.[9]

A study by Khemasuwan and colleagues[10] evaluated RV echocardiographic parameters after acute PE and showed that an elevated RVSP was associated with increased intensive care unit and in-hospital mortality. These results were similar to the findings demonstrated by Vitarelli and colleagues,[11] where an elevated RVSP correlated with more adverse outcomes in acute PE. On the contrary, low RVSP in the setting of PE may actually indicate the inability of the RV to mount higher pressures due to severe RV dysfunction and thereby pointing toward a worse prognosis.

Patients with evidence of right heart strain defined as increased RV to LV ratio greater than 0.9 or interventricular septal flattening and/or hemodynamic instability have a much higher mortality rate. Thus, early and accurate identification of this particular subset of patients, also known as intermediate risk PE (or submassive PE), is crucial. In a prospective clinical outcome study of 209 patients with acute PE, 31% of patients were identified to have echo evidence of RV dysfunction and were hemodynamically stable when compared with 47% of normotensive patients without evidence of RV dysfunction.[2] The group with RV dysfunction had a higher in-hospital mortality rate (5% vs none) and a 10% rate of PE-related shock.[2] In the acute setting, the use of echocardiography can be quick and valuable in triaging these patients.

CHRONIC PULMONARY EMBOLISM

Chronic PE develops in patients who have incomplete resolution of thrombus after an acute PE as a result of aberrant fibrinolytic mechanisms. This leads to the transformation of acute thrombus into a fibrotic lesion adherent to the vascular intima, and it also can lead to vascular remodeling of other pulmonary vessels due to changes in flow distribution and increased shear forces on the nonoccluded vessels. It has also been hypothesized that small vessel remodeling can occur due to release of mediators from platelets and endothelial cells leading to pulmonary vascular arteriopathy.[12,13] The presence of these chronic lesions and associated vascular occlusion causes increased pulmonary vascular resistance and increased PA pressures, an entity known as chronic thromboembolic pulmonary hypertension (CTEPH). The incidence of CTEPH varies from 1% to 5% after acute PE, with some studies suggesting as high as 8% incidence of CTEPH in patients after acute PE.[14,15] It has also been demonstrated that the RVSP can remain elevated up to 6 months after an acute submassive PE, which can lead to further RV remodeling. In a prospective study of patients with submassive PE who were treated with heparin, about 27% of the patients continued to have persistently elevated RVSP and echocardiographic findings consistent with pulmonary hypertension.[16]

The diagnosis of CTEPH can be challenging, given that the onset of symptoms occurs over time, with persistence of dyspnea sometimes incorrectly attributed to the previous PE. A careful clinical history, aided by echocardiography, can provide valuable data to prompt appropriate clinical suspicion for CTEPH. In patients with CTEPH, there are often changes of chronic RV volume and/or pressure overload, as well as evidence of elevated PASP. Patients are then referred for confirmatory diagnosis with ventilation-perfusion scan, right heart catheterization, and pulmonary angiography.

BEDSIDE ECHOCARDIOGRAPHY IN PULMONARY EMBOLISM

Although unable to diagnose PE itself, TTE can identify other causes of dyspnea, including pericardial effusions, cardiac tamponade, focal wall motion abnormalities, LV dysfunction, and various valvular disorders. Furthermore, TTE can be used to risk stratify patients who have a documented PE. The benefits of TTE in the evaluation of PE include its high sensitivity and specificity for right heart dysfunction, the safety of noninvasive imaging, the low cost associated with performance and interpretation, and the wide availability of bedside ultrasound.

Transesophageal echocardiography (TEE) has a limited role in the diagnostic evaluation of a patient with acute PE. TEE provides 100% specificity for the diagnosis of high-risk PE in patients with RV dilatation.[17] However, the risks of conscious or general sedation in potentially hemodynamically unstable patients; the procedural risks of bleeding, oropharyngeal injury, and esophageal perforation in patients warranting therapeutic anticoagulation for PE; and the orchestration required to perform an invasive procedure limit its routine use in the evaluation of patients with suspected or confirmed PE. As such, the following sections will focus on the use and application of TTE.

Transthoracic Echocardiographic Views and Modes

There are 4 standard views that provide both structural and functional data in patients with PE. The parasternal long axis view is obtained by placing the ultrasound transducer near the sternum on the third or fourth left intercostal space, with the index mark directed toward the patient's right shoulder. Both ventricles, the left atrium, the mitral and aortic valves, and the aortic root are seen in this view (**Fig. 2**). The parasternal short axis view is obtained by clockwise rotation of the ultrasound transducer by 90° until the index mark is directed toward the patient's left shoulder (**Fig. 3**). Tilting the ultrasound transducer up and down produces views of the base and apex of the heart, respectively. Both ventricles, all 4 valves, and the main PA can be assessed in these views. The apical 4-chamber view is obtained by placing the ultrasound transducer near the mid-axillary line on the fifth left intercostal space. Both ventricles, both atria, and the mitral and tricuspid valves can be seen in this view (**Fig. 4**) as well as in the subcostal view. The subcostal view is obtained by placing the ultrasound transducer in the mid-upper epigastric region and pointing it toward the patient's left shoulder (**Fig. 5**). Counterclockwise rotation of the ultrasound transducer by 90° provides a view of the IVC.

There are 6 ultrasound modes in echocardiography. Two-dimensional (2D) mode is the default mode that produces cross-sectional images of cardiac structures moving in real time (see **Figs. 2–5**). In M-mode, a sampling line is placed along a specific plane of interest in 2D mode, and the movement of structures in that plane over a horizontal axis of time is depicted. M-mode allows for the measurement of structural movement over a specific time period. In pulse wave Doppler (PWD) mode, a sampling cursor is placed at a specific point of interest in 2D mode. Pulse Doppler signals are transmitted by the transducer, reflected by moving red blood cells, and received by the transducer. These pulses create a graphical representation of blood flow velocity and direction at the specific point of interest over a horizontal axis of time. In continuous wave Doppler mode, a sampling line is placed along a specific plane

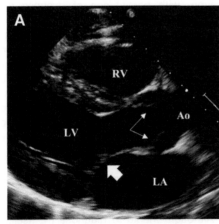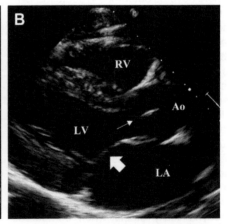

Fig. 2. Normal transthoracic echocardiogram in the parasternal long axis view demonstrating the right ventricle (RV), left ventricle (LV), aorta (Ao), left atrium (LA), mitral valve (*thick arrow*), and aortic valve (*thin arrow*) in the middle of systole (*A*) and the end of systole (*B*).

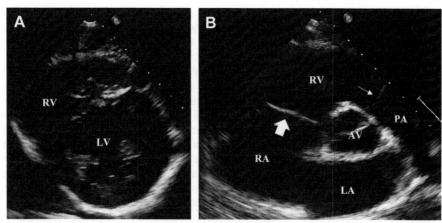

Fig. 3. Normal transthoracic echocardiogram in the parasternal short axis view at the mid-level (*A*) and at the base (*B*). The right ventricle (RV), left ventricle (LV), left atrium (LA), right atrium (RA), pulmonary artery (PA), pulmonic valve (*thin arrow*), tricuspid valve (*thick arrow*), and aortic valve (AV) can be visualized in these views.

of interest in 2D mode. Continuous Doppler signals are then used to create a graphical representation of blood flow velocity and direction along the specific plane of interest over a horizontal axis of time. In color flow Doppler mode, a sampling window is defined over a specific region of interest in 2D mode. Doppler signals are used to create a color map of blood flow velocity and direction, which is superimposed on the 2D images. Finally, in tissue Doppler imaging mode, a sampling cursor is placed at a specific site of interest in 2D mode. Doppler signals are used to create a graphical representation of tissue movement velocity and direction at the specific point of interest over a horizontal axis of time.

Acute Pulmonary Embolism

The echocardiographic assessment of RV chamber size, RV function, and PA hemodynamics is important for risk stratification in patients who present with acute PE. Echocardiographic evidence of RV dilatation, RV dysfunction, and

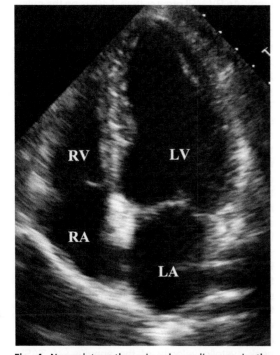

Fig. 4. Normal transthoracic echocardiogram in the apical 4-chamber view with the right ventricle (RV), left ventricle (LV), right atrium (RA), and left atrium (LA).

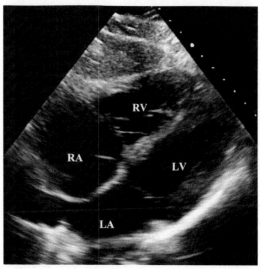

Fig. 5. Transthoracic echocardiogram in the subcostal view with the right ventricle (RV), left ventricle (LV), right atrium (RA), and left atrium (LA).

right heart thrombus is associated with worse prognosis.[2,18–29]

Assessment of right ventricular chamber size

RV chamber size can be assessed using 3 linear dimensions in the apical 4-chamber view at the end of diastole. The RV basal and mid-cavity dimensions are defined as the maximal diameters in the basal third of the RV and the mid-third of the RV, respectively.[7] The longitudinal dimension is defined as the distance from the RV apex to the plane of the tricuspid valve annulus.[7] Based on these dimensions, the RV chamber size can be categorized as normal or dilated. In acute PE, pressure overload from increased pulmonary vascular resistance leads to RV dilatation (**Fig. 6**). Multiple studies have demonstrated that RV dilatation is associated with poor prognosis in patients with acute PE.[18–21] In fact, an RV to LV basal diameter ratio greater than 0.9 is a sign of submassive PE and was an inclusion criterion for ultrasound-assisted catheter-directed thrombolytic therapy in recent studies.[21–23]

Assessment of global right ventricular systolic function

There are several quantitative methods to assess global RV systolic function. First, the RV fractional area change (FAC) can be calculated by dividing

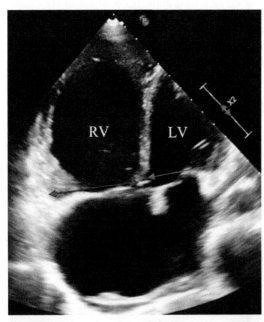

Fig. 6. Transthoracic echocardiogram in the apical 4-chamber view demonstrating right ventricular (RV) dilatation. The RV basal diameter (*red arrow*) is greater than the left ventricular (LV) basal diameter (*blue arrow*), depicting an RV to LV diameter ratio greater than 1.

the difference between the RV end-diastolic area (EDA) and the RV end-systolic area (ESA) by the RV EDA and multiplying this value by 100%, or [RV FAC = (RV EDA–RV ESA)/RV EDA × 100%].[7] These areas are determined by tracing the RV endocardium at the end of diastole and systole in the apical 4-chamber view. An RV FAC less than 35% is considered abnormal RV systolic function.[7] Alternatively, the rate of pressure rise over time (dP/dt) in the RV can be used to quantitate RV systolic function. It is determined by measuring the time required for the TR jet velocity to increase from 1 to 2 m per second in the continuous wave Doppler mode and dividing 12 mm Hg by this specific time interval.[7] Based on the simplified Bernoulli equation, 12 mm Hg represents the increase in pressure when the TR jet velocity increases from 1 m per second (4 mm Hg) to 2 m per second (16 mm Hg).[7] An RV dP/dt less than 400 mm Hg per second is considered to be consistent with abnormal RV systolic function.[5] Finally, the RV myocardial performance index (MPI) quantifies RV systolic function through the ratio of isovolumetric time divided by ejection time.[7] The RV MPI is determined by measuring the tricuspid closure-opening time in the pulse Doppler mode or pulse tissue Doppler mode, measuring the ejection time, and dividing the difference between these times by the ejection time.[7] An RV MPI greater than 0.40 using the pulse Doppler method and 0.55 using the pulse tissue Doppler method correlates with abnormal RV systolic function.[7]

Assessment of regional right ventricular systolic function

There are several methods to assess regional RV systolic function in patients with acute PE. First, the tricuspid valve annulus can be interrogated in the apical 4-chamber view to further assess RV function. The tricuspid annular plane systolic excursion (TAPSE) measures RV longitudinal function. The TAPSE can be obtained by entering M-mode, placing the cursor through the lateral annulus of the tricuspid valve and measuring the longitudinal displacement of the annulus at peak systole.[7] A TAPSE less than 17 mm represents RV systolic dysfunction[7] (**Fig. 7**A). Alternatively, the tricuspid annular systolic velocity (TASV) measures RV tissue movement. The TASV can be obtained by entering the pulsed tissue Doppler mode, placing the pulse cursor on the lateral annulus of the tricuspid valve and measuring peak systolic velocity of the annulus.[7] A TASV less than 10 cm per second indicates decreased RV tissue movement and, thereby, abnormal RV systolic function[7] (**Fig. 7**B). Both TAPSE and

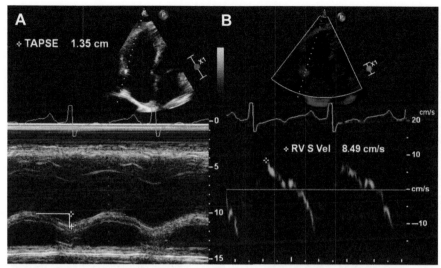

Fig. 7. Transthoracic echocardiograms in the apical 4-chamber view demonstrating regional right ventricular (RV) systolic dysfunction. (*A*) This M-mode of the lateral tricuspid annulus with a tricuspid annular plane systolic excursion (TAPSE) less than 1.7 cm indicates RV systolic dysfunction. (*B*) This tissue Doppler imaging mode of the lateral tricuspid annulus with a TASV less than 10 cm per second also indicates RV systolic dysfunction.

TASV assume that the displacement of a single RV segment represents the function of the entire RV. Despite this assumption, they have high specificity for RV dysfunction and are simple parameters that can be routinely obtained with all modern ultrasound machines.[7]

In addition, acute PE typically causes acute RV pressure overload, which can lead to flattening of the interventricular septum during systole (**Fig. 8**).[7] Under normal RV pressures, the septum contracts toward the center of the LV during systole and moves away from the center of the LV into the RV cavity during diastole. In the setting of acute RV pressure overload, the elevated RV pressures lead to displacement of the septum into the LV cavity during systole, flattening of the septum, and deformation of the LV cavity into a D-shape. Finally, patients with acute PE may have McConnell sign, which is the akinesis of the RV mid-free wall with normal contraction of the apex[24] (**Fig. 9**). This distinct echocardiographic pattern of regional RV dysfunction has 77% sensitivity and 94% specificity for the diagnosis of acute PE.[24]

Visualization of right heart thrombus

In rare instances, free-floating right heart thrombus can be identified on echocardiography. The reported incidence of right heart thrombus detected on TTE in large registry studies ranges from 2% to 5%.[29–31] A recent systematic review and meta-analysis demonstrated a 16.7% mortality rate among patients with right heart thrombus on echocardiography, compared with a 4.4% mortality rate among those who did not have right heart thrombus on echocardiography in the setting of acute PE.[32]

Assessment of pulmonary artery hemodynamics

Pulmonary artery hemodynamics can be useful in the evaluation of acute PE. The PASP, PA diastolic

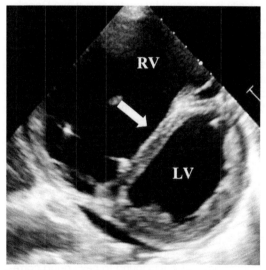

Fig. 8. Transthoracic echocardiogram in the parasternal short axis view demonstrating septal flattening during systole as a result of acute RV pressure overload. During systole, the elevated RV pressures from acute PE exceed the LV filling pressures and cause flattening of the interventricular septum (*white arrow*) with a D-shaped LV cavity.

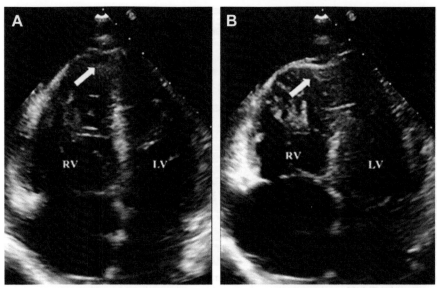

Fig. 9. Transthoracic echocardiograms in the apical 4-chamber view demonstrating McConnell's sign. In contrast to the akinesis of the RV free lateral wall throughout the cardiac cycle, the apical wall (*white arrow*) relaxes during diastole (*A*) and contracts during systole (*B*).

pressure (PADP), and mean PA pressure can be estimated from TTE.

As stated previously, the PASP is equivalent to the RVSP in the absence of a significant gradient across the RV outflow tract, pulmonary valve, or proximal pulmonary arteries. Based on the simplified Bernoulli equation, the RVSP is estimated using the TR jet peak velocity.[7] The TR jet peak velocity is assessed by continuous wave Doppler mode in 3 views: the apical 4-chamber view, the parasternal short axis view at the level of the aortic valve, and the RV inflow view. Given that TR can seem minimal in one angle and significant in another angle, all 3 views should be interrogated by continuous wave Doppler and the TR jet with the highest peak velocity should be used[7] (**Fig. 10**A). The RA pressure is estimated based on the IVC diameter and the presence of more than 50% IVC collapsibility with inspiration.[7] The IVC is best visualized in the subcostal view (**Fig. 10**B). PASP estimates greater than 40 mm Hg are consistent with pulmonary hypertension.[7]

Based on the simplified Bernoulli equation, the PADP estimate is the sum of the RA pressure and 4 times the square of the end-diastolic pulmonary regurgitant velocity.[7] This estimate based on echocardiography was found to have good correlation with invasive right heart catheter–based hemodynamics in a small prospective study.[33] However, this estimate is not routinely used because of the low detection rate of pulmonary regurgitation by continuous wave Doppler. Even if it is detected, the pulmonary regurgitant velocity

is frequently underestimated by continuous wave Doppler.[33]

The mean PA pressure can be estimated by 2 methods: first, by determining the sum of one-third of the PASP and two-thirds of the PADP, or [mean PA pressure = (1/3 PASP) + (2/3 PADP)] and[7] second, by determining the RV outflow tract acceleration time (AT), which is the time from the initial QRS complex to the peak systolic velocity in the RV outflow tract. This can be performed via PWD mode in the parasternal short axis view at the level of the base by placing the pulse wave cursor in the RV outflow tract, measuring the AT, and then subtracting the product of 0.45 and the AT from 79, or [mean PA pressure = 79 - (0.45 x AT)].[7] Mean PA pressure estimates greater than 25 mm Hg are consistent with pulmonary hypertension.[7] It should be emphasized that echocardiography cannot take the place of direct invasive measurement of pulmonary arterial hemodynamics by right heart catheterization when clinically indicated.

Chronic Thromboembolic Disease

The presence of chronic PA obstruction from unresolved acute thromboembolism usually leads to persistently elevated PA pressures and increased pulmonary vascular resistance. In particular, patients with CTEPH have elevated PA pressures with PASP estimates greater than 40 mm Hg and mean PA pressure estimates greater than 25 mm Hg, both of which can be assessed by echocardiography.[7,34]

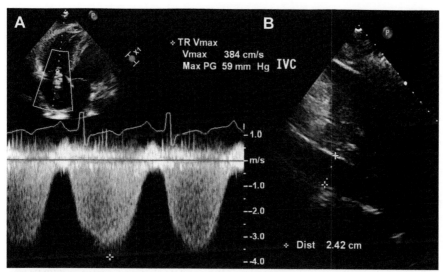

Fig. 10. Transthoracic echocardiograms used to estimate the PASP. (*A*) Apical 4-chamber view demonstrating severe tricuspid regurgitation with a jet peak velocity of 3.84 cm per second. (*B*) Subcostal view demonstrating a distended IVC diameter of 2.42 cm with no inspiratory collapsibility.

In the setting of chronically elevated PA pressures, patients with CTEPH may have a dilated main PA.[35] The main PA is best visualized in the parasternal short axis view at the level of the base; the main PA diameter can be assessed just distal to the pulmonic valve. A main PA diameter greater than 2.1 cm is considered abnormal.

Similar to those with acute PE, many patients with CTEPH have echocardiographic evidence of RV dilatation, RV dysfunction, and interventricular septal flattening. However, in contrast to those with acute PE, patients with CTEPH can develop chronic RV pressure overload leading to compensatory RV hypertrophy. RV free wall thickness can be measured in the parasternal long axis view or subcostal view; a value greater than 0.5 cm reflects RV hypertrophy.[7]

Finally, patients with CTEPH can have abnormal LV diastolic function.[36,37] LV diastolic function can be assessed by determining the mitral inflow patterns using PWD in the apical 4-chamber view. Normal LV diastolic function is associated with a tall early filling velocity (E wave) followed by a shorter atrial kick velocity (A wave) **(Fig. 11A)**. Patients with CTEPH have an impaired LV relaxation pattern that is associated with reversal of this mitral inflow pattern—that is, a short E wave followed by a taller A wave **(Fig. 11B)**. This impaired LV relaxation has been shown to reverse following pulmonary thromboendarterectomy.[37] The proposed mechanism for LV diastolic function in CTEPH is thought to be from LV compression due to RV enlargement, a thickened interventricular septum from RV hypertrophy, and interventricular septal

bowing in the setting of chronic pressure overload.[36,37]

APPLICATION OF BEDSIDE ECHOCARDIOGRAPHY IN ACUTE PULMONARY EMBOLISM
Risk Stratification

Early risk stratification is critical to the appropriate management of patients with acute PE. Based on their clinical presentation, patients with acute PE can be classified into the following risk categories:

1. Massive or high-risk PE: patients who are hemodynamically unstable, with systolic blood pressure less than 90 mm Hg over a period of more than 15 minutes, requiring intravenous vasopressor support or cardiac arrest in the setting of acute PE or syncope.
2. Submassive or intermediate-risk PE
   i. Intermediate high-risk: patients who are hemodynamically stable with both RV dysfunction and elevated cardiac biomarkers such as cardiac troponin and/or natriuretic peptide.
   ii. Intermediate low-risk: patients who are hemodynamically stable with either RV dysfunction or elevated cardiac markers.

Bedside echocardiography provides the clinician the opportunity to assess RV function and identify patients who are at increased risk of mortality. In fact, the American College of Chest Physicians and the American Heart Association have articulated management recommendations for

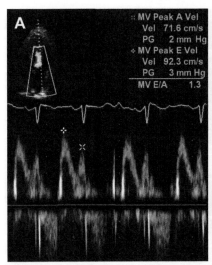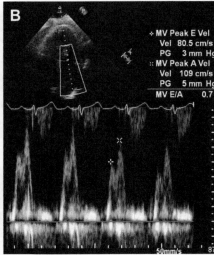

Fig. 11. Transthoracic echocardiograms demonstrating (*A*) normal LV diastolic function and (*B*) LV impaired relaxation seen in chronic thromboembolic pulmonary hypertension.

acute PE based on appropriate risk stratification with the use of echocardiography as a tool for assessing RV function.[38,39]

Pulmonary Embolism Response Team

The PE response team (PERT) is a novel system of care for acute PE that is currently being implemented in an increasing number of medical centers. The PERT uses a multidisciplinary team that consists of specialists from cardiology, interventional cardiology, pulmonary and critical care medicine, vascular surgery, and interventional radiology.[40] The activation of a PERT leads to rapid risk stratification and management of patients with acute PE using history, physical examination, laboratory data, imaging, and, importantly, bedside echocardiography. The objective of a PERT is to provide rapid evaluation and initiation of treatment in patients with massive versus submassive PE by activating different specialties that are needed to manage the patient, ideally within 90 minutes of activation of the PE alert. A recent longitudinal single-center study demonstrated that this multidisciplinary approach provided efficient, organized, and evidence-based care for patients with high-risk and intermediate-risk PE.[35] In this setting, bedside echocardiography plays a key role in directing the acute management of these patients.

BENEFITS AND RISKS OF BEDSIDE ECHOCARDIOGRAPHY

The benefits of bedside echocardiography include the wide availability, safety, and low cost of ultrasound; the ease and speed of image acquisition; and the high sensitivity and specificity for a broad range of clinical disorders. The only significant risk of bedside echocardiography is inaccurate image acquisition, analysis, and/or interpretation. Given that it can potentially affect the management of patients, bedside echocardiography should be performed by individuals who are properly trained and credentialed. Clinicians who are not properly trained and credentialed in echocardiography should be trained in the performance of a focused cardiac ultrasound to answer a specific question with a preestablished image acquisition protocol. In fact, the American Society of Echocardiography has distinguished the focused cardiac ultrasound from a formal echocardiogram and has published guidelines on the use of focused cardiac ultrasound by individuals who are not formally trained and certified to perform echocardiography.[41]

SUMMARY

In conclusion, bedside echocardiography can be a valuable tool in the evaluation and risk stratification of patients with acute and chronic PE. In patients with acute submassive or massive PE, echocardiography can demonstrate RV dilatation, RV systolic dysfunction, interventricular septal flattening/bowing, and elevated PA pressures. These echocardiographic findings can help identify patients who have an intermediate risk of mortality and would benefit from thrombolytic therapy. A minority of patients with acute PE may develop CTEPH with echocardiographic evidence of elevated PA pressures, a dilated main PA, RV hypertrophy with dilatation and systolic dysfunction, and impaired LV relaxation. The effectiveness, safety, and wide availability of bedside echocardiography empower the clinician to evaluate and risk stratify patients with acute and chronic PE in a robust manner.

REFERENCES

1. Goldhaber SZ, Visani L, De Rosa M. Acute pulmonary embolism: clinical outcomes in the International Cooperative Pulmonary Embolism Registry (ICOPER). Lancet 1999;353:1386–9.

2. Grifoni S, Olivotto I, Cecchini P, et al. Short-term clinical outcome of patients with acute pulmonary embolism, normal blood pressure, and echocardiographic right ventricular dysfunction. Circulation 2000;101: 2817–22.

3. Cohen DM, Winter M, Lindenauer PK, et al. Echocardiogram in the evaluation of hemodynamically stable acute pulmonary embolism: national practices and clinical outcomes. Ann Am Thorac Soc 2018;15(5): 581–8.

4. Haddad F, Hunt SA, Rosenthal DN, et al. Right ventricular function in cardiovascular disease, part 1: anatomy, physiology, aging, and functional assessment of the right ventricle. Circulation 2008;117: 1436–48.

5. Dell'Italia LJ. Anatomy and physiology of the right ventricle. Cardiol Clin 2012;30:167–87.

6. Guyton AC, Lindsey AW, Gilluly JJ. The limits of right ventricular compensation following acute increase in pulmonary circulatory resistance. Circ Res 1954;2: 326–32.

7. Rudski LG, Lai WW, Afilalo J, et al. Guidelines for the echocardiographic assessment of the right heart in adults: a report from the American Society of Echocardiography endorsed by the European Association of Echocardiography, a registered branch of the European Society of Cardiology, and the Canadian Society of Echocardiography. J Am Soc Echocardiogr 2010;23:685–713.

8. Brennan JM, Blair JE, Goonewardena S, et al. Reappraisal of the use of inferior vena cava for estimating right atrial pressure. J Am Soc Echocardiogr 2007; 20:857–61.

9. Shafiq Q, Moukarbel GV, Gupta R, et al. Practical echocardiographic approach for risk stratification of patients with acute pulmonary embolism. J Echocardiogr 2016;14:146–55.

10. Khemasuwan D, Yingchoncharoen T, Tunsupon P, et al. Right ventricular echocardiographic parameters are associated with mortality after acute pulmonary embolism. J Am Soc Echocardiogr 2015;28: 355–62.

11. Vitarelli A, Barilla F, Capotosto L, et al. Right ventricular function in acute pulmonary embolism: a combined assessment by three-dimensional and speckle-tracking echocardiography. J Am Soc Echocardiogr 2014;27:329–38.

12. Galie N, Kim NH. Pulmonary microvascular disease in chronic thromboembolic pulmonary hypertension. Proc Am Thorac Soc 2006;3:571–6.

13. Lang I. Chronic thromboembolic pulmonary hypertension: a distinct disease entity. Eur Respir Rev 2015;24:246 52.

14. Guerin L, Couturaud F, Parent F, et al. Prevalence of chronic thromboembolic pulmonary hypertension after acute pulmonary embolism. Prevalence of CTEPH after pulmonary embolism. Thromb Haemost 2014;112:598–605.

15. Pengo V, Lensing AW, Prins MH, et al. Incidence of chronic thromboembolic pulmonary hypertension after pulmonary embolism. N Engl J Med 2004;350: 2257–64.

16. Kline JA, Steuerwald MT, Marchick MR, et al. Prospective evaluation of right ventricular function and functional status 6 months after acute submassive pulmonary embolism: frequency of persistent or subsequent elevation in estimated pulmonary artery pressure. Chest 2009;136:1202–10.

17. Krivec B, Voga G, Zuran I, et al. Diagnosis and treatment of shock due to massive pulmonary embolism: approach with transesophageal echocardiography and intrapulmonary thrombolysis. Chest 1997;112: 1310–6.

18. Quiroz R, Kucher N, Schoepf UJ, et al. Right ventricular enlargement on chest computed tomography: prognostic role in acute pulmonary embolism. Circulation 2004;109:2401–4.

19. Schoepf UJ, Kucher N, Kipfmueller F, et al. Right ventricular enlargement on chest computed tomography: a predictor of early death in acute pulmonary embolism. Circulation 2004;110:3276–80.

20. Scridon T, Scridon C, Skali H, et al. Prognostic significance of troponin elevation and right ventricular enlargement in acute pulmonary embolism. Am J Cardiol 2005;96:303–5.

21. Fremont B, Pacouret G, Jacobi D, et al. Prognostic value of echocardiographic right/left ventricular end-diastolic diameter ratio in patients with acute pulmonary embolism: results from a monocenter registry of 1,416 patients. Chest 2008;133: 358–62.

22. Kucher N, Boekstegers P, Muller OJ, et al. Randomized, controlled trial of ultrasound-assisted catheter-directed thrombolysis for acute intermediate-risk pulmonary embolism. Circulation 2014;129:479–86.

23. Piazza G, Hohlfelder B, Jaff MR, et al. A prospective, single-arm, multicenter trial of ultrasound-facilitated, catheter-directed, low-dose fibrinolysis for acute massive and submassive pulmonary embolism: the SEATTLE II Study. JACC Cardiovasc Interv 2015;8: 1382–92.

24. McConnell MV, Solomon SD, Rayan ME, et al. Regional right ventricular dysfunction detected by echocardiography in acute pulmonary embolism. Am J Cardiol 1996;78:469–73.

25. Holley AB, Cheatham JG, Jackson JL, et al. Novel quantitative echocardiographic parameters in acute PE. J Thromb Thrombolysis 2009;28:506–12.

26. Kjaergaard J, Schaadt BK, Lund JO, et al. Quantitative measures of right ventricular dysfunction by echocardiography in the diagnosis of acute non-massive pulmonary embolism. J Am Soc Echocardiogr 2006;19:1264–71.

27. Coutance G, Cauderlier E, Ehtisham J, et al. The prognostic value of markers of right ventricular dysfunction in pulmonary embolism: a meta-analysis. Crit Care 2011;15:R103.

28. Kreit JW. The impact of right ventricular dysfunction on the prognosis and therapy of normotensive patients with pulmonary embolism. Chest 2004;125:1539–45.

29. Barrios D, Rosa-Salazar V, Jimenez D, et al. Right heart thrombi in pulmonary embolism. Eur Respir J 2016;48:1377–85.

30. Torbicki A, Galie N, Covezzoli A, et al. Right heart thrombi in pulmonary embolism: results from the international cooperative pulmonary embolism registry. J Am Coll Cardiol 2003;41:2245–51.

31. Kukla P, McIntyre WF, Koracevic G, et al. Relation of atrial fibrillation and right-sided cardiac thrombus to outcomes in patients with acute pulmonary embolism. Am J Cardiol 2015;115:825–30.

32. Barrios D, Rosa-Salazar V, Morillo R, et al. Prognostic significance of right heart thrombi in patients with acute symptomatic pulmonary embolism: systemic review and meta-analysis. Chest 2017;151:409–16.

33. Masuyama T, Kodama K, Kitabatake A, et al. Continuous-wave Doppler echocardiographic detection of pulmonary regurgitation and its application to noninvasive estimation of pulmonar artery pressure. Circulation 1986;74:484–92.

34. Moser KM, Spragg RG, Utley J, et al. Chronic thrombotic obstruction of major pulmonary arteries. Ann Intern Med 1983;99:299–304.

35. Liu M, Ma Z, Guo X, et al. Computed tomographic pulmonary angiography in the assessment of severity of chronic thromboembolic pulmonary hypertension and right ventricular dysfunction. Eur J Radiol 2011;80:e462–9.

36. Mahmud E, Raisinghani A, Hassankhani A, et al. Correlation of left ventricular diastolic filling characteristics with right ventricular overload and pulmonary artery pressure in chronic thromboembolic pulmonary hypertension. J Am Coll Cardiol 2002;40:318–24.

37. Gurudevan SV, Malouf PJ, Auger WR, et al. Abnormal left ventricular diastolic filling in chronic thromboembolic pulmonary hypertension: true diastolic dysfunction or left ventricular underfilling? J Am Coll Cardiol 2007;49:1334–9.

38. Jaff MR, McMurtry S, Archer SL, et al. Management of massive and submassive pulmonary embolism, iliofemoral deep vein thrombosis, and chronic thromboembolic pulmonary hypertension: a scientific statement from the American Heart Association. Circulation 2011;123:1788–830.

39. Kearon C, Akl EA, Ornelas J, et al. Antithrombotic therapy for VTE disease: CHEST guideline and expert panel report. Chest 2016;149:315–52.

40. Kabrhel C, Rosovsky R, Channick R, et al. A multidisciplinary pulmonary embolism response team: initial 30-month experience with a novel approach to delivery of care to patients with submassive and massive pulmonary embolism. Chest 2016;150:384–93.

41. Spencer KT, Kimura BJ, Korcarz CE, et al. Focused cardiac ultrasound: recommendations from the American Society of echocardiography. J Am Soc Echocardiogr 2013;26:567–81.

Management of Low-Risk Pulmonary Embolism

Ebtesam Attaya Islam, MD, PhD[a], Richard E. Winn, MD, MS[b,c], Victor Test, MD[d],*

KEYWORDS

- Pulmonary embolism • Diagnosis • PE risks stratification • Low-risk PE • Subsegmental PE
- Incidental PE • Medical management • Outpatient

KEY POINTS

- The stratification of patients into risk strata can be complicated and involves assessment of the accuracy of the diagnosis of pulmonary embolism as well as objective clinical factors.
- Although clinical gestalt is effective in identifying high-risk patients with pulmonary embolism, the identification of intermediate-risk and low-risk patients can be accurately derived by the combination of biomarkers, imaging, and risk stratification scoring systems or criteria.
- Once patients have been identified as low risk, candidates of outpatient management can be identified by evaluation of bleeding risk, cardiopulmonary reserve, patient adherence, and capabilities.
- Subsegmental pulmonary embolism can be challenging to diagnose because of the difficulty of imaging. Management decision requires close examination of imaging quality and criteria, pretest probability, presence of deep venous thrombosis, bleeding risk, and other risk factors.
- Incidental pulmonary embolism is not an uncommon problem. It is typically managed in the same manner as symptomatic pulmonary embolism with anticoagulation after assessment of bleeding risks.

INTRODUCTION

Pulmonary embolism (PE) occurs when thrombi form in deep veins or the right atrium and then embolize to the pulmonary artery. PE is closely linked with deep venous thrombosis (DVT) and should be considered a different manifestation of the same disorder: venous thromboembolism (VTE).[1] Classically, 90% of emboli originate from proximal lower extremity venous thrombosis.[2] In patients with a high probability of PE, DVT was detected in 48.6%.[3] Indicators of DVT include lower extremity findings, such as edema, leg and calf tenderness, erythema, venous cords, and Homan signs. Because of the nonspecific symptoms of PE and VTE, there can be substantial delays in seeking medical attention.[4]

PE is a leading cause of morbidity and mortality in the United States, and between 5% and 10% of hospital deaths are attributable to PE.[5] From 1998 to 2005, the number of patients discharged from US hospitals with a diagnosis of PE increased from 126,546 to 229,637.[5] Over this period of time, the hospital case fatality rate decreased from 12.3% to 8.2% (P<.001).[5] The length of stay decreased, but hospital charges for these patients increased nearly 100% (P<.001). In the United States, 300,000 deaths occur annually from acute episodes of PE.[6] The incidence rates reported for

[a] Department of Internal Medicine, Division of Pulmonary and Critical Care Medicine, Texas Tech University Health Sciences Center, 3601 4th Street, Stop 9410, Lubbock, TX 79430, USA; [b] Infectious Diseases, Texas Tech University Health Sciences Center, 3601 4th Street, Lubbock, TX 79430, USA; [c] Pulmonary Medicine Division, Texas Tech University Health Sciences Center, 3601 4th Street, Lubbock, TX 79430, USA; [d] Pulmonary and Critical Care Medicine, Texas Tech University Health Sciences Center, 3601 4th Street, Stop 9410, Lubbock, TX 79430, USA
* Corresponding author.
E-mail address: Victor.test@ttuhsc.edu

Clin Chest Med 39 (2018) 561–568
https://doi.org/10.1016/j.ccm.2018.04.013
0272-5231/18/© 2018 Elsevier Inc. All rights reserved.

PE (with or without DVT) range from 29 to 78 per 100,000 person-years.[7,8] Because of the disease being underrecognized or misdiagnosed, most deaths are discovered on autopsy[9,10] even with numerous diagnostic tests and treatment modalities.[5,11] However, the risk of death decreases with diagnosis and effective treatment.[12] PE can present along a spectrum from the asymptomatic individual incidentally diagnosed to patients presenting with cardiogenic shock.[13]

The diagnosis of acute PE is ultimately guided by the clinician's index of suspicion for the disease and augmented by diagnostic tests. The recognition of the signs and symptoms of PE is the most important initial diagnostic step. A careful clinical history and physical is crucial to identify the patients at risk and to assess the pretest probability. In a review of the Prospective Investigation of Pulmonary Embolism Diagnosis (PIOPED I) data, dyspnea is the most common symptom followed by pleuritic chest pain, cough, lower extremity edema, hemoptysis, palpitations, wheezing, and anginalike pain,[14] with pleuritic chest pain and hemoptysis occurring more commonly in the setting of pulmonary infarction.[1,14] However, pulmonary infarction does not occur often because of the dual circulation from the bronchial and pulmonary arteries.[13] Nonspecific symptoms and signs, such as tachycardia, tachypnea, and fever, should also be considered as signs of PE. In Stein and Henry's[14] study, tachypnea is the most common physical examination finding followed by crackles, tachycardia, and increased pulmonic heart tone. Other examination findings were found in between 6% and 14% of patients and include evidence of DVT, fever greater than 38.5°C, diaphoresis, wheezing, and a pleural friction rub.[14]

Based on symptoms as well as comorbidities, patients can be classified as low, intermediate, or high risk. With the advent of the multidetector computed tomography (CT) scanners, the sensitivity of detecting PEs has increased, with increased detection of subsegmental and incidental PEs. The diagnosis and management of these issues are discussed.

CLINICAL SUSPICION AND CLINICAL DECISION RULES

The clinician's suspicion of PE and DVT assists in making the diagnosis. Numerous studies have demonstrated failures or delays in the diagnosis of PE lead to the increase in morbidity and mortality.[15–19] More patients are undergoing evaluation with imaging for PE, but the diagnostic yield of these tests can be as low as 3.1% in the absence of clinical prediction rules.[20]

RISK STRATIFICATION AND PRETEST PROBABILITY

Patients can be stratified into low, moderate, or high-risk categories using structured clinical prediction rules or by empirical assessment for diagnostic pretest probability.[21] Structured clinical prediction rules standardize the approach to pretest assessment of probability and remove the variability found in clinical practice. There are numerous clinical prediction scores, including the Wells Score, Simplified Wells Score, Geneva Score, Revised Geneva Score, Simplified Revised Geneva Score, Pulmonary Embolism Rule Out Criteria, and other scoring systems.[21–35] The most commonly used and validated scores include the Wells Score, Simplified Wells Score, and the Geneva scores.[27] These scoring systems can be used with high sensitivity D dimer to further stratify patients and limit the number of diagnostic imaging.[35,36]

LOW-RISK PULMONARY EMBOLISM

PEs are usually categorized into low, intermediate, or high risk; these are based on the criteria that are outlined in this section. Patients with hypotension, marked impairment of oxygenation, and syncope are classified as high risk.[22] Intermediate-risk patients are hemodynamically stable but could have end-organ damage, such as cardiac ischemia, right heart strain, and/or encephalopathy.[22] Hemodynamically stable patients without end-organ damage are categorized as low-risk PE.[22] Low-risk PE is defined by the American College of Cardiology as acute PE without clinical markers defining massive or submassive PE.[37] However, clinicians may view low-risk PE and recurrent VTE differently and may classify patients based on a cancer diagnosis and its staging. Prandoni and colleagues[38] classified patients without malignancy as low risk, whereas intermediate-risk patients had local or recently resected cancer and those with locally advanced or distant metastases were considered high risk. Patients with low-risk PE have a 1-year survival rate of more than 95%, whereas those with high-risk PE have a 40% mortality rate within 90 days.[22,39]

Different scores have been developed so patients with low-risk PE can be assessed for safe outpatient management. The Pulmonary Embolism Severity Index (PESI) and Hestia are two examples. The PESI (**Table 1**) was developed as a clinical prediction rule to classify patients with PE into classes of increasing mortality.[40]

These classes are divided into 5 groups based on a point system.[40,41] The original score

Table 1		
Pulmonary Embolism Severity Index criteria		
Demographics	**Comorbid Illness**	**Clinical Findings**
Age	Cancer	Pulse
Sex	Heart failure	Systolic blood
	Chronic lung	pressure
	disease	Respiratory rate
		Temperature
		Altered mental
		status
		Arterial oxygen
		saturation

Adapted from Aujesky D, Obrosky DS, Stone RA, et al. Derivation and validation of a prognostic model for pulmonary embolism. Am J Respir Crit Care Med 2005;172(8):1041–6.

Table 2	
Hestia criteria	
Hemodynamically Unstable	Intravenous Pain Medications for >24 h
Thrombolysis or embolectomy necessary	Medical/social reason for treatment in the hospital
Active bleeding or high risk of bleeding	Creatinine clearance <20 mL/min
Oxygen supplementation to maintain oxygen saturation >90% required for >24 h	Documented history of heparin-induced thrombocytopenia
PE diagnosed during anticoagulation treatment	Severe liver impairment
Pregnant?	

Adapted from Zondag W, Vingerhoets LM, Durian MF, et al. Hestia criteria can safely select patients with pulmonary embolism for outpatient treatment irrespective of right ventricular function. J Thromb Haemost 2013;11(4):686–92.

is divided into 5 classes, with class one being very low risk with less than 65 points; class 5 is very high risk with greater than 125 points.[40] Those patients classified as class I and II are considered safe to treat at home. The simple PESI (sPESI) is based on 6 variables, including age greater than 80 years, cancer, chronic lung or heart disease, heart rate, systolic blood pressure less than 100 mm Hg, and oxygen saturation less than 90%. Patients with any one of these 6 criteria that is positive are considered high-risk patients and should not be sent home to be treated, but rather be treated as inpatients. Dentali and colleagues[42] found that sPESI has comparable accuracy compared with the PESI at 3 months and 6 months. However, the accuracy at 1 year was better for the original PESI in comparison with the sPESI.[42]

The Hestia score is another score to assess for low-risk PE. Again, like the PESI criteria, the Hestia scoring is based on 11 criteria (**Table 2**).[43] Like the sPESI, even one answer *yes* to any of the criteria eliminates outpatient management.

SUBSEGMENTAL PULMONARY EMBOLISM

O'Connell[44] lists 4 main locations for PEs, main, lobar, segmental, or subsegmental, based on the most proximal pulmonary arterial segment involved. Multi-detector-row CT (MDCT) scanners improved resolution, increased sensitivity, and provided thinner slices; smaller arteries are seen, including subsegmental pulmonary arteries.[45–47] It is difficult to define the subsegmental branch, as it is unclear when the vessel becomes subsegmental and the term is used to denote a distal branch, with its significance being unclear.

The increased usage of CT pulmonary angiography has led to a 5.4% increase in the diagnosis for subsegmental PE (SSPE).[48] The investigators showed the increase from the single-detector CT was 4.7%, 7.1% with the 4 detectors, 6.9% with 16 detectors, and 15.0% with the MDCT 64 detector,[49] in contrast to a high probability from a V/Q scan; 1% are SSPEs.[50] The investigators of PIOPED I showed that 6% of patients had SSPEs with pulmonary angiography,[50,51] whereas a low-probability read on the V/Q scan had 17% of patients with PEs in the subsegmental arteries.

However, caution must be used when analyzing imaging from CT angiography. Increased sensitivity is accompanied by increased pitfalls.[52] These pitfalls include but are not limited to breathing artifact, insufficient enhancement of the pulmonary arteries due to missed bolus or bolus mistiming, streak artifacts, and obesity, which can reduce the sensitivity for smaller thrombi.[50,52] Despite the increase in the diagnosis of PE with CT angiography, the mortality and fatality rates are the same.[53,54] The American College of Chest Physicians' (ACCP) recent guidelines on antithrombotic therapy recommend the following criteria to help confirm that the diagnosis of SSPE is correct: (1) high-quality pulmonary angiogram with adequate opacification; (2) multiple intraluminal filling defects; (3) defects involving more proximal subsegmental arteries; (4) defects seen on more than one image; (5) defects surrounded by contrast rather than appearing to be adherent to the arterial walls; (6) defects seen on more than one projection; (7) symptomatic patients; (8) a high clinical pretest probability for PE; and (9) elevated D dimer.[55] These criteria are guides and are not used as a scoring system[55] (**Figs. 1–3**).

Rezaie[56] discusses that true SSPE is likely to come from a small DVT and that many of these so-called SSPEs are false-positive overcalls by the radiologist. After review of almost 1000 CT angiograms with 174 that were initially read as positive, the investigator found a false-positive rate of 26% overall with 46% among solitary PEs, 27% among segmental PEs, and 59% among SSPEs.[57] This finding further illustrates the difficulty of the treatment of SSPEs (see later discussion).

INCIDENTAL PULMONARY EMBOLISM

As noted with SSPEs, the increased frequency of incidental PEs (IPEs) has been reported with the advent of CT scanners. When a PE is found on a CT scan unexpectedly, performed for reasons other than evaluating PEs, this is referred to as an IPE.[44] O' Connell[44] refers to those patients without identifiable risk factors as patients with IPE.[44] IPEs are most often found in patients with oncological issues being staged for cancer,[58,59] trauma patients,[60] and evaluation of symptoms, with 3.6% found in cancer staging.[44] One study found that IPEs were highest in those patients with breast cancer.[61] Those IPEs found in patients with malignancies were highest at 71.1% in the lower lobe of the right pulmonary artery and least (15.2%) in the lingula of the left pulmonary artery.[61] Interestingly, although these patients were getting CT scans for staging and IPEs were found, O'Connell found 54% of patients with cancer had complained of fatigue.[62] These clots may not be IPEs due to the complaint of fatigue; but physicians may be attributing this complaint to the malignancy, cytopenias, or chemotherapy rather than IPE.[44]

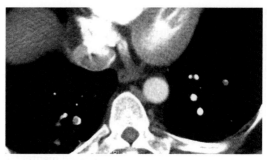

Fig. 2. SSPE, right lower lobe posteriorly, left lower lobe laterally.

MANAGEMENT OF LOW-RISK PULMONARY EMBOLISM

The identification of patients at low risk for recurrent VTE and death from VTE has been well studied over the last decade. Traditionally, patients with VTE, including DVT and PE, were managed with parenteral anticoagulation with unfractionated heparin with transition to warfarin regardless of risk and required several days in the hospital as an essential management requirement. With the advent of the low-molecular-weight heparins and the development of direct oral anticoagulants, investigation into strategies for outpatient management of PE have been performed.

Outpatient management of PE is based on the ability to stratify patients in terms of risk for recurrent VTE, bleeding, and death. Clinical factors, comorbidities, and psychosocial factors are considered when assessing patients for outpatient management of PE. Traditionally, patients had to meet rigid criteria for outpatient discharge. Clinical factors to consider include risk stratification scores and other factors, such as hypoxemia, tachycardia, right heart strain on imaging, near-syncope/syncope, and coexisting DVT.[58] Comorbidities that have been considered in the assessment for outpatient management include

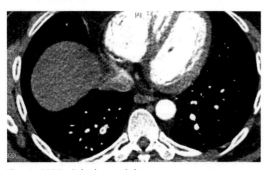

Fig. 1. SSPE, right lower lobe.

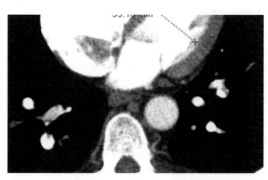

Fig. 3. SSPE, right lower lobe posteriorly, left lower lobe.

an alternative diagnosis that requires inpatient care; active bleeding; risk of bleeding, including cirrhosis, abnormal coagulation, renal insufficiency, and recent major surgery; pregnancy; cerebrovascular disease; recent gastrointestinal bleeding; and thrombocytopenia.[58] Psychosocial issues considered in the decision to pursue outpatient management include adequate social support, factors that may result in medical nonadherence, and access to prompt clinical follow-up.[58]

After assessment of these factors, patients can be assessed by several scoring instruments to determine their risk from acute VTE. The PESI, sPESI, and the Hestia criteria and are used to identify very-low-risk patients who do not have features that make them intermediate or high risk.

In a study, patients who met the criteria for outpatient management of PE by the PESI risk class I and II were assessed for short-term (5 days) and medium-term adverse outcomes after stratification based on these relative contraindications.[63] The patients with relative contraindications had a higher percentage of admission compared with the patients without relative contraindications who had longer hospital stays (median stay 59.5 hours compared with 37.0 hours [P<.01]). In addition, the major 30-day outcome events were more likely in the group with contraindications (5.9% vs 1.8%, P<.05). These events included recurrent VTE events (3 with relative contraindications to 2 with no relative contraindications), major bleeding (4 to 3), and all-cause mortality (2 to 0).[63]

The PESI and the sPESI have been assessed for the ability to safely stratify patients according to risk in acute PE. In addition, the PESI score has been used in a randomized trial to assess outpatient safety. Aujesky and colleagues[64] used the PESI score for low-risk class I, II as criteria for randomization to outpatient therapy with low-molecular-weight heparin with transition to a vitamin K antagonist or as an inpatient with identical therapy in 344 patients. After 90 days, there was no difference in deaths or recurrent VTE in the two groups.[64] There were 3 (1.8%) patients with major bleeding in the outpatient group and none in the inpatient group by 90 days (P = .086).[64]

Zondag and colleagues[65] used the Hestia criteria in a study to assess the feasibility of outpatient management of PE. In this initial study, 297 patients were assessed with the Hestia criteria and placed in an outpatient treatment group (treated initially with low-molecular-weight heparin) and followed to assess for recurrent VTE, major bleeding, and death over 3 months. Six patients

(2%) had recurrent VTE, 2 patients (0.7%) had major bleeding, and 3 patients died (1%, none from recurrent VTE).[65] A subsequent follow-up study used the Hestia criteria to assess 496 patients with acute PE, and 275 were treated as outpatients based on their Hestia criteria.[43] There were no adverse events during the follow-up in the outpatient group compared with 4.5% of the patients who were treated in the hospital (P<.001).[43] The sensitivity and negative predictive value for the Hestia criteria for adverse outcomes were 100%.[43]

In summary, the outpatient management of low-risk patients with PE as determined by clinical assessment, scoring systems, and evaluation with clinical tests, such as pro–b-type natriuretic peptide, troponin I, and imaging, can be used safely.[55] An assessment of bleeding risk either clinically or with a formal scoring system should be considered when selecting patients for outpatient management as well as an assessment of the patients' capabilities, adherence, and ability to achieve prompt follow-up evaluation.

SEGMENTAL AND SUBSEGMENTAL PULMONARY EMBOLISM

Isolated segmental and SSPE present a significant diagnostic challenge with regard to the accuracy of the diagnosis, as noted earlier. Pretest probability plays a key determining factor in the approach to this problem, and clinical scoring systems may be helpful particularly in conjunction with the D dimer in patients who were classified as low risk to have a PE. The presence of more than one abnormality, the presence of DVT, and the absence of an alternative diagnosis are clinical factors that would suggest the need for anticoagulation. Outcome data in these patients are sparse. Carrier and colleagues[49] published a meta-analysis in 2010 whereby 22 articles were reviewed. They found in this meta-analysis that the rate of SSPE was between 4.7% and 9.4% depending on the type of CT scanner.[49] Of the patients who were untreated, the percentage of recurrent VTE on CT angiography at 3 months was 0.9% to 1.1% depending on the CT scanner.[49] A subsequent study by Goy and colleagues[66] assessed management of patients with SSPE in a retrospective fashion and found that 15% of PEs were subsegmental. Anticoagulation was received in 52.4% of patients with SSPE.[66] At the conclusion of the study, there was an increase in serious bleeding in the group who received anticoagulation but no difference in recurrent thrombosis with or without anticoagulation.[66]

In contrast, a study in 2013 evaluated 748 patients with PE of whom 116 (16%) had SSPE.[67]

They were assessed for 3-month outcomes for recurrent VTE and mortality.[67] No difference was found between proximal PE and SSPE in these two outcomes.[67] The ACCP's recent guidelines make the following recommendations regarding therapy in patients with SSPE: If SSPE is confirmed on high-quality imaging (as defined earlier) and there is no evidence for proximal DVT, surveillance is recommended if the risk of recurrence is thought to be low (no chronic or reversible risk factors, such as recent hospitalization, immobility, active malignancy, recent surgery) and patients have adequate cardiopulmonary reserve and the absence of severe symptoms that cannot be attributed to another disorder.[55] If these conditions are not met, then patients should be placed on anticoagulation.[55]

INCIDENTAL PULMONARY EMBOLISM

The management of IPE remains challenging. In noncancer patients, previous studies have been equivocal in terms of outcome.[68–70] The data in patients with cancer strongly suggest that patients with IPE who are treated have a significant benefit in terms of decreased thrombotic events and improved mortality. Published guidelines from the American College of Physicians (did not update a previous recommendation from 2012) and the National Comprehensive Cancer Network recommend treatment in patients with IPE similarly to symptomatic PE.[71,72]

SUMMARY

The definition of low-risk PE is defined by presentation, evaluation of biomarkers and imaging, and stratification scoring. The management of low-risk PE is complicated and involves careful assessment of risks, benefits, as well as psychosocial support for patients and caregivers.

REFERENCES

1. Islam E, Test V. The diagnosis of acute pulmonary embolism. The Southwest Respiratory and Critical Care Chronicles 2014;2(8):21–30.
2. Stein PD, Terrin ML, Hales CA, et al. Clinical, laboratory, roentgenographic, and electrocardiographic findings in patients with acute pulmonary embolism and no pre-existing cardiac or pulmonary disease. Chest 1991;100(3):598–603.
3. Perrier A, Roy PM, Aujesky D, et al. Diagnosing pulmonary embolism in outpatients with clinical assessment, D-dimer measurement, venous ultrasound, and helical computed tomography: a multicenter management study. Am J Med 2004;116(5):291–9.
4. Elliott CG, Goldhaber SZ, Jensen RL. Delays in diagnosis of deep vein thrombosis and pulmonary embolism. Chest 2005;128(5):3372–6.
5. Park B, Messina L, Dargon P, et al. Recent trends in clinical outcomes and resource utilization for pulmonary embolism in the United States: findings from the nationwide inpatient sample. Chest 2009; 136(4):983–90.
6. Heit J, Cohen A, Anderson F Jr. Estimated annual number of incident and recurrent, non-fatal and fatal venous thromboembolism (VTE) events in the U.S.Heit, JA, AT Cohen, and FA Anderson Jr.; for the VTE Impact Assessment Group. Blood 2005; 106(11) [abstract: #910:267a].
7. Silverstein MD, Heit JA, Mohr DN, et al. Trends in the incidence of deep vein thrombosis and pulmonary embolism: a 25-year population-based study. Arch Intern Med 1998;158(6):585–93.
8. Heit JA. Epidemiology of venous thromboembolism. Nat Rev Cardiol 2015;12(8):464–74.
9. Ryu JH, Olson EJ, Pellikka PA. Clinical recognition of pulmonary embolism: problem of unrecognized and asymptomatic cases. Mayo Clin Proc 1998;73(9):873–9.
10. Pulido T, Aranda A, Zevallos MA, et al. Pulmonary embolism as a cause of death in patients with heart disease: an autopsy study. Chest 2006;129(5):1282–7.
11. Wood KE. Major pulmonary embolism: review of a pathophysiologic approach to the golden hour of hemodynamically significant pulmonary embolism. Chest 2002;121(3):877–905.
12. Carson JL, Kelley MA, Duff A, et al. The clinical course of pulmonary embolism. N Engl J Med 1992;326(19):1240–5.
13. Tapson VF. Acute pulmonary embolism. N Engl J Med 2008;358(10):1037–52.
14. Stein PD, Henry JW. Clinical characteristics of patients with acute pulmonary embolism stratified according to their presenting syndromes. Chest 1997;112(4):974–9.
15. Dalen JE, Alpert JS. Natural history of pulmonary embolism. Prog Cardiovasc Dis 1975;17(4):259–70.
16. Dalen JE. Pulmonary embolism: what have we learned since Virchow? Natural history, pathophysiology, and diagnosis. Chest 2002;122(4):1440–56.
17. Lilienfeld DE, Chan E, Ehland J, et al. Mortality from pulmonary embolism in the United States: 1962 to 1984. Chest 1990;98(5):1067–72.
18. Clagett GP, Anderson FA Jr, Heit J, et al. Prevention of venous thromboembolism. Chest 1995;108(4 Suppl):312S–34S.
19. Anderson FA Jr, Wheeler HB, Goldberg RJ, et al. A population-based perspective of the hospital incidence and case-fatality rates of deep vein thrombosis and pulmonary embolism. The Worcester DVT Study. Arch Intern Med 1991;151(5):933–8.

20. Hoo GW, Wu CC, Vazirani S, et al. Does a clinical decision rule using D-dimer level improve the yield of pulmonary CT angiography? AJR Am J Roentgenol 2011;196(5):1059–64.

21. Penaloza A, Verschuren F, Meyer G, et al. Comparison of the unstructured clinician gestalt, the wells score, and the revised Geneva score to estimate pretest probability for suspected pulmonary embolism. Ann Emerg Med 2013;62(2):117–24.e2.

22. Corrigan D, Prucnal C, Kabrhel C. Pulmonary embolism: the diagnosis, risk-stratification, treatment and disposition of emergency department patients. Clin Exp Emerg Med 2016;3(3):117–25.

23. Heit JA, Sobell JL, Li H, et al. The incidence of venous thromboembolism among factor V Leiden carriers: a community-based cohort study. J Thromb Haemost 2005;3(2):305–11.

24. Poort SR, Rosendaal FR, Reitsma PH, et al. A common genetic variation in the 3'-untranslated region of the prothrombin gene is associated with elevated plasma prothrombin levels and an increase in venous thrombosis. Blood 1996; 88(10):3698–703.

25. British Thoracic Society Standards of Care Committee Pulmonary Embolism Guideline Development Group. British Thoracic Society guidelines for the management of suspected acute pulmonary embolism. Thorax 2003;58(6):470–83.

26. Belohlavek J, Dytrych V, Linhart A. Pulmonary embolism, part I: epidemiology, risk factors and risk stratification, pathophysiology, clinical presentation, diagnosis and nonthrombotic pulmonary embolism. Exp Clin Cardiol 2013;18(2):129–38.

27. Moores LK, King CS, Holley AB. Current approach to the diagnosis of acute nonmassive pulmonary embolism. Chest 2011;140(2):509–18.

28. Gibson NS, Sohne M, Kruip MJ, et al. Further validation and simplification of the Wells clinical decision rule in pulmonary embolism. Thromb Haemost 2008;99(1):229–34.

29. Douma RA, Gibson NS, Gerdes VE, et al. Validity and clinical utility of the simplified Wells rule for assessing clinical probability for the exclusion of pulmonary embolism. Thromb Haemost 2009;101(1): 197–200.

30. Le Gal G, Righini M, Roy PM, et al. Prediction of pulmonary embolism in the emergency department: the revised Geneva score. Ann Intern Med 2006;144(3): 165–71.

31. Klok FA, Kruisman E, Spaan J, et al. Comparison of the revised Geneva score with the Wells rule for assessing clinical probability of pulmonary embolism. J Thromb Haemost 2008;6(1):40–4.

32. Ceriani E, Combescure C, Le Gal G, et al. Clinical prediction rules for pulmonary embolism: a systematic review and meta-analysis. J Thromb Haemost 2010;8(5):957–70.

33. Douma RA, Mos IC, Erkens PM, et al. Performance of 4 clinical decision rules in the diagnostic management of acute pulmonary embolism: a prospective cohort study. Ann Intern Med 2011;154(11):709–18.

34. Wells PS, Anderson DR, Rodger M, et al. Derivation of a simple clinical model to categorize patients probability of pulmonary embolism: increasing the models utility with the SimpliRED D-dimer. Thromb Haemost 2000;83(3):416–20.

35. Bokobza J, Aubry A, Nakle N, et al. Pulmonary embolism rule-out criteria vs D-dimer testing in low-risk patients for pulmonary embolism: a retrospective study. Am J Emerg Med 2014;32(6):609–13.

36. Raja AS, Greenberg JO, Qaseem A, et al. Evaluation of patients with suspected acute pulmonary embolism: best practice advice from the clinical guidelines committee of the american college of physicians. Ann Intern Med 2015;163(9):701–11.

37. Jaff MR, McMurtry MS, Archer SL, et al. Management of massive and submassive pulmonary embolism, iliofemoral deep vein thrombosis, and chronic thromboembolic pulmonary hypertension: a scientific statement from the American Heart Association. Circulation 2011;123(16):1788–830.

38. Prandoni P, Lensing AW, Piccioli A, et al. Recurrent venous thromboembolism and bleeding complications during anticoagulant treatment in patients with cancer and venous thrombosis. Blood 2002; 100(10):3484–8.

39. Kucher N, Rossi E, De Rosa M, et al. Massive pulmonary embolism. Circulation 2006;113(4):577–82.

40. Aujesky D, Obrosky DS, Stone RA, et al. Derivation and validation of a prognostic model for pulmonary embolism. Am J Respir Crit Care Med 2005;172(8): 1041–6.

41. Jimenez D, Aujesky D, Moores L, et al. Simplification of the pulmonary embolism severity index for prognostication in patients with acute symptomatic pulmonary embolism. Arch Intern Med 2010;170(15): 1383–9.

42. Dentali F, Riva N, Turato S, et al. Pulmonary embolism severity index accurately predicts long-term mortality rate in patients hospitalized for acute pulmonary embolism. J Thromb Haemost 2013;11(12): 2103–10.

43. Zondag W, Vingerhoets LM, Durian MF, et al. Hestia criteria can safely select patients with pulmonary embolism for outpatient treatment irrespective of right ventricular function. J Thromb Haemost 2013; 11(4):686–92.

44. O'Connell C. How I treat incidental pulmonary embolism. Blood 2015;125(12):1877–82 [quiz: 2009].

45. Jha S. The road to overdiagnosis: the case of subsegmental pulmonary embolism. Acad Radiol 2015;22(8):985–7.

46. Patel S, Kazerooni EA, Cascade PN. Pulmonary embolism: optimization of small pulmonary artery

visualization at multi-detector row CT. Radiology 2003;227(2):455–60.

47. Novelline R. Squire's fundamentals of radiology. 6th edition. Cambridge (England): Harvard University Press; 2004.

48. Carrier M, Righini M, Le Gal G. Symptomatic sub-segmental pulmonary embolism: what is the next step? J Thromb Haemost 2012;10(8):1486–90.

49. Carrier M, Righini M, Wells PS, et al. Subsegmental pulmonary embolism diagnosed by computed tomography: incidence and clinical implications. A systematic review and meta-analysis of the management outcome studies. J Thromb Haemost 2010; 8(8):1716–22.

50. Stein PD, Henry JW. Prevalence of acute pulmonary embolism in central and subsegmental pulmonary arteries and relation to probability interpretation of ventilation/perfusion lung scans. Chest 1997;111(5):1246–8.

51. Investigators P. Value of the ventilation/perfusion scan in acute pulmonary embolism. Results of the prospective investigation of pulmonary embolism diagnosis (PIOPED). JAMA 1990;263(20):2753–9.

52. Aviram G, Levy G, Fishman JE, et al. Pitfalls in the diagnosis of acute pulmonary embolism on spiral computer tomography. Curr Probl Diagn Radiol 2004;33(2):74–84.

53. Wiener RS, Schwartz LM, Woloshin S. Time trends in pulmonary embolism in the United States: evidence of overdiagnosis. Arch Intern Med 2011; 171(9):831–7.

54. DeMonaco NA, Dang Q, Kapoor WN, et al. Pulmonary embolism incidence is increasing with use of spiral computed tomography. Am J Med 2008; 121(7):611–7.

55. Kearon C, Akl EA, Ornelas J, et al. Antithrombotic therapy for VTE disease: CHEST guideline and expert panel report. Chest 2016;149(2):315–52.

56. Rezaie S. Best case ever: low risk pulmonary embolism. In: Helman A, editor. https://emergencymedicinecases.com/best-case-ever-low-risk-pulmonary-embolism/2016. Accessed May 25, 2018.

57. Hutchinson BD, Navin P, Marom EM, et al. Overdiagnosis of pulmonary embolism by pulmonary CT angiography. AJR Am J Roentgenol 2015;205(2):271–7.

58. Klok FA, Huisman MV. Management of incidental pulmonary embolism. Eur Respir J 2017;49(6) [pii: 1700275].

59. Storto ML, Di Credico A, Guido F, et al. Incidental detection of pulmonary emboli on routine MDCT of the chest. AJR Am J Roentgenol 2005;184(1):264–7.

60. Schultz DJ, Brasel KJ, Washington L, et al. Incidence of asymptomatic pulmonary embolism in moderately to severely injured trauma patients. J Trauma 2004;56(4):727–31 [discussion: 731–23].

61. Deniz MA, Deniz ZT, Adin ME, et al. Detection of incidental pulmonary embolism with multi-slice computed tomography in cancer patients. Clin Imaging 2017;41:106–11.

62. O'Connell CL, Boswell WD, Duddalwar V, et al. Unsuspected pulmonary emboli in cancer patients: clinical correlates and relevance. J Clin Oncol 2006;24(30):4928–32.

63. Vinson DR, Drenten CE, Huang J, et al. Impact of relative contraindications to home management in emergency department patients with low-risk pulmonary embolism. Ann Am Thorac Soc 2015;12(5):666–73.

64. Aujesky D, Roy PM, Verschuren F, et al. Outpatient versus inpatient treatment for patients with acute pulmonary embolism: an international, open-label, randomised, non-inferiority trial. Lancet 2011; 378(9785):41–8.

65. Zondag W, Mos IC, Creemers-Schild D, et al. Outpatient treatment in patients with acute pulmonary embolism: the Hestia Study. J Thromb Haemost 2011; 9(8):1500–7.

66. Goy J, Lee J, Levine O, et al. Sub-segmental pulmonary embolism in three academic teaching hospitals: a review of management and outcomes. J Thromb Haemost 2015;13(2):214–8.

67. den Exter PL, Kroft LJ, van der Hulle T, et al. Embolic burden of incidental pulmonary embolism diagnosed on routinely performed contrast-enhanced computed tomography imaging in cancer patients. J Thromb Haemost 2013;11(8):1620–2.

68. Schramm D, Bach AG, Meyer HJ, et al. Thrombotic events as incidental finding on computed tomography in intensive care unit patients. Thromb Res 2016;141:171–4.

69. Gandhi R, Salonen D, Geerts WH, et al. A pilot study of computed tomography-detected asymptomatic pulmonary filling defects after hip and knee arthroplasties. J Arthroplasty 2012;27(5):730–5.

70. Sun JM, Kim TS, Lee J, et al. Unsuspected pulmonary emboli in lung cancer patients: the impact on survival and the significance of anticoagulation therapy. Lung Cancer 2010;69(3):330–6.

71. Kearon C, Akl EA, Comerota AJ, et al. Antithrombotic therapy for VTE disease: antithrombotic therapy and prevention of thrombosis, 9th ed: American College of Chest Physicians evidence-based clinical practice guidelines. Chest 2012; 141(2 Suppl):e419S–96S.

72. Streiff MB, Holmstrom B, Ashrani A, et al. Cancer-associated venous thromboembolic disease, version 1.2015. J Natl Compr Canc Netw 2015; 13(9):1079–95.

Aggressive Treatment of Intermediate-Risk Patients with Acute Symptomatic Pulmonary Embolism

David Jimenez, MD, PhD[d],*, Behnood Bikdeli, MD[b,c], Peter S. Marshall, MPH, MD[d], Victor Tapson, MD[e]

KEYWORDS

• Pulmonary embolism • Submassive • Intermediate-risk • Thrombolysis • Reperfusion • Prognosis

KEY POINTS

• Intermediate-risk pulmonary embolism (PE) is defined by hemodynamic stability but the presence of right ventricular dysfunction, myocardial injury, or both.
• Most patients with intermediate-risk PE who receive standard anticoagulation and monitoring have an excellent short-term prognosis.
• Accumulation of factors indicating worse outcomes from PE or early deterioration on standard anticoagulation might alter the risk–benefit assessment in favor of thrombolytic therapy before the development of hemodynamic instability.

INTRODUCTION

Pulmonary embolism (PE) remains a worldwide major health issue.[1] PE is the most common cause of vascular death after myocardial infarction and stroke, and is the leading preventable cause of death in hospitalized patients.[2] Although contemporary observational data indicate significant reductions in all-cause and PE-related mortality over time,[3,4] the overall short-term mortality rate continues to remain significant and many nonfatal long-term complications may arise. Guidelines recommend risk stratification of patients with acute symptomatic PE.[5,6] Early prognostication allows clinicians to better determine the level of care (eg, intensive care vs step-down, regular floor, or outpatient treatment) and associated ancillary therapies.

From this perspective, this article provides an overview of the current definition of intermediate-risk PE, followed by a discussion of the available treatments for these patients, focusing on

Disclosure Statements: None.
Declaration of Interests: D. Jimenez has nothing to disclose. B. Bikdeli is supported by the National Heart, Lung, and Blood Institute, National Institutes of Health (NIH), through grant number T32 HL007854. The content is solely the responsibility of the authors and does not necessarily represent the official views of the NIH. B. Bikdeli reports that he serves as an expert (on behalf of the plaintiff) for litigation related to inferior vena cava filters. The content of the current article is not directly related to that litigation.

[a] Respiratory Department, Hospital Ramón y Cajal and Medicine Department, Universidad de Alcalá (IRYCIS), Ctra. Colmenar Km. 9,100, Madrid 28034, Spain; [b] Division of Cardiology, Department of Medicine, Columbia University Medical Center, New York-Presbyterian Hospital, 622 West 168th Street, New York, NY 10032, USA; [c] Center for Outcomes Research and Evaluation (CORE), Yale University School of Medicine, 333 Cedar Street, New Haven, CT 06510, USA; [d] Section of Pulmonary, Critical Care and Sleep Medicine, Department of Medicine, Yale School of Medicine, 333 Cedar Street, New Haven, CT 06520-8057, USA; [e] Department of Medicine, Cedars-Sinai Medical Center, 8700 Beverly Boulevard, Los Angeles, CA 90048, USA
* Corresponding author.
E-mail address: djimenez.hrc@gmail.com

Clin Chest Med 39 (2018) 569–581
https://doi.org/10.1016/j.ccm.2018.04.011
0272-5231/18/© 2018 Elsevier Inc. All rights reserved.

thrombolytic therapy. Recently completed and ongoing clinical studies for the treatment of patients with intermediate-risk PE are included. Finally, a practical clinical algorithm that integrates risk stratification and management alternatives is provided.

DEFINITION OF INTERMEDIATE-RISK PULMONARY EMBOLISM

The definition of intermediate-risk (or submassive) PE has evolved over time (**Table 1**). The classic

definition of intermediate-risk PE is the presence of either right ventricular (RV) dysfunction or myocardial injury in acute PE without systemic hypotension (systolic blood pressure $\geq$90 mm Hg).[6] However, observational studies have suggested that concomitant use of blood biomarkers and imaging markers of RV dysfunction improve the prognostic value over use of either alone.[7–10] Scridon and colleagues[7] enrolled 141 subjects with acute PE and found that those with echocardiographic RV enlargement and elevated troponin

Table 1
Definitions used for stratification of pulmonary embolism

	Definition	Major Studies Using the Definition	Comment
Massive PE or ESC high	Persistent systolic hypotension (systolic blood pressure <90 mm Hg) or cardiogenic shock	Almost all studies	Initial appropriate management, including adequate use of intravenous fluids should be attempted before hypotension is attributed to acute PE
Submassive PE	Presence of RV dysfunction evidence by increased RV/LV ratio on CT or echocardiography	Tenecteplase or Placebo: Cardiopulmonary Outcomes at 3 Months (TOPCOAT) Ultrasound Accelerated Thrombolysis of Pulmonary Embolism (ULTIMA) AINEP Randomized Trial of Inhaled Nitric Oxide to Treat Acute Pulmonary Embolism (iNOPE)	Some studies have raised concerns about the prognostic utility of some of the echocardiographic factors, in isolation
Submassive PE	Defined by echocardiography or CT plus biomarkers	Pulmonary Embolism Thrombolysis Trial (PEITHO)	Mortality rate within the first 30 d after randomization of only 3.2% in the placebo group
Moderate PE	Defined by imaging findings	Moderate Pulmonary Embolism Treated with Thrombolysis (MOPETT)	Needs further validation on impact on prognosis
ESC intermediate-high	Absence of hypotension, positive PESI or sPESI but presence of RV dysfunction plus myocardial injury		Needs validation in a management study or RCT
ESC intermediate-low	Absence of hypotension, positive PESI or sPESI, but presence of RV dysfunction or myocardial injury or none		The difference in the risk of death in patients at intermediate to high and intermediate-low risk is not pronounced[46]

Abbreviations: AINEP, antiInflamatorios no esteroideos para la embolia pulmonar; ESC, European Society of Cardiology; LV, left ventricle; PESI, Pulmonary Embolism Severity Index; RCT, randomized controlled trial; RV, right ventricle; sPESI, simplified PESI.

levels had a 30-day all-cause mortality of 38%. In a study of 124 stable and unstable subjects with acute PE, the combination of echocardiography and cardiac troponin T (cTnT) had improved prognostic value compared with each test alone.[8] Accordingly, the European Society of Cardiology guidelines define intermediate-high patients with acute symptomatic PE as those who are hemodynamically stable and have myocardial injury and RV dysfunction.[5]

AGGRESSIVE TREATMENT OF INTERMEDIATE-RISK PULMONARY EMBOLISM

Thrombolytic therapy provides more rapid lysis of PE and more rapid restoration of pulmonary perfusion, with associated reduction in pulmonary artery pressure and resistance, and improvement in RV function, than anticoagulation alone.[11] In the past decade, several randomized controlled trials and meta-analyses have contributed to substantially clarify the optimal management of intermediate-risk PE (Table 2). These studies have focused on the use of full-dose systemic thrombolysis, low-dose systemic thrombolysis, and pharmacomechanical catheter-directed therapy.

Full-Dose Systemic Thrombolysis

The Tenecteplase or Placebo: Cardiopulmonary Outcomes at 3 Months (TOPCOAT) study sought to determine the efficacy and safety of tenecteplase in normotensive subjects with acute symptomatic PE and RV strain (determined by echocardiography or biomarkers).[12] These subjects were randomized to receive heparin plus weight-based tenecteplase or heparin plus placebo. The primary composite outcome included 5-day survival to hospital discharge without shock, intubation, or major hemorrhage; 90-day rate of normal RV function; 6-minute walk distance greater than 330 m; no dyspnea at rest; and no recurrent PE or deep vein thrombosis (DVT). After enrolling 83 subjects, the study was terminated early due to logistical constraints for the principal investigator. Despite being underpowered, the primary endpoint occurred significantly less frequently in subjects randomized to thrombolysis compared with the low-molecular-weight heparin (LMWH) (15% vs 37%, $P = .017$).[12]

The Pulmonary Embolism Thrombolysis Trial (PEITHO) was a randomized, double-blind trial that compared tenecteplase plus heparin with placebo plus heparin in normotensive subjects with intermediate-risk PE.[13] Eligible subjects had RV dysfunction or enlargement on echocardiography or computed tomography (CT), as well as

myocardial injury as indicated by a positive test for cardiac troponin I (cTnI) or cTnT. The primary outcome was death or hemodynamic collapse within 7 days after randomization. The main safety outcomes were major extracranial bleeding and ischemic or hemorrhagic stroke within 7 days after randomization. The results of the trial showed that thrombolytic therapy prevented hemodynamic decompensation (1.6% vs 5.0%, $P = .002$) but increased the risk of major bleeding (11.5% vs 2.4%, $P<.001$) and hemorrhagic stroke (2.0 vs 0.2%, $P = .003$). Interestingly, there was a trend toward greater major extracranial bleeding incidence in subjects older than 75 years of age than in those 75 years of age and younger with tenecteplase versus placebo treatment.

Since publication of these studies, several average effect meta-analyses have compared systematic thrombolytic therapy plus anticoagulation with anticoagulation alone in subjects with acute PE. Marti and colleagues[14] evaluated 15 trials comprising 2057 subjects with acute PE. After exclusion of studies that included high-risk PE, thrombolytic therapy was not associated with a significant reduction of overall mortality (odds ratio [OR] 0.64, 95% CI 0.35–1.17). Chatterjee and colleagues[15] identified 16 trials comprising 2115 subjects and performed subset analyses in the 1775 subjects with intermediate-risk PE. In the latter subgroup, thrombolysis was associated with lower mortality risk compared with standard anticoagulation (OR 0.48, 95% CI 0.25–0.92). In both meta-analyses, thrombolysis was associated with higher rates of major bleeding and intracranial hemorrhage compared with anticoagulation. In summary, these data indicate that the benefits of full-dose systemic thrombolytic therapy in unselected normotensive patients with acute PE are largely offset by the increase in bleeding complications. To the authors' knowledge, a patient-level meta-analysis from these trials does not exist, and pooled results per key clinical subgroups (eg, younger patients) remain unknown.

Low-Dose Systemic Thrombolysis

It has been hypothesized that a lower dose of a systemically administered thrombolytic drug might be effective in PE, with the additional benefit of enhancing its safety profile. The Moderate Pulmonary Embolism Treated with Thrombolysis (MOPETT) study was a prospective, controlled, randomized, single-center, open study that randomized 121 subjects with moderate PE to receive either 50 mg of tissue plasminogen activator (TPA) with anticoagulation or anticoagulation alone.[16] The primary outcomes were the development of

Table 2
Major randomized controlled trials for the treatment of intermediate-risk pulmonary embolism

Study	Definition of Intermediate-Risk PE	Subjects (N)	Intervention[a]	Control[a]	Age (y), Mean (Range or SD)	Follow-up (d)	Male (N), (%)	Primary Outcome	Effect	Comment
Meyer et al,[13] 2014	RV dysfunction (by echocardiography or CT) and elevated cTnI or cTnT	1005	Tenecteplase (30–50 mg)	Placebo	66.2 (15.3)	30	473 (47)	All-cause mortality or hemodynamic collapse within 7 d after randomization	OR 0.44 (95% CI 0.23–0.87, P = .02) in favor of tenecteplase	No change in mortality Significant increase in bleeding
Kline et al,[12] 2014	Echocardiographic RV dysfunction, or elevated cTnI or cTnT, or elevated BNP or NT-proBNP	83	Tenecteplase	Placebo	55.4 (14)	5	49 (59.0)	Composite of (1) death, circulatory shock requiring vasopressor support, need for intubation, or serious treatment-related adverse bleeding outcomes within 5 d posttreatment; and (2) VTE recurrence, poor functional capacity, or poor physical health-related quality of life within 90 d	37% placebo-treated and 15% tenecteplase-treated subjects had at least 1 adverse outcome (P = .02)	The trial was terminated prematurely

Study	Inclusion Criteria	N	Intervention	Control		N		Outcome	Results	Limitations
Sharifi et al,[16] 2013	Moderate PE (defined by radiologic thrombus burden) and ≥2 of the following: chest pain, tachypnea, tachycardia, dyspnea, cough, oxygen desaturation, or elevated jugular venous pressure	121	TPA (50 mg)	Placebo	Intervention: 58 (9) Control: 59 (10)	840	55 (45.5)	Incidence of pulmonary hypertension, and the composite of pulmonary hypertension and PE recurrence	Pulmonary hypertension: 16 vs 57%, $P<.001$ Composite: 16 vs 63%, $P<.001$	Unusually high rates of pulmonary hypertension as a surrogate endpoint
Kucher et al,[22] 2014	Echocardiographic RV/LV ratio >1.0	59	rTPA (10–20 mg through PA catheter)	Placebo	63 (14)	90	28 (47.5)	RV/LV ratio at 24 h vs baseline	CDT group: 1.28 vs 0.99, $P<.001$ Heparin group: 1.20 vs 1.17, $P = .31$	Not powered for clinical outcomes

Abbreviations: BNP, brain natriuretic peptide; CDT, catheter-directed thrombolysis; CT, computed tomography; cTnI, cardiac troponin I; NT-proBNP, N-terminal pro-brain natriuretic peptide; OR, odds ratio; rTPA, tissue plasminogen activator; VTE, venous thromboembolism.

[a] Patients also received standard anticoagulation.

pulmonary hypertension (ie, pulmonary artery systolic pressures ≥40 mm Hg) measured by echocardiography and a composite of pulmonary hypertension and recurrent PE at intermediate-term follow-up. In this trial, pulmonary hypertension developed less commonly in the thrombolysis group (16% vs 57%, P<.001). The study was not powered, however, for clinical endpoints and the difference for the rates of recurrent pulmonary emboli (0% vs 5%, P = .08) or death (1.6% vs 5%, P = .30) did not reach statistical significance. There were no bleeding complications with the low-dose thrombolysis.

A recent network meta-analysis evaluated 4 trials[17–20] (298 subjects) that compared low-dose to standard-dose thrombolysis.[21] In this meta-analysis, there was no statistically significant difference in overall mortality (OR 0.96, 95% CI 0.23–4.17) or major bleeding, although low-dose thrombolysis showed a nonsignificant trend toward reduced major bleeding events (OR 0.44, 95% CI 0.15–1.28), which needs to be confirmed in larger studies. Lack of statistical power might account for the nonsignificant results, as suggested by the wider CIs.

Pharmacomechanical Catheter-Directed Therapy

Catheter-directed thrombolysis (CDT) potentially offers the benefits of systemic thrombolysis while minimizing bleeding risk attributable to a lower dose of the thrombolytic agent. Furthermore, some forms of CDT also use ultrasound assistance, which is hypothesized to improve the clot resolution in the pulmonary vasculature. The Ultrasound Accelerated Thrombolysis of Pulmonary Embolism (ULTIMA) trial was the first randomized catheter intervention study for subjects with acute PE. It enrolled subjects with acute symptomatic PE with embolus located in at least 1 main or proximal lower lobe pulmonary artery and an RV-to–left ventricle (LV) ratio greater than or equal to 1 per bedside echocardiography.[22] This multicenter trial investigated whether ultrasound-assisted CDT was superior to anticoagulation alone in the reversal of RV dilatation in intermediate-risk PE subjects. The primary outcome was the difference in the RV-to-LV ratio from baseline to 24 hours. In the interventional group (30 subjects), the RV-to-LV ratio was reduced from 1.28 plus or minus 0.19 at baseline to 0.99 plus or minus 0.17 at 24 hours, respectively (P<.001); whereas in the control group (29 subjects) no significant decrease of the RV-to-LV ratio was observed at 24 hours (1.20 ± 0.14 vs 1.17 ± 0.20, respectively; P = .31). In both study groups, bleeding complications were rare, with 3

(10%) minor bleedings in the interventional group and 1 (3%) in the control group (P = .61). There was no major bleeding. The sample size was too small to demonstrate a change in mortality. The SEATTLE II study was a prospective, single-arm, multicenter study to assess the efficacy and safety of ultrasound-facilitated, catheter-directed, low-dose fibrinolysis to reverse RV dysfunction in a total of 150 subjects with CT-confirmed PE, symptoms for 14 days or less, and an RV-to-LV diameter ratio of at least 0.9.[23] Ultrasound-facilitated, catheter-directed, low-dose fibrinolysis decreased RV-to-LV diameter ratio (1.55 vs 1.13, respectively; P<.0001), reduced pulmonary hypertension (51.4 mm Hg vs 36.9 mm Hg, respectively; P<.0001), decreased anatomic thrombus burden (modified Miller Index score, 22.5 vs 15.8, respectively; P<.0001), and minimized major bleeding complications (16 moderate and 1 major bleedings in 15 subjects) in subjects with acute massive and submassive PE.

Indirect evidence suggests a low major bleeding rate following ultrasound-assisted thrombolysis (rate of major bleeding complications 3.6%, 95% CI 1.4%–7.2%) compared with full-dose systemic thrombolytic therapy[24]; however, this is likely higher than that seen with anticoagulation alone. Clinical outcome studies are warranted to confirm a favorable risk-to-benefit ratio.

CDT has several variants (**Table 3**). The balance of the available (published) data suggests that ultrasound-assisted thrombolysis does not increase thrombolytic efficacy when added to traditional CDT, and does not reduce the thrombolytic dose or shorten infusion times.[25,26]

Ongoing Studies

The Optimum Duration of Acoustic Pulse Thrombolysis Procedure in Acute Pulmonary Embolism (OPTALYSE PE) is yet to be published but included 101 subjects with acute proximal PE at 17 centers randomized to 1 of 4 cohorts (NCT02396758). All subjects received therapeutic anticoagulation along with ultrasound-assisted CDT. The first cohort received 4 mg of TPA over 2 hours. The second cohort received 4 mg of TPA over 4 hours. The third cohort received 6 mg of TPA over 6 hours. The fourth cohort received 12 mg of TPA over 6 hours. Preliminary results show that all cohorts saw a significant reduction in the main indicator of right heart strain from PE by approximately 23% to 26%, with a very low bleeding rate of 3%.

DS-1040B is an inhibitor of the activated form of thrombin-activatable fibrinolysis inhibitor (TAFIa). In a thrombus, TAFIa removes lysine residues at the carboxyterminal of fibrin degradation

Table 3
Catheter-directed therapies

Technique	Description
Thrombolysis	Catheter in main PA, thrombolytic infused Often combined with mechanical or ultrasound fragmentation to increase surface area of thrombus exposed to thrombolytic
Fragmentation	Breaking up large, central clot with catheter device (device rotated by operator) Fragments migrate distally Often combined with local thrombolysis
Embolectomy	Catheter directed to thrombus and manual suction used to remove thrombus
Balloon angioplasty	Compression of embolus Often combined with local thrombolysis
Percutaneous thrombectomy	Clot pulverized and removed via catheter by rotation of device or hydrodynamic vortex

Abbreviation: PA, pulmonary artery.

products, which prevents effective binding of plasminogen and TPA, resulting in impaired thrombolysis.[27] A phase 1b, double-blind, placebo-controlled, randomized, single-ascending dose, multicenter study is assessing the safety, efficacy, tolerability, pharmacokinetics, and pharmacodynamics of DS-1040B in subjects with acute intermediate risk PE (NCT02923115).

The Recombinant Human Prourokinase to Treat Acute Pulmonary Embolism (ERUPTE) trial will randomize subjects with a high risk (massive) or intermediate risk (submassive PE) to low-dose (40 mg) recombinant human prourokinase or to alteplase (100 mg if weight ≥65 kg, 1.5 mg/kg if weight <65 kg) (NCT03108833). The primary outcome will be the change in the CT-assessed Qanadli score from baseline to 48 hours.

The primary aim of the Efficacy and Safety of Half Dose Alteplase Added to Heparin in Patients with Moderate Pulmonary Embolism (MONALYSE) open-label trial is to evaluate whether a mid-dose (safe dose) of alteplase, in addition to standard treatment with LMWH, is effective to reduce RV dysfunction, pulmonary hypertension, and

recurrent PE within the first 7 and 30 days after randomization of subjects with intermediate-risk PE (NCT02604238).

Close Monitoring of Intermediate-Risk Pulmonary Embolism

Patients with intermediate-risk PE could benefit from monitoring for deterioration. An important finding of the PEITHO trial was that rescue thrombolytic therapy appeared to be of benefit in patients who developed cardiovascular collapse after initially being treated with anticoagulant therapy alone. Of the 499 subjects who received placebo in this trial, 25 (5.0%) experienced hemodynamic decompensation 1.79 plus or minus 1.60 days after randomization. Persistent hypotension or a drop in blood pressure was recorded in 18 subjects, vasopressors were administered to 14 subjects, and 5 subjects in the placebo group required cardiopulmonary resuscitation. Twenty-three of these subjects received open-label thrombolysis and only 2 of them died (success of rescue thrombolysis, 91%).

Pulmonary Embolism Response Teams

Given the relative frequency of PE and the complexity of decision-making for advanced therapies for PE, including for those with intermediate-risk PE, multiple groups have recently developed PE response teams (PERTs)[28] that coordinate management and interventions for these critical and complicated patients. A recent study showed that 91% of the PERT activations in the Weill Cornell Medical College came from subjects with submassive (intermediate-risk) PE.[28] Future studies will address whether PERTs improve clinical outcomes and are cost-effective.

ADDITIONAL OR ALTERNATIVE TREATMENT STRATEGIES

Additional treatment strategies for patients with acute PE may include use of inferior vena cava (IVC) filters.[29] The overall body of evidence for the efficacy and safety of IVC filters for prevention of PE is slim.[30] Temporary use of IVC filters in patients receiving thrombolytic therapy appears interesting but is not yet supported by solid data. Such treatment should not be used in unselected patients with intermediate-risk PE. It might, however, be considered in a minority of high-risk patients on a case-by-case basis after multidisciplinary discussions (see previous discussion of PERTs).

The inflammatory response associated with acute PE contributes to the development of RV dysfunction.[31–33] Nonsteroidal antiinflammatory drugs might facilitate the reversal of PE-associated RV dysfunction.[34] Jimenez and colleagues[35] randomly assigned 34 normotensive subjects who had acute PE associated with echocardiographic RV dysfunction and normal systemic blood pressure to receive intravenous diclofenac (2 doses of 75 mg in the first 24 hours after diagnosis) or intravenous placebo. All subjects received standard anticoagulation with subcutaneous LMWH and an oral vitamin K antagonist. The study stopped prematurely due to slow recruitment. The intention-to-treat analysis showed persistent RV dysfunction at 48 hours in 59% (95% CI 33%–82%) of the diclofenac group and in 76% (95% CI 50%–93%) of the placebo group, a difference that did not reach statistical significance. Similar proportions (35%) of subjects in the diclofenac and placebo groups had persistent RV dysfunction at 7 days. Major bleeding occurred in none of subjects in the diclofenac group and in 5.9% of subject in the placebo group.

Interest has arisen in use of pulmonary arterial vasodilators (eg, inhaled nitric oxide [NO], oral phosphodiesterase inhibitors) in the treatment of acute PE.[36,37] Vasodilator drugs could affect hypoxic vasoconstriction, platelet activation, and release of vasoactive mediators (eg, endothelin thromboxane). Theoretically, vasodilator treatment would lower the pulmonary artery pressure and unload the RV. Because PE causes acute RV overload by both mechanical obstruction and pulmonary vasospasm, Kline and colleagues[38] tested if adjunctive inhaled NO gas would improve RV function and viability in acute PE (NCT 01939301). They conducted a 4-hospital, randomized, double-blind, placebo-controlled trial. Seventy-eight eligible normotensive subjects with acute PE and RV dysfunction received either oxygen plus 50 parts per million nitrogen (placebo) or oxygen plus 50 parts per million NO for 24 hours. At 24 hours, 5 of the 38 (13%) subjects treated with placebo and 9 of the 38 (24%) subjects treated with NO reached the primary composite endpoint ($P = .375$), which required a normal RV on echocardiography and a plasma troponin T concentration less than 14 pg/mL. The secondary endpoint required a blood brain natriuretic peptide concentration less than 90 pg/mL and a Borg dyspnea score less than or equal to 2, and it was reached in 34% with placebo and 13% of the NO ($P = .11$) group.

REDEFINITION OF INTERMEDIATE-RISK PULMONARY EMBOLISM

Among PE patients without hypotension, it is still not possible to confidently identify those who will derive net benefit from thrombolytic therapy. One of the important findings of the PEITHO trial was that the combination of RV dysfunction and myocardial injury might be insufficient for identifying normotensive patients with acute PE at a high-risk for short-term PE-related complications (mortality rate within the first 30 days after randomization of 3.2% in the placebo group).[13] For this reason, several prognostic scoring systems (eg, PROTECT multimarker index, FAST score, and Bova score) exist for identification of patients with PE who have an intermediate risk to a high risk for short-term PE-related adverse events. The PROTECT study derived (n = 848) and validated (n = 529) a multimarker prognostication that consisted of a clinical prognostic rule (ie, simplified Pulmonary Embolism Severity Index, brain natriuretic peptide, cTnI, and complete compression ultrasound testing for concomitant DVT) for hemodynamically stable patients diagnosed with acute symptomatic PE in the emergency department.[39] A 30-day complicated course was defined as death from any cause, hemodynamic collapse (need for cardiopulmonary resuscitation, systolic blood pressure <90 mm Hg for at least 15 minutes, need for catecholamine administration, or need for thrombolysis) and/or adjudicated recurrent PE. The positive predictive value of the PROTECT score for the prediction of a complicated course was 25.8% (95% CI 10.4%–41.2%) in the derivation cohort and 21.2% (95% CI 9.0%–38.9%) in the validation cohort.

The FAST score includes heart-type fatty acid binding protein (H-FABP), heart rate, and syncope.[40] A prospective cohort study that enrolled 271 normotensive subjects with acute PE assessed the validity of the FAST score for accurately identifying intermediate-high PE subjects. In this study, a FAST score greater than or equal to 3 points had a positive predictive value of 22% (95% CI 14%–33%) for 30-day complications (ie, all-cause death or at least any of the following major complications: (1) need for administration of vasopressors to maintain adequate tissue perfusion and prevent or treat cardiogenic shock, (2) mechanical ventilation, or (3) cardiopulmonary resuscitation).

The Bova score consisted of a heart rate of 110 or more beats per minute, systolic blood pressure 90 to 100 mm Hg, RV dysfunction, and elevated cardiac troponin.[41] The model identified 3 stages (I, II, and III) with 30-day PE-related complication rates of 4.2%, 10.8%, and 29.2%, respectively. A recent study demonstrated that the Bova score shows good reproducibility and evidence of validity for identification of intermediate-risk to high-risk patients with acute symptomatic PE.[42]

A recent study compared the performance of a modified FAST score (ie, using high-sensitivity cTnT instead of H-FABP) and the Bova score for risk stratification of 388 consecutive normotensive subjects with acute symptomatic PE.[43] The primary endpoint was defined as PE-related death, need for mechanical ventilation, cardiopulmonary resuscitation, or the administration of vasopressors during the first month after the diagnosis of acute PE. Although the modified FAST score identified a significantly higher proportion of subjects (111 out of 388, 28.6%, 95% CI 24.2%–33.4%) in the intermediate-high class compared with the Bova score (63 out of 388, 16.2%, 95% CI 12.7%–20.3%), the positive predictive values regarding the primary endpoint were similar (FAST score, 19%, 95% CI 13%–27%; Bova score 19%, 95% CI 11%–30%). Ideally, future studies should enroll subjects with these refined criteria to determine the net benefit in select subgroups. In the interim, subgroup analyses of the published large trials (eg, PEITHO) or pooled subject-level analyses from these studies can clarify which of the existing scores provide better discrimination about intermediate-risk patients who derive benefit from thrombolytic therapy.

A PRACTICAL TREATMENT APPROACH

In hemodynamically stable patients with acute symptomatic PE, presence of syncope, tachycardia, mild hypotension (which remains ≥90 mm Hg), an increase in jugular venous pressure, severe respiratory insufficiency (arterial oxyhemoglobin saturation <90%), or early signs of shock (among others) may prompt the order of echocardiography and cardiac biomarkers of myocardial injury (ie, cTnI or cTnI) (**Fig. 1**). The authors suggest the use of echocardiography instead of CT to assess RV function in normotensive patients with acute symptomatic PE.[44] Patients who have myocardial injury and RV dysfunction should receive standard anticoagulation and be monitored for short-term deterioration, which might prompt activation of PERT for rapid and individualized care. In these patients, evidence of severe RV dysfunction and myocardial injury, accumulation of prognostic factors (eg, syncope,[40] concomitant DVT,[45] elevated lactate levels,[46] severe respiratory insufficiency) indicating poor prognosis from PE, or subtle hemodynamic changes (eg, increasing heart rate or persistent downtrend of systolic blood pressure) might alter the risk–benefit assessment in favor of thrombolytic therapy before the development of frank hemodynamic instability (**Table 4**). For patients who require thrombolytic therapy and do not have a high risk of bleeding, full-dose systemic thrombolytic therapy should be preferred over low-dose systemic thrombolytic therapy or CDT.

SUMMARY

Management of patients with intermediate-risk PE is complicated by the various definitions, paucity of data for certain interventions, and uncertain

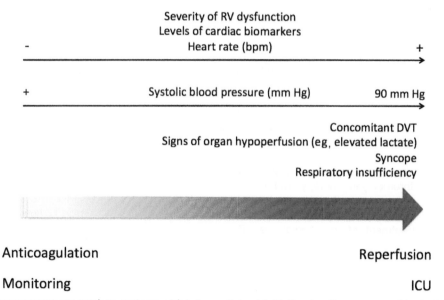

Fig. 1. A management approach to patients with intermediate-risk (defined as the presence of both RV dysfunction and myocardial injury) pulmonary embolism. Accumulation of factors indicating poor prognosis (*right side*) may alter the risk–benefit assessment in favor of thrombolytic therapy before the development of hemodynamic instability. bpm, beats per minute; ICU, intensive care unit.

Table 4
Pulmonary embolism markers of severity

	Markers (Study)	Comment
Clinical prognostic scores	PESI[47]	Identification of low-risk PE Validated in an RCT[48]
	Simplified PESI[49]	Identification of low-risk PE Not validated in an RCT
	Hestia criteria[50]	Identification of low-risk PE Validated in a management study[48]
	RIETE score[51]	Identification of low-risk PE Not validated in an RCT
	Bova score[41]	Identification of intermediate-risk PE Not validated in an RCT
	FAST score[40]	Identification of intermediate-risk PE Not validated in an RCT
RV enlargement or dysfunction	ECG[52] Echocardiogram[53] CT[54] BNP or NT-proBNP[55] Adrenomodullin[56]	Identification of intermediate-risk PE Limited usefulness, in isolation
Clot burden	Concomitant DVT[45] D-dimer[57] CT-assessed thrombus load[58]	Identification of intermediate-risk PE Limited usefulness, in isolation
Myocardial injury	cTnI or cTnT[59] hsTnT[60] H-FABP[61]	Identification of intermediate-risk PE Limited usefulness, in isolation
Kidney injury	Cystatin C[62]	Lacks large validation No well-defined role for identification of intermediate-risk PE
Organ hypoperfusion	Lactate[46] Copeptin[63]	Lacks large validation No well-defined role for identification of intermediate-risk PE

Abbreviations: BNP, brain natriuretic peptide; ECG, electrocardiogram; hsTnT, high-sensitivity troponin T; RIETE, Registro Informatizado de la Enfermedad Tromboembólica.

guideline recommendations. Although evidence suggests that most patients with intermediate-risk PE who receive standard anticoagulation and monitoring have an excellent short-term prognosis, the increased severity of vital signs and markers of RV dysfunction and myocardial injury, factors indicating poor prognosis from PE, or early deterioration on standard anticoagulation might alter the risk–benefit assessment in favor of thrombolytic therapy before the development of hemodynamic instability. PERTs may provide rapid multidisciplinary assessment and optimal treatment of intermediate-risk PE patients.

REFERENCES

1. Naess IA, Christiansen SC, Romundstad P, et al. Incidence and mortality of venous thrombosis: a population-based study. J Thromb Haemost 2007; 5:692–9.

2. Heit JA. The epidemiology of venous thromboembolism in the community. Arterioscler Thromb Vasc Biol 2008;28:370–2.

3. Jimenez D, de Miguel J, Guijarro R, et al. Trends in the management and outcomes of acute pulmonary embolism: analysis from the RIETE registry. J Am Coll Cardiol 2016;67:162–70.

4. Minges KE, Bikdeli B, Wang Y, et al. National trends in pulmonary embolism hospitalization rates and outcomes for adults aged ≥65 years in the United States (1999 to 2010). Am J Cardiol 2015;116:1436–42.

5. Konstantinides SV, Torbicki A, Agnelli G, et al, Authors/Task Force Members. 2014 ESC Guidelines on the diagnosis and management of acute pulmonary embolism: the task force for the diagnosis and management of acute pulmonary embolism of the European Society of Cardiology (ESC) endorsed by the European Respiratory Society (ERS). Eur Heart J 2014;35:3033–73.

6. Jaff MR, McMurtry MS, Archer SL, et al, American Heart Association Council on Cardiopulmonary,

Critical Care, Perioperative and Resuscitation; American Heart Association Council on Peripheral Vascular Disease; American Heart Association Council on Arteriosclerosis, Thrombosis and Vascular Biology. Management of massive and sub-massive pulmonary embolism, iliofemoral deep vein thrombosis and chronic thromboembolic pulmonary hypertension: a scientific statement from the American Heart Association. Circulation 2011;123: 1788–830.

7. Scridon I, Scridon C, Skali H, et al. Prognostic signif-icance of troponin elevation and right ventricular enlargement in acute pulmonary embolism. Am J Cardiol 2005;96:303–5.

8. Binder L, Pieske B, Olschewski M, et al. N-terminal pro-brain natriuretic peptide or troponin testing fol-lowed by echocardiography for risk stratification of acute pulmonary embolism. Circulation 2005;112: 1573–9.

9. Jiménez D, Aujesky D, Moores L, et al. Combina-tions of prognostic tools for identification of high-risk normotensive patients with acute symptomatic pulmonary embolism. Thorax 2011;66:75–81.

10. Kucher N, Wallmann D, Carone A, et al. Incremental prognostic value of troponin I and echocardiogra-phy in patients with acute pulmonary embolism. Eur Heart J 2003;24:1651–6.

11. Tapson VF. Thrombolytic therapy in acute pulmonary embolism. Curr Opin Cardiol 2012;27:585–91.

12. Kline JA, Nordenholz KE, Courtney DM, et al. Treat-ment of submassive pulmonary embolism with ten-ecteplase or placebo: cardiopulmonary outcomes at 3 months: multicenter double-blind, placebo-controlled randomized trial. J Thromb Haemost 2014;12:459–68.

13. Meyer JA, Vicaut E, Danays T, et al, PEITHO Inves-tigators. Fibrinolysis for patients with intermediate-risk pulmonary embolism. N Engl J Med 2014;370: 1402–11.

14. Marti C, John G, Konstantinides S, et al. Systemic thrombolytic therapy for acute pulmonary embolism: a systematic review and meta-analysis. Eur Heart J 2015;36:605–14.

15. Chatterjee S, Chakraborty A, Weinberg I, et al. Throm-bolysis for pulmonary embolism and risk of all-cause mortality, major bleeding, and intracranial hemor-rhage: a meta-analysis. JAMA 2014;311:2414–21.

16. Sharifi M, Bay C, Skrocki L, et al, "MOPETT" Investi-gators. Moderate pulmonary embolism treated with thrombolytics (from the 'MOPETT' trial). Am J Cardiol 2013;111:273–7.

17. Goldhaber SZ, Agnelli G, Levine MN. Reduced dose bolus alteplase vs conventional alteplase infusion for pulmonary embolism thrombolysis. An interna-tional multicenter randomized trial. The Bolus Alte-plase Pulmonary Embolism Group. Chest 1994; 106:718–24.

18. Sors H, Pacouret G, Azarian R, et al. Hemodynamic effects of bolus vs 2-h infusion of alteplase in acute massive pulmonary embolism. A randomized controlled multicenter trial. Chest 1994;106:712–7.

19. Wang C, Zhai Z, Yang Y, et al. China Venous Throm-boembolism (VTE) Study Group. Efficacy and safety of low dose recombinant tissue-type plasminogen activator for the treatment of acute pulmonary throm-boembolism: a randomized, multicenter, controlled trial. Chest 2010;137:254–62.

20. Abdelsamad AA, El-Morsi AS, Mansour AE. Efficacy and safety of high dose versus low dose streptokinase for treatment of submassive pul-monary embolism. Egypt Heart J 2011;63:67–72.

21. Jimenez D, Martin-Saborido C, Muriel A, et al. Effi-cacy and safety outcomes of recanalization proced-ures in patients with acute symptomatic pulmonary embolism: systematic review and network meta-analysis. Thorax 2018;73(5):464–71.

22. Kucher N, Boekstegers P, Muller OJ, et al. Randomized, controlled trial of ultrasound-assisted catheter-directed thrombolysis for acute intermediate-risk pulmonary embolism. Circulation 2014;129:479–86.

23. Piazza G, Hohlfelder B, Jaff MR, et al. A prospective, single-arm, multicenter trial of ultrasound-facilitated, catheter-directed, low-dose fibrinolysis for acute massive and submassive pulmonary embolism: the SEATTLE II Study. JACC Cardiovasc Interv 2015;8: 1382–92.

24. Engelberger RP, Kucher N. Ultrasound-assisted thrombolysis for acute pulmonary embolism: a systematic review. Eur Heart J 2014;35:758–64.

25. Engelberger RP, Spirk D, Willenberg T, et al. Ultra-sound-assisted versus conventional catheter-directed thrombolysis for acute iliofemoral deep vein thrombosis. Circ Cardiovasc Interv 2015;8 [pii: e002027].

26. Liang NL, Avgerinos ED, Marone LK, et al. Equivalent outcomes between ultrasound-assisted thrombolysis and standard catheter-directed thrombolysis for the treatment of acute pulmonary embolism. J Vasc Surg Venous Lymphat Disord 2015;3:120–1.

27. DS-1040b Global Investigator's Brochure Version 4.0, 2016.

28. Sista AK, Friedman OA, Dou E, et al. A Pulmonary Em-bolism Response Team's initial 20 month experience treating 87 patients with submassive and massive pul-monary embolism. Vasc Med 2017. https://doi.org/10.1177/1358863X17730430. 1358863X17730430.

29. Bikdeli B, Bikdeli B. Updates on advanced therapies for acute pulmonary embolism. Int J Cardiovasc Pract 2016;1:47–50.

30. Bikdeli B, Chatterjee S, Desai N, et al. Inferior vena caval filters to prevent pulmonary embolism: systematic review and meta-analysis of efficacy and safety. J Am Coll Cardiol 2017;70:1587–97.

31. Watts JA, Gellar MA, Obraztsova M, et al. Role of inflammation in right ventricular damage and repair following experimental pulmonary embolism in rats. Int J Exp Pathol 2008;89:389–99.

32. Watts JA, Zagorski J, Gellar MA, et al. Cardiac inflammation contributes to right ventricular dysfunction following experimental pulmonary embolism in rats. J Mol Cell Cardiol 2006;41:296–307.

33. Watts J, Marchick MR, Kline JA. Right ventricular heart failure from pulmonary embolism: key distinctions from chronic pulmonary hypertension. J Card Fail 2010;16:250–9.

34. Watts JA, Gellar MA, Stuart LK, et al. Proinflammatory events in right ventricular damage during pulmonary embolism: effects of treatment with ketorolac in rats. J Cardiovasc Pharmacol 2009;54:246–52.

35. Jimenez D, Nieto R, Corres J, et al. Diclofenac for reversal of right ventricular dysfunction in acute normotensive pulmonary embolism: a pilot study. Thromb Res 2017;162:1–6.

36. Capellier G, Jacques T, Balvay P, et al. Inhaled nitric oxide in patients with pulmonary embolism. Intensive Care Med 1997;23:1089–92.

37. Szold O, Khoury W, Biderman P, et al. Inhaled nitric oxide improves pulmonary functions following massive pulmonary embolism: a report of four patients and review of the literature. Lung 2006;184:1–5.

38. Kline JA, Hall CL, Jones AE, et al. Randomized trial of inhaled nitric oxide to treat acute pulmonary embolism: the iNOPE trial. Am Heart J 2017;186:100–10.

39. Jimenez D, Kopecna D, Tapson V, et al, on behalf of the PROTECT investigators. Derivation and validation of multimarker prognostication for normotensive patients with acute symptomatic pulmonary embolism. Am J Respir Crit Care Med 2014;189:718–26.

40. Dellas C, Tschepe M, Seeber V, et al. A novel H-FABP and fast prognostic score for risk assessment of normotensive pulmonary embolism. Thromb Haemost 2014;111:996–1003.

41. Bova C, Sanchez O, Prandoni P, et al. Identification of intermediate-risk patients with acute symptomatic pulmonary embolism. Eur Respir J 2014;44:694–703.

42. Fernandez C, Bova C, Sanchez O, et al. Validation of a model for identification of patients at intermediate to high risk for complications associated with acute symptomatic pulmonary embolism. Chest 2015;148:211–8.

43. Hobhom L, Hellenkamp K, Hasenfuß G, et al. Comparison of risk assessment strategies for not-high-risk pulmonary embolism. Eur Respir J 2016;47:1170–8.

44. Barrios D, Morillo R, Lobo JL, et al, PROTECT Investigators. Assessment of right ventricular function in acute pulmonary embolism. Am Heart J 2017;185:123–9.

45. Jiménez D, Aujesky D, Díaz G, et al, RIETE Investigators. Prognostic significance of deep vein thrombosis in patients presenting with acute symptomatic pulmonary embolism. Am J Respir Crit Care Med 2010;181:983–91.

46. Vanni S, Nazerian P, Bova C, et al. Comparison of clinical scores for identification of patients with pulmonary embolism at intermediate-high risk of adverse clinical outcome: the prognostic role of plasma lactate. Intern Emerg Med 2017;12:657–65.

47. Aujesky D, Obrosky DS, Stone RA, et al. Derivation and validation of a prognostic model for pulmonary embolism. Am J Respir Crit Care Med 2005;172:1041–6.

48. Aujesky D, Roy PM, Verschuren F, et al. Outpatient versus inpatient treatment for patients with acute pulmonary embolism: an international, open-label, randomised, non-inferiority trial. Lancet 2011;378:41–8.

49. Jiménez D, Aujesky D, Moores L, et al, RIETE Investigators. Simplification of the Pulmonary Embolism Severity Index for prognostication in patients with acute symptomatic pulmonary embolism. Arch Intern Med 2010;170:1383–9.

50. Zondag W, Mos IC, Creemers-Schild D, et al, Hestia Study Investigators. Outpatient treatment in patients with acute pulmonary embolism: the Hestia study. J Thromb Haemost 2011;9:1500–7.

51. Maestre A, Trujillo-Santos J, Riera-Mestre A, et al, RIETE Investigators. Identification of low-risk patients with acute symptomatic pulmonary embolism for outpatient therapy. Ann Am Thorac Soc 2015;12:1122–9.

52. Qaddoura A, Digby GC, Kabali C, et al. The value of electrocardiography in prognosticating clinical deterioration and mortality in acute pulmonary embolism: a systematic review and meta-analysis. Clin Cardiol 2017. https://doi.org/10.1002/clc.22742.

53. Sanchez O, Trinquart L, Colombet I, et al. Prognostic value of right ventricular dysfunction in patients with hemodynamically stable pulmonary embolism: a systematic review. Eur Heart J 2008;29:1569–77.

54. Trujillo-Santos J, den Exter PL, Gomez V, et al. Computed tomography-assessed right ventricular dysfunction and risk stratification of patients with acute non-massive pulmonary embolism: systematic review and meta-analysis. J Thromb Haemost 2013;11:1823–32.

55. Pieralli F, Olivotto I, Vanni S, et al. Usefulness of bedside testing for brain natriuretic peptide to identify right ventricular dysfunction and outcome in normotensive patients with acute pulmonary embolism. Am J Cardiol 2006;97:1386–90.

56. Pedowska-Włoszek J, Kostrubiec M, Kurnicka K, et al. Midregional proadrenomedullin (MR-proADM)

in the risk stratification of patients with acute pulmonary embolism. Thromb Res 2013;132: 506–10.

57. Lobo JL, Zorrilla V, Aizpuru F, et al, RIETE Investigators. D-dimer levels and 15-day outcome in acute pulmonary embolism. Findings from the RIETE Registry. J Thromb Haemost 2009;7: 1795–801.

58. Furlan A, Aghayev A, Chang CC, et al. Short-term mortality in acute pulmonary embolism: clot burden and signs of right heart dysfunction at CT pulmonary angiography. Radiology 2012;265:283–93.

59. Becattini C, Vedovati MC, Agnelli G. Prognostic value of troponins in acute pulmonary embolism: a meta-analysis. Circulation 2007;116:427–33.

60. Lankeit M, Jiménez D, Kostrubiec M, et al. Predictive value of the high-sensitivity troponin T assay and the simplified Pulmonary Embolism Severity Index in hemodynamically stable patients with acute pulmonary embolism: a prospective validation study. Circulation 2011;124:2716–24.

61. Bajaj A, Rathor P, Sehgal V, et al. Risk stratification in acute pulmonary embolism with heart-type fatty acid-binding protein: a meta-analysis. J Crit Care 2015;30:1151.e1-7.

62. Kostrubiec M, Łabyk A, Pedowska-Włoszek J, et al. Neutrophil gelatinase-associated lipocalin, cystatin C and eGFR indicate acute kidney injury and predict prognosis of patients with acute pulmonary embolism. Heart 2012;98:1221–8.

63. Hellenkamp K, Schwung J, Rossmann H, et al. Risk stratification of normotensive pulmonary embolism: prognostic impact of copeptin. Eur Respir J 2015; 46:1701–10.

An Update on the "Novel" and Direct Oral Anticoagulants, and Long-Term Anticoagulant Therapy

Mia Djulbegovic, MD[a], Alfred Ian Lee, MD, PhD[b],*

KEYWORDS

- Venous thromboembolism • Direct oral anticoagulant (DOAC) • P-glycoprotein transport • CYP3A4
- Idarucizumab • Thrombin time • Anti-Xa level • Andexanet-alfa

KEY POINTS

- For treatment of acute venous thromboembolism, direct oral anticoagulants are comparable to vitamin K antagonists in efficacy and have similar or improved bleeding profiles.
- For secondary venous thromboembolism prevention, extended anticoagulation with direct oral anticoagulants at full or reduced dosing is safe and effective.
- The utility of direct oral anticoagulants in certain patient populations, such as geriatric patients, or those with renal impairment, antiphospholipid syndrome, bariatric surgery, or cancer-associated thrombosis, is uncertain.
- A variety of laboratory tests are available to monitor direct oral anticoagulant activity.
- In patients on direct oral anticoagulants who experience major bleeding, various interventions, including specific drug antidotes, can be used.

INTRODUCTION

Venous thromboembolism (VTE), encompassing deep venous thrombosis and pulmonary embolism, is a common cause of morbidity and mortality and also recurs frequently. Annually, up to 1 in 120 people develop VTE, approximating the incidence of stroke.[1] The mainstay of VTE treatment is anticoagulation. Direct oral anticoagulants (DOAC), low-molecular-weight heparins (LMWH), fondaparinux, and vitamin K antagonists (VKA) are all reasonable treatment options with comparable efficacy and favorable bleeding risk profiles. Guidelines from the American College of Chest Physicians (ACCP) recommend DOACs over VKAs, and VKAs over LMWH, in hemodynamically stable patients without active cancer.[2] In real-world practice, however, such decisions must be tailored on an individual patient basis because different clinical scenarios will guide the use of different anticoagulants.[3]

Patients who present with VTE in the setting of a reversible thrombotic risk factor are generally anticoagulated for no more than 3 months because of a low risk of VTE recurrence thereafter (Fig. 1).[2,4] For patients with unprovoked VTE occurring in the absence of an identifiable thrombotic risk factor, the duration of anticoagulation varies, and the decision-making process can be complex.[5] In this article, the authors provide an evidence-based

Disclosure Statement: The authors have no disclosures.
[a] Traditional Internal Medicine Residency Program, Department of Internal Medicine, Yale School of Medicine, 333 Cedar Street, New Haven, CT 06520, USA; [b] Section of Hematology, Department of Internal Medicine, Yale School of Medicine, 333 Cedar Street, New Haven, CT 06520, USA
* Corresponding author.
E-mail address: alfred.lee@yale.edu

Clin Chest Med 39 (2018) 583–593
https://doi.org/10.1016/j.ccm.2018.04.010
0272-5231/18/© 2018 Elsevier Inc. All rights reserved.

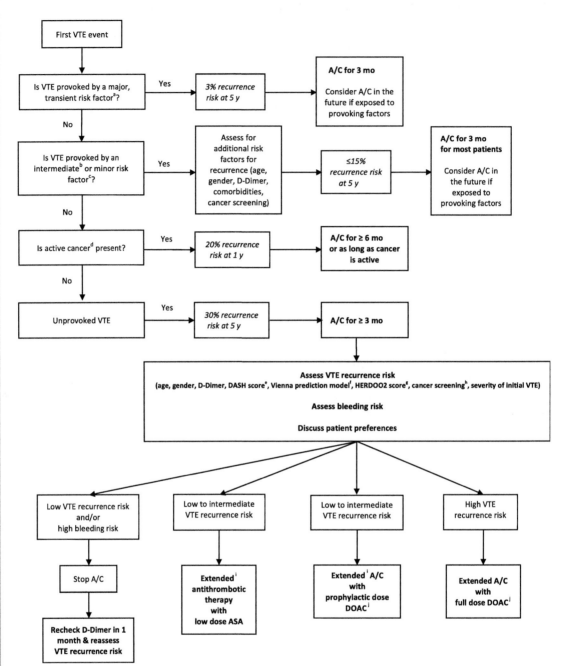

Fig. 1. Algorithm to determine duration of anticoagulation after a first VTE event. The rationale for this approach is based on the risk of recurrence after discontinuation of anticoagulation (italicized text boxes). This algorithm applies for most patients but should not replace clinical judgment. Patient preferences, comorbidities, and bleeding risk should also be incorporated into any decision regarding anticoagulation. A/C, anticoagulation; ASA, aspirin. [a] Major, transient risk factors include surgery, trauma, or prolonged immobilization. [b] Intermediate, transient risk factors include pregnancy, the postpartum state, and use of hormone replacement (estrogen or testosterone) or oral contraceptives. [c] Minor, transient risk factors include prolonged travel >4 hours or bed rest >3 days. [d] Active cancer includes untreated or relapsed malignancy, or recent treatment for malignancy. [e] DASH score includes D-dimer (measured after discontinuing anticoagulation), age, sex, and hormone exposure. [f] Vienna prediction model includes gender, location of the first VTE event, and D-dimer (measured after discontinuing anticoagulation). [g] HERDOO2 score incorporates hyperpigmentation, edema, leg redness, D-dimer (measured while on anticoagulation), obesity, and older age. [h] Cancer screening in VTE includes an expanded age-appropriate cancer screening consisting of mammography and Papanicolaou smears in women, prostate

approach to the use of DOACs in VTE, focusing on acute VTE and secondary VTE prevention. They also discuss the use of DOACs in specialized VTE populations, therapeutic monitoring, and the development and use of antidotes for major bleeding.

OVERVIEW OF DIRECT ORAL ANTICOAGULANTS

The DOACs include the factor Xa inhibitors apixaban, betrixaban, edoxaban, and rivaroxaban, and the direct thrombin inhibitor dabigatran. Apixaban, dabigatran, edoxaban, and rivaroxaban are all used in acute VTE and prevention of VTE after orthopedic surgery. Betrixaban is used for prevention of VTE in hospitalized patients and is not discussed further in this review.[6] A summary of the available DOACs used in acute VTE and secondary VTE prevention, their dosing regimens, pharmacokinetics, and other clinical pearls is provided in **Table 1**.

In general, the bleeding risks of DOACs are similar to or better than VKA.[3,7–10] DOACs are associated with less intracranial hemorrhage than VKA.[9,11] The risk of gastrointestinal bleeding (GIB) appears to be similar when all DOACs together are compared with VKA, although individually, dabigatran and rivaroxaban may carry higher risks of GIB than warfarin.[3,12] An increase in GIB among elderly patients has been specifically reported for dabigatran versus other DOACs or VKA.[13]

DOACs have fewer drug-drug interactions (DDI) than VKAs. The most important DDIs are between DOACs and agents that affect P-glycoprotein (P-gp) transport because of the dependence of DOACs on P-gp-mediated intestinal absorption. In addition, rivaroxaban and apixaban are partially metabolized by CYP3A4, so agents that affect the activity of this enzyme may alter levels of these specific DOACs. A short list of common medications that affect P-gp or CYP3A4 activity is included in the legend of **Table 1**.

The half-lives of the different DOACs are short compared with VKA, with rivaroxaban demonstrating the shortest half-life (5–9 hours). Clearance of DOACs is dependent in part on renal function. In patients with significant renal impairment, some clinicians favor apixaban over other DOACs because renal elimination may be lower with this agent.[14] However, large-scale studies of the different DOACs in VTE patients with severe renal impairment have not been conducted, so the true efficacy and safety of these agents in advanced or end-stage renal disease are unknown. Interestingly, in studies of atrial fibrillation, efficacy of edoxaban is decreased in patients with very high creatinine clearance (CrCl),[15] although this has not been specifically reported for VTE.

OVERVIEW OF ANTICOAGULATION IN VENOUS THROMBOEMBOLISM

An algorithm for determining the overall anticoagulation plan in VTE patients is shown in **Fig. 1**. For patients with a provoked VTE due to a major, reversible thrombotic risk factor (eg, surgery, trauma, or prolonged immobilization), the risk of VTE recurrence is sufficiently low that anticoagulation is usually stopped after 3 months. For patients with VTE due to an intermediate or minor thrombotic risk factor (eg, pregnancy, exogenous estrogen exposure, prolonged travel, or bed rest), the risk of VTE recurrence, although higher than for VTE due to a major thrombotic risk factor, is still low, such that 3 months of anticoagulation are generally advised, pending an assessment of additional risk factors for VTE recurrence. Patients with cancer-associated VTE usually continue anticoagulation for at least 6 months or as long as their cancer is active owing to a very high risk of VTE recurrence in the setting of active malignancy.

For patients with unprovoked VTE, at least 3 months of anticoagulation are advised. A comprehensive assessment of additional risk factors for VTE recurrence should be performed, taking into account patient age, gender, D-dimer levels (typically measured after discontinuation of anticoagulation), cancer screening, the severity of the initial VTE event, and other patient comorbidities, in addition to patient preference and bleeding risk (see **Fig. 1**). The results of this assessment are used to determine whether to stop anticoagulation entirely, transition to a reduced form of extended antithrombotic therapy (eg, with low-dose aspirin[16,17] or a low-dose DOAC[18–21]), or continue with full-dose anticoagulation.

DIRECT ORAL ANTICOAGULANTS IN ACUTE VENOUS THROMBOEMBOLISM

Four major randomized clinical trials showed similar efficacies for each of the individual DOACs

---

cancer screening in men, and colorectal cancer screening, as well as symptom-directed evaluations for occult malignancy. [i] Extended anticoagulation refers to long-term, or indefinite, anticoagulation (ie, with no scheduled stop date). [j] Relative contraindications to DOACs include (but are not limited to) hemodynamic instability, active cancer, antiphospholipid syndrome, and end-stage renal disease (although pharmacokinetic studies suggest that prophylactic dose apixaban might be safe in the latter).

Table 1
General properties of direct oral anticoagulants

	Apixaban	Dabigatran	Edoxaban	Rivaroxaban
Target	Xa	IIa (Thrombin)	Xa	Xa
Acute VTE dosing	10 mg BID × 7 d, then 5 mg BID	150 mg BID (start after 5–10 d of parenteral anticoagulation)	60 mg QD (start after 5–10 d of parenteral anticoagulation)	15 mg BID × 21 d, then 20 mg QD
Extended anticoagulation dosing	5 mg BID (full dose) or 2.5 mg BID (prophylactic dose)	150 mg BID	60 mg QD	20 mg QD (full dose) or 10 mg QD (prophylactic dose)
Renal dosing	Consider dose reduction to 2.5 mg BID if CrCl <25 (based on expert opinion, not empirically studied) Preferred DOAC in ESRD requiring HD (based on expert opinion, not empirically studied)	Avoid if CrCl ≤30 mL/min (not empirically studied) Avoid coadministration of P-gp inhibitor if CrCl is 30–50 mL/min	Contraindicated if CrCl >95 mL/min (reduced efficacy) 30 mg QD if CrCl is between 15 and 50 mL/min	Avoid if CrCl ≤30 mL/min
Geriatric dosing	No dose adjustment	No dose adjustment mandated, but extreme caution is advised in patients of age ≥75 y (increased bleeding risk)	No dose adjustment	In older adults with CrCl 30–50 mL/min, consider dose reduction (specific dose adjustment not provided)
Administration	Without regard to meals	Without regard to meals	Without regard to meals	Administer 20-mg dose with meals Administer 10-mg dose without regard to meals

Half-life	12 h	12–17 h	10–14 h	5–9 h
Drug-drug interactions	P-gp inducers may decrease apixaban concentration P-gp inhibitors may increase apixaban concentration CYP3A4 inducers may decrease apixaban concentration CYP3A4 inhibitors may increase apixaban concentration	P-gp inducers may decrease dabigatran concentration P-gp inhibitors may increase dabigatran concentration PPIs decrease dabigatran absorption and plasma level by 30%–40%	P-gp inducers may decrease edoxaban concentration P-gp inhibitors may increase edoxaban concentration	P-gp inducers may decrease rivaroxaban concentration P-gp inhibitors may increase rivaroxaban concentration CYP3A4 inducers may decrease rivaroxaban concentration CYP3A4 inhibitors may increase rivaroxaban concentration
Bleeding risk	May have lower bleeding risk than other DOACs	Greater GIB risk compared with VKA and other DOACs, particularly in elderly patients	Comparable to other DOACs	May have greater GIB risk compared with VKA
Side effects		Dyspepsia, gastritis (35%)		
Reversal agent	Andexanet (not yet approved)	Idarucizumab	Andexanet (not yet approved)	Andexanet (not yet approved)

Abbreviations: BID, twice daily; ESRD, end-stage renal disease; QD, once daily.
Lexicomp Online, Hudson, Ohio; Wolters Kluwer Clinical Drug Information; used for pharmacokinetic data (2018).

compared with VKA in reducing the risk of recurrent VTE after an acute VTE event.[22–25] For acute VTE treatment, all DOACs require some form of a loading dose (see **Table 1**). Rivaroxaban and apixaban each use 1 to 3 weeks of high-intensity dosing upfront (for rivaroxaban, 15 mg twice daily × 3 weeks, then 20 mg once daily; for apixaban, 10 mg twice daily × 1 week, then 5 mg twice daily). Use of dabigatran and edoxaban should be preceded by 5 to 10 days of parenteral anticoagulation in the form of heparin or LMWH.

The efficacy and safety data of DOACs coupled with their ease of use have prompted many clinicians and some consensus groups (eg, ACCP) to favor DOACs over VKA for treatment of acute VTE in patients who do not have cancer or other absolute or relative contraindications to their use.[2,3,7–9,26] A small amount of early data also suggests that medication adherence and/or persistence may be improved with some DOACs compared with VKA.[27] However, the utility of DOACs in several specialized VTE populations is uncertain, and in many situations, other anticoagulants may be favored (see later discussion).

DIRECT ORAL ANTICOAGULANTS IN SECONDARY VENOUS THROMBOEMBOLISM PREVENTION

For patients with a high risk of recurrent VTE who are candidates for extended anticoagulation, there are several treatment options (see **Fig. 1**). Two major studies evaluated the use of low-dose aspirin 100 mg once daily for secondary VTE prevention[16,17]; one demonstrated a mild reduction in recurrent VTE, whereas the other showed no change in recurrent VTE but a favorable benefit in overall cardiovascular outcomes. A few older studies compared low-dose versus full-dose warfarin (targeting an international normalized ratio [INR] of 1.5–2 or 2–3, respectively) in extended thromboprophylaxis, with somewhat divergent results.[28,29]

The current body of evidence suggests that for nonpregnant adults without active cancer, DOACs at either full or prophylactic dose are likely the best option for secondary VTE prevention. In separate randomized clinical trials of secondary VTE prophylaxis, each of which compared a DOAC at full or reduced dosing (apixaban 2.5 mg twice daily, dabigatran 150 mg twice daily, rivaroxaban 10 mg once daily) with various permutations of VKA, low-dose aspirin, and/or placebo, DOACs were as effective as VKA and more effective than aspirin in reducing the risk of recurrent VTE, with bleeding risks comparable to low-dose aspirin and lower than VKA.[18–21] Standard and network meta-analyses support these observations and

suggest that the different DOACs may be interchangeable in this regard.[26,30] A post hoc analysis of patients enrolled on the Hokusai-VTE study comparing edoxaban to VKA for acute VTE suggested that extended thromboprophylaxis with edoxaban may also be effective.[19]

Based on these data, for patients with unprovoked VTE who warrant extended antithrombotic therapy but are deemed to have a low risk of VTE recurrence, low-dose aspirin may be appropriate (see **Fig. 1**). For patients with an intermediate risk of VTE recurrence, dose-reduced apixaban (2.5 mg twice daily) or dose-reduced rivaroxaban (10 mg once daily) is acceptable. For patients with a high risk of VTE recurrence, continuation of full-dose anticoagulation is recommended.

DIRECT ORAL ANTICOAGULANTS IN SPECIAL POPULATIONS

Certain patient populations were excluded from the original randomized controlled trials of DOACs. The appropriateness of DOACs in these types of patients is therefore uncertain.

- *Renal insufficiency*: Patients with severe renal impairment (CrCl <25–30 mL/min) were excluded from all of the major trials of DOACs in VTE. For VTE patients with modest renal impairment (CrCl 30–50 mL/min), meta-analyses suggest that efficacy and bleeding risks of apixaban, dabigatran, and rivaroxaban are similar to VKA and other anticoagulants.[31,32] Apixaban may have lower renal clearance than other DOACs[14] and is often preferred by clinicians in patients with modest renal impairment, although clinical data in support of this are lacking. Pharmacokinetic studies in atrial fibrillation suggest that apixaban may also be used in dialysis, although the numbers of patients in those studies were small.[33,34] Recommended doses of the different DOACs in patients with renal impairment are listed in **Table 1**.
- *Geriatrics*: A meta-analysis of elderly patients (aged ≥75) with VTE on clinical trials of apixaban, dabigatran, edoxaban, or rivaroxaban showed similar efficacy and bleeding risks of these agents compared with VKA, although GIB risk was higher with dabigatran.[13] No specific dose adjustments are recommended for any of the DOACs in treatment of geriatric patients with VTE, although extreme caution is advised with dabigatran in the elderly (see **Table 1**).
- *Antiphospholipid syndrome (APS)*: Warfarin is widely accepted as the standard of care in

APS.[35] A randomized controlled trial, the RAPS (rivaroxaban in APS) study, compared rivaroxaban with warfarin in APS patients and found similar rates of thrombosis.[36] However, most patients in the RAPS study were lower-risk patients with "single-positive" disease (ie, positive for only one of the 3 antiphospholipid antibody tests of lupus anticoagulant, anticardiolipin antibodies, or beta-2 glycoprotein-1 antibodies), and biochemical markers of coagulation activity differed somewhat from clinical outcomes.[37] Hence, at present, DOACs are not generally advised in APS except in select patients with single-positive disease.

- *Thrombophilia*: Some, but not all, of the major clinical trials of DOACs in acute VTE and secondary VTE prevention excluded patients with known heritable thrombophilias. In the studies that did not exclude such patients, heritable thrombophilias were found in only a small percentage of the study populations. Because of this, some clinicians avoid using DOACs in patients with certain heritable thrombophilias, although most investigators think that they are safe for use in such patients based on collective experience and case reports.[38]
- *Obesity*: About 15% to 30% of patients on the major clinical trials of DOACs in VTE were obese. Efficacy and safety outcomes in these studies appeared to be largely independent of body mass, although other pharmacokinetic studies reported reduced drug concentrations for at least some of the DOACs in obese patients.[39] Guidelines from the International Society of Thrombosis and Haemostasis advise against the use of DOACs in patients weighing greater than 120 kg or with a body mass index of greater than 40 kg/m^2 unless peak and trough drug levels can be measured for confirmation.
- *Bariatric surgery*: Apixaban is absorbed in the small intestine, dabigatran in the lower stomach and duodenum, edoxaban in the proximal small intestine, and rivaroxaban in the stomach.[40] Bariatric surgery would therefore be expected to alter DOAC drug levels, although data about this are limited. Pharmacokinetic studies suggest reduced absorption specifically of rivaroxaban after sleeve gastrectomy or gastric banding,[41] but efficacy and safety studies are lacking. At present, most investigators avoid using DOACs in patients who have undergone bariatric surgery unless peak and trough drug levels can be measured.
- *Cancer-associated VTE*: LMWH has been widely accepted as the standard of care in patients with VTE due to cancer, based on the seminal CLOT trial, which showed a reduction in recurrent VTE in cancer-VTE patients treated with dalteparin rather than VKA.[42] A small percentage of patients with cancer were included in some of the major clinical trials of DOACs in VTE, and subgroup analyses of those patients suggested comparable efficacy of DOACs and other anticoagulants.[43] Memorial Sloan Kettering Cancer Center (MSKCC) treated a large cohort of VTE patients with cancer with rivaroxaban and found risks of recurrent VTE and bleeding to be similar to historical controls of LMWH[44]; in the MSKCC study, patients with gastrointestinal or genitourinary lesions were excluded, and those aged ≥75 were given a reduced dose of rivaroxaban (10 mg twice daily × 3 weeks, then 15 mg once daily). Preliminary data from the SELECT-D trial of rivaroxban versus dalteparin in cancer-VTE showed comparable efficacy of the 2 anticoagulants but an increased risk in clinically relevant nonmajor bleeding in rivaroxaban-treated patients.[45] A recent randomized clinical trial of edoxaban versus dalteparin in cancer VTE showed comparable efficacy of the 2 agents in terms of recurrent VTE, although edoxaban was associated with a slight increase in major bleeding, mostly because of upper GIB.[46] The general sense from all of these studies is that DOACs may be reasonable to use in select patients with cancer-VTE, but caution should be used in patients with gastrointestinal or genitourinary lesions, or those on immunosuppression because of the risk of drug interactions.

LABORATORY MONITORING OF DIRECT ORAL ANTICOAGULANTS

The DOACs were developed to allow for fixed dose administration in most patients without a need for therapeutic monitoring. However, in some situations (eg, renal impairment, geriatrics, obesity, or gastric bypass), laboratory monitoring can be useful. DOACs frequently affect prothrombin time (PT), INR, and/or partial thromboplastin time (PTT), with Xa inhibitors preferentially affecting the PT and INR and dabigatran preferentially affecting the PTT.[47,48] Hence, in patients on an Xa inhibitor or dabigatran, a prolonged PT/INR or PTT, respectively, can be a useful surrogate for the presence of the drug, although normal coagulation studies do not exclude DOAC activity.

Dabigatran, as a direct thrombin inhibitor, prolongs the thrombin time (TT). This test is exquisitely sensitive to even minute amounts of dabigatran and can therefore be used to determine the drug's presence. To measure dabigatran activity, a dilute TT, ecarin clotting time, or ecarin chromogenic assay may be used, all of which demonstrate linear correlations with dabigatran drug concentration. For the Xa inhibitors, drug activity is best measured using an anti-Xa level, which is proportional to drug concentration. Quest Diagnostics offers measurements of dabigatran and Xa inhibitor drug concentrations based on dilute TT and anti-Xa level, respectively, although the reliability and applicability of these assays for clinical use have not been rigorously studied.

REVERSAL OF DIRECT ORAL ANTICOAGULANTS

Despite the favorable bleeding profiles of DOACs, the occurrence of major bleeding in patients on these drugs can sometimes be difficult to manage owing to lack of ready access to techniques for measuring and reversing drug activity. Treatments for such patients are shown in **Fig. 2** and may

include activated charcoal, dialysis, platelet or plasma transfusions, tranexamic acid, desmopressin, recombinant factor VIIa, or 4-factor prothrombin complex concentrate, depending on the clinical circumstances and the specific DOAC used.[49,50] Although a universal approach to major bleeding with DOACs has not been definitively established, outcomes of patients on DOACs with major bleeding historically have been better than VKA,[51] perhaps owing to the short half-lives of the DOACs.

The recent development of antidotes for specific DOACs has improved the care of patients on these agents who bleed. For patients on dabigatran, idarucizumab, a humanized monoclonal antibody against dabigatran, will reverse TT, dilute TT, ecarin clotting time, and PTT within minutes of administration.[52] Idarucizumab is administered in two 5-g intravenous boluses separated by ≤15 minutes and is US Food and Drug Administration (FDA)-approved for patients on dabigatran who have life-threatening bleeding or require an emergent, invasive intervention. In some patients who receive idarucizumab, an initial

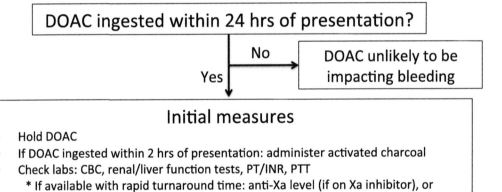

Fig. 2. Management of acute bleeding on DOACs. CBC, complete blood count; DDAVP, desmopressin; PCC, prothrombin complex concentrate.

improvement in coagulation parameters is sometimes followed by an increase in these laboratory values 12 to 24 hours later, which may reflect migration of excess dabigatran from extravascular into intravascular spaces; administration of a second dose of idarucizumab to such patients rapidly corrects their coagulation studies, although the clinical implications of this are uncertain.

For patients on Xa inhibitors, andexanet-alfa, an Xa decoy molecule that binds and inactivates Xa inhibitors, will normalize the anti-Xa level within minutes of administration.[53] Andexanet-alfa is currently under Priority Review by the FDA.

SUMMARY

Over the past several years, DOACs have revolutionized anticoagulation management in VTE owing to their ease of use and favorable outcomes. In comparison to traditional anticoagulants such as VKA, DOACs demonstrate similar efficacy and bleeding risks in treatment of acute VTE, although dabigatran may be associated with an increased risk of GIB in elderly patients. Multiple studies have also demonstrated a definitive role for DOACs in secondary prevention of recurrent VTE when used at full or reduced dosing. Efficacy and safety studies are lacking for certain patient populations such as those with severe renal impairment, APS, obesity, bariatric surgery, and cancer-associated VTE, although emerging data may be encouraging. Laboratory studies to estimate DOAC concentrations exist, but their validity in clinical decision-making is still under investigation. The development of specific antidotes such as andexanet-alfa or idarucizumab should further improve safety profiles and offer greater patient and provider confidence in the use of the DOACs in VTE treatment.

REFERENCES

1. Heit JA, Spencer FA, White RH. The epidemiology of venous thromboembolism. J Thromb Thrombolysis 2016;41:3–14.

2. Kearon C, Akl EA, Ornelas J, et al. Antithrombotic therapy for VTE disease: CHEST guideline and expert panel report. Chest 2016;149(2):315–52.

3. Burnett AE, Mahan CE, Vazquez SR, et al. Guidance for the practical management of the direct oral anticoagulants (DOACs) in VTE treatment. J Thromb Thrombolysis 2016;41(1):206–32.

4. Anderson FA, Spencer FA. Risk factors for venous thromboembolism. Circulation 2003;107(23 suppl 1):I9–16.

5. Tosetto A, Iorio A, Marcucci M, et al. Predicting disease recurrence in patients with previous unprovoked venous thromboembolism: a proposed prediction score (DASH). J Thromb Haemost 2012; 10(6):1019–25.

6. Cohen AT, Harrington RA, Goldhaber SZ, et al. Extended thromboprophylaxis with betrixaban in acutely ill medical patients. N Engl J Med 2016; 375(6):534–44.

7. van der Hulle T, den Exter PL, Kooiman J, et al. Meta-analysis of the efficacy and safety of new oral anticoagulants in patients with cancer-associated acute venous thromboembolism. J Thromb Haemost 2014;12(7):1116–20.

8. Mantha S, Ansell J. Indirect comparison of dabigatran, rivaroxaban, apixaban and edoxaban for the treatment of acute venous thromboembolism. J Thromb Thrombolysis 2015;39(2):155–65.

9. van Es N, Coppens M, Schulman S, et al. Direct oral anticoagulants compared with vitamin K antagonists for acute venous thromboembolism: evidence from phase 3 trials. Blood 2014;124(12):1968–75.

10. Yeh CH, Gross PL, Weitz JI. Evolving use of new oral anticoagulants for treatment of venous thromboembolism. Blood 2014;124(7):1020–8.

11. Eikelboom J, Merli G. Bleeding with direct oral anticoagulants vs warfarin: clinical experience. Am J Med 2016;129(11S):S33–40.

12. Sherwood MW, Nessel CC, Hellkamp AS, et al. Gastrointestinal bleeding in patients with atrial fibrillation treated with rivaroxaban or warfarin: ROCKET AF trial. J Am Coll Cardiol 2015;66(21):2271–81.

13. Sharma M, Cornelius VR, Patel JP, et al. Efficacy and harms of direct oral anticoagulants in the elderly for stroke prevention in atrial fibrillation and secondary prevention of venous thromboembolism: systematic review and meta-analysis. Circulation 2015;132(3): 194–204.

14. Mavrakanas T, Bounameaux H. The potential role of new oral anticoagulants in the prevention and treatment of thromboembolism. Pharmacol Ther 2011; 130(1):46–58.

15. Giugliano RP, Ruff CT, Braunwald E, et al. Edoxaban versus warfarin in patients with atrial fibrillation. N Engl J Med 2013;369(22):2093–104.

16. Becattini C, Agnelli G, Schenone A, et al. Aspirin for preventing the recurrence of venous thromboembolism. N Engl J Med 2012;366(21):1959–67.

17. Brighton TA, Eikelboom JW, Mann K, et al. Low-dose aspirin for preventing recurrent venous thromboembolism. N Engl J Med 2012;367(21):1979–87.

18. Agnelli G, Buller HR, Cohen A, et al. Apixaban for extended treatment of venous thromboembolism. N Engl J Med 2013;368(8):699–708.

19. Raskob G, Ageno W, Cohen AT, et al. Extended duration of anticoagulation with edoxaban in patients with venous thromboembolism: a post-hoc analysis of the Hokusai-VTE study. Lancet Haematol 2016;3(5):e228–36.

20. Schulman S, Kearon C, Kakkar AK, et al. Extended use of dabigatran, warfarin, or placebo in venous thromboembolism. N Engl J Med 2013;368(8): 709–18.

21. Weitz JI, Lensing AW, Prins MH, et al. Rivaroxaban or aspirin for extended treatment of venous thromboembolism. N Engl J Med 2017;376:1211–2222.

22. Agnelli G, Buller HR, Cohen A, et al. Oral apixaban for the treatment of acute venous thromboembolism. N Engl J Med 2013;369(9):799–808.

23. Hokusai VTEl, Buller HR, Decousus H, et al. Edoxaban versus warfarin for the treatment of symptomatic venous thromboembolism. N Engl J Med 2013; 369(15):1406–15.

24. Investigators E, Bauersachs R, Berkowitz SD, et al. Oral rivaroxaban for symptomatic venous thromboembolism. N Engl J Med 2010;363(26):2499–510.

25. Schulman S, Kearon C, Kakkar AK, et al. Dabigatran versus warfarin in the treatment of acute venous thromboembolism. N Engl J Med 2009;361(24): 2342–52.

26. Sterne JA, Bodalia PN, Bryden PA, et al. Oral anticoagulants for primary prevention, treatment and secondary prevention of venous thromboembolic disease, and for prevention of stroke in atrial fibrillation: systematic review, network meta-analysis and cost-effectiveness analysis. Health Technol Assess 2017;21(9):1–386.

27. Abdou JK, Auyeung V, Patel JP, et al. Adherence to long-term anticoagulation treatment, what is known and what the future might hold. Br J Haematol 2016;174(1):30–42.

28. Kearon C, Ginsberg JS, Kovacs MJ, et al. Comparison of low-intensity warfarin therapy with conventional-intensity warfarin therapy for long-term prevention of recurrent venous thromboembolism. N Engl J Med 2003;349(7):631–9.

29. Ridker PM, Goldhaber SZ, Danielson E, et al. Long-term, low-intensity warfarin therapy for the prevention of recurrent venous thromboembolism. N Engl J Med 2003;348(15):1425–34.

30. Djulbegovic M, Lee AI. Direct oral anticoagulants for the prevention of recurrent venous thromboembolism: a systematic review & network meta-analysis. Blood 2017;130:4721.

31. Harel Z, Sholzberg M, Shah PS, et al. Comparisons between novel oral anticoagulants and vitamin K antagonists in patients with CKD. J Am Soc Nephrol 2014;25(3):431–42.

32. Sardar P, Chatterjee S, Herzog E, et al. Novel oral anticoagulants in patients with renal insufficiency: a meta-analysis of randomized trials. Can J Cardiol 2014;30(8):888–97.

33. Wang X, Tirucherai G, Marbury TC, et al. Pharmacokinetics, pharmacodynamics, and safety of apixaban in subjects with end-stage renal disease on hemodialysis. J Clin Pharmacol 2016;56(5):628–36.

34. Mavrakanas TA, Samer CF, Nessim SJ, et al. Apixaban pharmacokinetics at steady state in hemodialysis patients. J Am Soc Nephrol 2017;28(7):2241–8.

35. Erkan D, Aguiar CL, Andrade D, et al. 14th International Congress on Antiphospholipid Antibodies: task force report on antiphospholipid syndrome treatment trends. Autoimmun Rev 2014;13(6): 685–96.

36. Cohen H, Hunt BJ, Efthymiou M, et al. Rivaroxaban versus warfarin to treat patients with thrombotic antiphospholipid syndrome, with or without systemic lupus erythematosus (RAPS): a randomised, controlled, open-label, phase 2/3, non-inferiority trial. Lancet Haematol 2016;3(9):e426–36.

37. Urbanus RT. Rivaroxaban to treat thrombotic antiphospholipid syndrome. Lancet Haematol 2016; 3(9):e403–4.

38. Skelley JW, White CW, Thomason AR. The use of direct oral anticoagulants in inherited thrombophilia. J Thromb Thrombolysis 2017;43(1):24–30.

39. Martin K, Beyer-Westendorf J, Davidson BL, et al. Use of the direct oral anticoagulants in obese patients: guidance from the SSC of the ISTH. J Thromb Haemost 2016;14(6):1308–13.

40. Martin KA, Lee CR, Farrell TM, et al. Oral anticoagulant use after bariatric surgery: a literature review and clinical guidance. Am J Med 2017;130(5): 517–24.

41. Rottenstreich A, Barkai A, Arad A, et al. The effect of bariatric surgery on direct-acting oral anticoagulant drug levels. Thromb Res 2018;163:190–5.

42. Lee AY, Levine MN, Baker RI, et al. Low-molecular-weight heparin versus a coumarin for the prevention of recurrent venous thromboembolism in patients with cancer. N Engl J Med 2003;349(2):146–53.

43. Prins MH, Lensing AW, Brighton TA, et al. Oral rivaroxaban versus enoxaparin with vitamin K antagonist for the treatment of symptomatic venous thromboembolism in patients with cancer (EINSTEIN-DVT and EINSTEIN-PE): a pooled subgroup analysis of two randomised controlled trials. Lancet Haematol 2014;1(1):e37–46.

44. Mantha S, Laube E, Miao Y, et al. Safe and effective use of rivaroxaban for treatment of cancer-associated venous thromboembolic disease: a prospective cohort study. J Thromb Thrombolysis 2017;43(2):166–71.

45. Young A, Marshall A, Thirlwall J, et al. Anticoagulation therapy in selected cancer patients at risk of recurrence of venous thromboembolism: results of the select-D™ pilot trial. Blood 2017;130:625.

46. Raskob GE, van Es N, Verhamme P, et al. Edoxaban for the treatment of cancer-associated venous thromboembolism. N Engl J Med 2018;378(7): 615–24.

47. Cuker A, Husseinzadeh H. Laboratory measurement of the anticoagulant activity of edoxaban: a

systematic review. J Thromb Thrombolysis 2015; 39(3):288–94.

48. Cuker A, Siegal DM, Crowther MA, et al. Laboratory measurement of the anticoagulant activity of the non-vitamin K oral anticoagulants. J Am Coll Cardiol 2014;64(11):1128–39.

49. Majeed A, Agren A, Holmstrom M, et al. Management of rivaroxaban- or apixaban-associated major bleeding with prothrombin complex concentrates: a cohort study. Blood 2017;130(15):1706–12.

50. Schulman S, Ritchie B, Nahirniak S, et al. Reversal of dabigatran-associated major bleeding with activated prothrombin concentrate: a prospective cohort study. Thromb Res 2017;152:44–8.

51. Hylek EM, Held C, Alexander JH, et al. Major bleeding in patients with atrial fibrillation receiving apixaban or warfarin: the ARISTOTLE trial (Apixaban for Reduction in Stroke and Other Thromboembolic Events in Atrial Fibrillation): predictors, characteristics, and clinical outcomes. J Am Coll Cardiol 2014;63(20):2141–7.

52. Pollack CV Jr, Reilly PA, Eikelboom J, et al. Idarucizumab for dabigatran reversal. N Engl J Med 2015; 373(6):511–20.

53. Siegal DM, Curnutte JT, Connolly SJ, et al. Andexanet alfa for the reversal of factor Xa inhibitor activity. N Engl J Med 2015;373(25): 2413–24.

Hypercoagulability in Pulmonary Hypertension

Isabel S. Bazan, MD*, Wassim H. Fares, MD, MSC

KEYWORDS

- Pulmonary arterial hypertension • Hypercoagulability • Thromboembolism • Anticoagulation
- Pulmonary hypertension • Pulmonary embolism • Right heart failure • Right ventricle

KEY POINTS

- Patients with pulmonary arterial hypertension are at increased risk of developing thrombi.
- There are known and suspected pathways that contribute to the hypercoagulability in patients with pulmonary arterial hypertension.
- The benefit of anticoagulation and antiplatelet therapy is not known in this patient population.
- Hypercoagulability is an etiology and a consequence of pulmonary hypertension.

INTRODUCTION

Pulmonary hypertension (PH) is defined as increased pressure in the pulmonary circulation, defined by convention and consensus as a mean pulmonary artery pressure of at least 25 mm Hg at rest.[1] The World Health Organization (WHO) has classified PH into 5 major groups: pulmonary arterial hypertension (PAH), PH caused by left heart disease, PH caused by lung disease or chronic hypoxia, PH caused by chronic thromboembolic disease, and a miscellaneous group.[2,3] PAH is a clinical condition that falls under WHO group 1, and can be idiopathic (IPAH), heritable (HPAH), caused by drugs and toxins (DTPAH), or associated with several other conditions (APAH) including connective tissue disease, congenital heart disease, HIV infection, or portal hypertension. PAH is characterized by molecular and pathologic alterations in the pulmonary circulation that result primarily in progressive vascular remodeling of the pulmonary arteries, increased pulmonary vascular resistance, and eventually right heart failure and death.[4,5] These alterations

are caused by several inflammatory, metabolic, and cellular changes that ultimately result in occlusive lesions, in situ thromboses, and plexiform lesions, that are all representative of the pathologic findings of PAH.[4,6,7] There is evidence of pro-thrombotic pathobiology which suggests an increased hypercoagulable state in PAH patients. Based on limited evidence, anticoagulation therapy is recommended in certain PH patients; however, the degree of hypercoagulability and benefit of anticoagulant therapy are not known.

PATHOPHYSIOLOGY OF PULMONARY ARTERIAL HYPERTENSION

PAH is characterized by excessive vasoconstriction of the distal pulmonary arteries (although the vasculopathy is not strictly limited to the pulmonary arterial system[8]). This is related to endothelial dysfunction and smooth muscle cell hypertrophy and proliferation (that at least in part is related to abnormal function or expression of potassium channels on smooth muscle cells), which leads to impaired production of vasodilator and

Disclosure Statement: The authors have no financial or commercial conflicts of interest to disclose. No funding was used for this article.

Section of Pulmonary, Critical Care and Sleep Medicine, Yale School of Medicine, 300 Cedar Street, PO Box 208057, New Haven, CT 06520-8057, USA

* Corresponding author. Section of Pulmonary, Critical Care and Sleep Medicine, Yale School of Medicine, 300 Cedar Street, TAC-441 South, PO Box 208057, New Haven, CT 06520-8057.

E-mail address: isabel.bazan@yale.edu

Clin Chest Med 39 (2018) 595–603

https://doi.org/10.1016/j.ccm.2018.04.005

antiproliferative agents such as nitric oxide and prostacyclin, as well as overexpression of vaso-constrictor and proliferative substances such as thromboxane A2 and endothelin-1.[5] Other path-ways and molecules, including serotonin,[9] have also been implicated in the pathogenesis of PAH. Activation of the endothelin pathway has been demonstrated in both plasma and lung tissue of PAH patients.[10] Although it is unclear whether increased endothelin-1 is a cause or consequence of PAH, it is known that endothelin-1 causes vaso-constrictive and mitogenic effects by binding to pulmonary vascular smooth muscle cells.[11] Endo-thelin receptor antagonists are efficacious in improving symptoms, exercise capacity, hemody-namics, and time to clinical worsening in PAH patients.[12,13]

The nitric oxide and cyclic guanosine mono-phosphate (cGMP) pathway is also important in the pathogenesis of PAH. Inhibition of cGMP destruction by phosphodiesterase type 5 (PDE-5) inhibitors results in pulmonary vasodila-tion. PDE-5 inhibitors also have antiproliferative ef-fects.[14] PDE-5 inhibitors and guanylate cyclase stimulators are approved for the treatment of PAH and have shown to varying degrees benefits in hemodynamics, exercise capacity, and time to clinical worsening as with endothelin receptor antagonists.[2,15]

The third pathway that has been a major thera-peutic target for PAH is the prostacyclin pathway. Prostacyclin is predominantly produced by endo-thelial cells, and it induces potent vasodilation. It also inhibits platelet aggregation, and has cytopro-tective and antiproliferative effects.[16] PAH patients have a reduction in prostacyclin synthase expres-sion in pulmonary arteries and prostacyclin urinary metabolites.[17] Synthetic analogs of prostacyclins have been developed that share similar pharma-codynamic effects of prostacyclin.[18-20] Efficacy of prostanoids is also seen in APAH and CTEPH (although currently not approved for CTEPH).[21-23]

A common feature in all forms of PAH is the vascular remodeling of the distal region of pulmo-nary arteries. This pathologic remodeling results in the formation of a layer of myofibroblasts and extracellular matrix between the endothelium and the internal elastic lamina, termed the neointima. The cellular processes underlying the musculariza-tion of the usually nonmuscular distal arteries is incompletely understood, but the adventitial fibro-blast is thought to be the first cell activated to proliferate and synthesize matrix proteins in response to a pulmonary hypertensive stimulus.[24] Upregulation of matrix metalloproteinases occurs, and these metalloproteinases are involved in the migration of the adventitial fibroblasts into the

media layer. PAH is also associated with alter-ations of proliferation and apoptosis, resulting in thickened and obstructive pulmonary arteries.[5]

Endothelial cells also play a key role in vascular remodeling. Disorganized endothelial cell prolifer-ation leads to the formation of plexiform lesions that are characteristic of PAH. The initiating stim-ulus that results in abnormal endothelial prolifera-tion is not known, but may be hypoxia, shear stress, inflammation, response to drug or toxin, or a combination of these with a background ge-netic/genomic susceptibility. Defects in growth-suppressive genes have been reported in plexi-form lesions, including growth factors such as platelet-derived growth factor, fibroblast growth factor, transforming growth factor beta (TGFβ), and bone morphogenic proteins.[2,25]

Inflammation also contributes to the pathogen-esis of PAH. Pathologic specimens of patients with PAH show an accumulation of perivascular in-flammatory cells including macrophages, dendritic cells, T and B lymphocytes, and mast cells. There is also an increased level of circulating cytokines and chemokines.[26-28] The role of inflammation is particularly noted in certain groups of PAH including HIV APAH and connective tissue disease APAH. Interestingly, patients with systemic lupus erythematosus APAH have improved on immuno-suppressive therapy, emphasizing the role of inflammation in this subset of patients.[29-31] The pathogenesis of PH in patients with sickle cell dis-ease (WHO group 5 PH) is also linked to inflamma-tion, as elevated inflammatory markers and levels of cytokines and chemokines are associated with worse hemodynamics and poorer clinical out-comes.[32,33] Mitochondrial dysfunction has also been shown to be pathologic in PAH.[34]

Pathologically, PAH results in medial hypertro-phy, intimal proliferative and fibrotic changes, adventitial thickening, plexiform lesions, and thrombotic lesions in the distal pulmonary arteries. Thrombi are present in both the small distal pulmo-nary arteries and in proximal elastic pulmonary arteries.[2]

HYPERCOAGULABILITY IN PULMONARY ARTERIAL HYPERTENSION

There is a high prevalence of vascular thrombotic lesions found postmortem in patients with IPAH, as described in several studies.[35-38] These in situ thromboses may be caused by abnormalities in the coagulation cascade, endothelial cells, and/or platelets. Reduced plasma fibrinolysis was first re-ported in1973.[39] Since then, studies have shown that PAH patients have elevated plasma levels of fibrinopeptide A- and D-dimers,[5] and 1 study found increased levels of fibrinogen and decreased fibrinolytic response in patients with IPAH, comparable to that of patients with CTEPH.[40] Fibrinopeptide A is generated when thrombin cleaves fibrinogen, suggesting an elevated level of plasma thrombin activity, and indeed studies have shown increased thrombin activity in treatment-naïve PAH patients.[41]

Procoagulant activity and fibrinolytic function of the pulmonary artery endothelium are also altered. This dysfunction is reflected by the increased levels of von Willebrand factor and plasminogen activator inhibitor type-1 in the plasma of PAH patients. Plasminogen activator inhibitor was found in much higher concentrations in arterial blood than in mixed venous blood, suggesting intrapulmonary production.[42] Additionally, shear stress of blood flow toward vessel walls generates a thrombogenic surface, resulting in thrombotic lesions. The effect of shear stress and vessel injury can be seen in other types of PH as well, suggesting that the prothrombotic state is not unique to PAH.[5]

Tissue factor is a transmembrane glycoprotein that initiates the coagulation cascade, and it is thought to play a role in angiogenesis and cancer metastasis.[43–45] Tissue factor binds to factor VII to catalyze the activation of factor X, leading to the generation of thrombin and the formation of a fibrin clot. Tissue factor expression is sensitive to changes in blood flow, hypoxia, growth factors such as platelet-derived growth factor, and chemokines. One study found that tissue factor was upregulated in the diseased vessels of PAH patients.[46] Another study found tissue factor-expressing endothelial microparticles in the circulation of PAH patients.[47] Tissue factor expression may be a key contributor to the formation of in situ thromboses.

There is growing evidence that the interaction between platelets, and the arterial wall may contribute to functional and structural alterations in the pulmonary vessels. Apart from their known role in coagulation, platelets release procoagulant, vasoactive, and mitogenic mediators in response to vascular abnormalities, such as thromboxane A2, platelet-activating factor, serotonin, platelet-derived growth factor, TGFb, and VEGF.[9,35,40] Thromboxane A2, which stimulates the activation of new platelets and increases platelet aggregation, is increased in PAH patients, with a corresponding reduction in prostacyclin metabolites.[48] Abnormal platelet aggregation has been described in in vitro, in vivo, and human studies.[49–51] PAH patients have higher levels of megakaryocyte-stimulating hormone thrombopoietin, and 1 study found that the pulmonary vasculature seemed to

be the site of production of thrombopoietin.[52] Increased platelet production, activation, and aggregation may lead to a vicious cycle that contributes to thrombosis (Fig. 1). It is unclear whether thrombosis and platelet dysfunction are causes or consequences of PAH; however, the overarching evidence seems to be pointing toward an underlying pathology of hypercoagulability as a contributing etiology to PAH, and it gets worse as PAH and right heart dysfunction ensue.

In addition to the previously mentioned pathophysiologic abnormalities, patients with PAH may also be at increased risk for venous thromboembolism (VTE). PAH can cause significant dyspnea with exertion, and right heart failure can result in peripheral edema, both of which can lead a patient to be immobile.[2] Additionally, heart failure alone is an independent risk factor for VTE.[53]

CHRONIC THROMBOEMBOLIC PULMONARY HYPERTENSION

CTEPH results from the chronic obstruction of pulmonary arteries due to thromboembolic disease. Usually, acute pulmonary emboli are resorbed by local fibrinolysis, with complete restoration of the pulmonary arterial bed.[54] CTEPH arises when prior acute pulmonary emboli for unknown reasons do not completely resorb. These unresolved clots then undergo fibrosis into an organized clot, ultimately leading to mechanical obstruction of the pulmonary arteries.[2,54] This obstruction causes the release of inflammatory and vasculotropic mediators, resulting in vascular remodeling. Microvascular disease is also thought to occur, which can be related to shear stress in nonobstructed areas, postcapillary remodeling related to bronchial-to-pulmonary venous shunting, pressure, and inflammation.[54] Low blood flow states are created as a result of obstructed arteries and can result in the in situ thromboses, related to those of PAH. Thrombophilic factors such as antiphospholipid antibodies, lupus anticoagulant, protein S and C deficiency, activated protein C resistance including factor V Leiden mutation, prothrombin gene mutation, antithrombin III deficiency, and elevated factor VIII have been statistically associated with approximately one-a third of CTEPH patients.[2] Obstruction of pulmonary arteries and secondary remodeling of small, peripheral pulmonary vessels most likely contribute to elevated total pulmonary resistance.[8,55–57]

Pathologically, organized thrombi are tightly attached to the medial layer in the elastic pulmonary arteries, and subsequently replace normal intima. The thrombi occlude the lumen or form different grades of stenosis, webs, and/or bands.

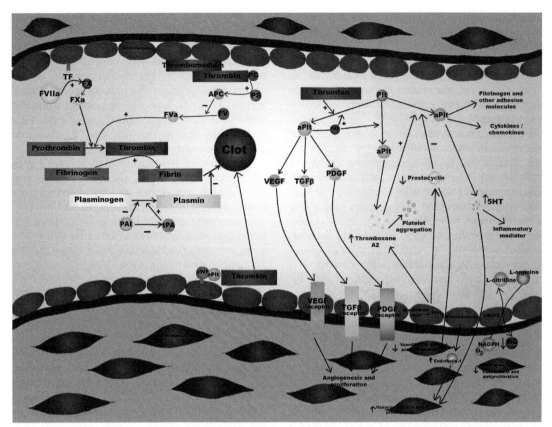

Fig. 1. Summary of hypercoagulable pathways in pulmonary arterial hypertension. This figure depicts a schematic of the pulmonary artery, with the combined known and suspected pathways that contribute to hypercoagulability in PAH. This figure is not comprehensive or inclusive of all known hypercoagulability pathways implicated in PAH. A condensed version of the coagulation cascade is shown, and in PAH, tissue factor (TF) is increased, resulting in increased thrombin, fibrin, and formation of clot. Plasminogen activator inhibitor (PAI) is also increased, decreasing clot inhibitors. Decreased thrombomodulin reduces inhibition of the clot formation. There are also more activated platelets in patients with PAH, and the effects of activated platelets are shown, including increased inflammatory mediators, vasoconstriction, platelet aggregation and prothrombotic factors, fibrinogen, and other adhesion molecules. Activated platelets stimulate growth factors, resulting in proliferation and angiogenesis. Finally, the prostacyclin, endothelin-1, and nitric oxide pathways are shown, highlighting their differential effects on vasoconstriction and proliferation, and are the primary targets of the currently available treatments for PAH. 5HT, serotonin; APC, activated protein C; aPlt, activated platelet; cGMP, cyclic guanosine monophosphate; eNOS, endothelial nitric oxide synthase; FV, factor V; FVa, activated factor V; FVIIa, activated factor VII; FX, factor X; FXa, activated factor X; GTP, guanosine triphosphate; NADPH, nicotinamide adenine dinucleotide phosphate hydrogenase; O2, oxygen; PAI, plasminogen activator inhibitor; PC, protein C; PDGF, platelet-derived growth factor; PGH2, prostaglandin H2; Plt, platelet; PS, protein S; TF, tissue factor; TGFβ, transforming growth factor β; tPA, tissue plasminogen activator; VEGF, vascular endothelial growth factor; vWF, von Willebrand factor.

Collateral vessels from the systemic circulation (bronchial, costal, diaphragmatic, and coronary arteries) can grow to attempt reperfusion of areas distal to the obstructed territories. The microvascular changes that occur in occluded and nonoccluded areas are similar to those seen in PAH, although plexiform lesions are uncommon.[2,58]

It is estimated that 1% to 4% of acute pulmonary embolism survivors develop CTEPH within 2 years from their first embolic event.[55,59,60]

Anywhere from 25% to 50% of CTEPH patients do not have a past medical history of pulmonary embolism or deep vein thrombosis.[55,61] It is suspected that thrombotic and/or inflammatory lesions exist in the pulmonary vasculature, resulting in the formation of thromboses and vascular remodeling without a clinically evident acute thromboembolic event. Conditions that cause chronic inflammatory states such as myeloproliferative disorders and inflammatory bowel disease and postsplenectomy patients have been associated with the development of CTEPH.[62] Unlike all other forms of PH, patients with CTEPH are potentially curable via a pulmonary endarterectomy.[63] The feasibility and success of this surgery depend on the surgical accessibility of thromboembolic residues and the underlying comorbidities of the patient.[63,64] However, even with successful removal of chronic clots, some patients continue to have PH postoperatively. It is speculated that persistent PH is partly due to the remodeled microvasculature.[58] Balloon pulmonary angioplasty has also been gaining momentum in CTEPH management; however, its exact role is yet to be determined, as its technique, strategy, and catheters are rapidly evolving.[65]

ANTICOAGULATION AND PULMONARY HYPERTENSION

Currently, anticoagulation is recommended for patients with IPAH, HPAH, and DTPAH. According to the 2015 European Society of Cardiology and the European Respiratory Society guidelines, anticoagulation is a class IIb recommendation, meaning that its usefulness and efficacy are not well established, but it may be considered (**Table 1**).[2] There have been some retrospective and observational single-center studies that have shown survival benefit in patients who get anticoagulation with warfarin.[36,66] These early studies were done prior to the available PAH-targeted therapies.[36,66–68] More recent randomized control trials and registry data have been inconclusive. For example, in 2014, the Comparative, Prospective Registry of Newly Initiated Therapies for Pulmonary Hypertension (COMPERA) registry examined the survival rates of PAH patients based on use of anticoagulation. It found that in the subgroup of IPAH patients, there was a significant improvement in 3-year survival.[69] A major caveat to the COMPERA registry is that the median age of this population receiving anticoagulation was 70 years, and it does not reflect the typical demographics of the PAH population.

In contrast, the Registry to Evaluate Early and Long-term PAH Disease Management (REVEAL) compared the survival of IPAH patients on warfarin with those who have never been anticoagulated, and found no difference in survival.[70] These limited and inconclusive data likely reflect the heterogeneity of PAH patients. Clinical use of anticoagulation in IPAH patients is widely variable and provider dependent. It is generally recommended that in the absence of contraindications, patients on long-term intravenous prostanoid analogues

Table 1
Summary of evidence for anticoagulation by World Health Organization groups

WHO Group		Class of Recommendation[a]
1 PAH	IPAH	IIb
	HPAH	IIb
	DTPAH	IIb
	CTD-PAH	III
	Porto-PH	III
	HIV-PAH	Unknown
	CHD-PAH	Unknown
2 PH caused by left heart disease		Unknown
3 PH caused by lung disease/ chronic hypoxia		Unknown
4 CTEPH		I
5 Miscellaneous		Unknown

Abbreviations: CHD-PAH, congenital heart disease-pulmonary arterial hypertension; CTD-PAH, connective tissue disease-pulmonary arterial hypertension; CTEPH, chronic thromboembolic pulmonary hypertension; DTPAH, drugs/toxins induced pulmonary arterial hypertension; HIV-PAH, HIV-induced pulmonary arterial hypertension; HPAH, heritable pulmonary arterial hypertension; IPAH, idiopathic pulmonary arterial hypertension; PH, pulmonary hypertension; porto-PH, portopulmonary hypertension.

[a] Class of recommendation. Class I recommendation: is recommended/indicated (evidence and/or general agreement that a given treatment of procedure is beneficial, useful, effective). Class IIa recommendation: should be considered (conflicting evidence with weight of evidence/opinion in favor of usefulness/efficacy). Class IIb: may be considered (conflicting evidence with usefulness/efficacy less well established). Class III: is not recommended (evidence or general agreement that given treatment is not useful/effective, and in some cases may be harmful).

Data from Galiè N, Humbert M, Vachiery JL, et al. 2015 ESC/ERS guidelines for the diagnosis and treatment of pulmonary hypertension. The joint task force for the diagnosis and treatment of pulmonary hypertension of the European Society of Cardiology (ESC) and the European Respiratory Society (ERS) endorsed by: Association for European Paediatric and Congenital Cardiology (AEPC), International Society for Heart and Lung Transplantation (ISHLT). Eur Heart J 2015:37(1);67–119.

should receive anticoagulation therapy because of the risk of catheter-associated thrombosis.[2]

The potential benefits of anticoagulation for patients with APAH is even less clear. A subgroup analysis of from the REVEAL registry found that patients with systemic sclerosis APAH had an increased mortality when treated with warfarin.[70] The COMPERA registry also found to have other forms of APAH including those associated with connective tissue diseases, congenital heart disease, and portopulmonary hypertension, had no survival benefit with anticoagulation.[69] Specific to congenital heart disease APAH, the use of anticoagulation in patients with Eisenmenger syndrome is controversial. These patients have a high incidence of pulmonary artery thrombosis and stroke, but also have an elevated risk of hemorrhage and hemoptysis.[71] Although there are no data to guide this clinical dilemma, the authors' own practice is to avoid anticoagulation in congenital heart disease APAH. Hemoptysis is also a known complication of patients with IPAH and CTEPH, with prevalence varying from 1% to 6%,[72] and it can limit the use of anticoagulation. Because many patients with portopulmonary hypertension have coagulopathy and thrombocytopenia, they have an elevated bleeding risk; anticoagulation is not recommended in these patients, although it has not been studied.

The preferred treatment for patients with CTEPH, as mentioned previously, is a pulmonary endarterectomy. Supplemental medical therapy for CTEPH includes anticoagulation, as well as diuretics and supplemental oxygen if needed for heart failure or hypoxemia, respectively. Although there are no studies comparing indefinite anticoagulation to no therapy or a shorter duration of anticoagulation, data extrapolated from treatment of acute and recurrent venous thromboembolism have led to the recommendation of lifelong anticoagulation for CTEPH patients, even after successful surgical intervention. The placement of routine inferior vena cava filter placement in this patient population is not justified by evidence.[2]

The role of direct oral anticoagulants (DOACs) for any group of PH is unknown. Several studies have shown that DOACs are at least as effective as warfarin for the management of venous thromboembolism and atrial fibrillation, and some have shown a reduction in bleeding and mortality.[73,74] DOACs have not yet been studied in people with PAH, but in a monocrotaline-induced PAH rat model, rivaroxaban attenuated the increase in right ventricular systolic pressure and right ventricular hypertrophy caused by monocrotaline.[75] Although the generalizability of this to people is limited, it does warrant further investigation into the role of DOACs in PAH.

Since dysregulated platelets have been identified in the pathophysiology of PAH, antiplatelet therapy has been studied. However, although some studies have shown reduction in thromboxane A2 levels and reduction in platelet activation markers with aspirin, none have shown any improvement in exercise tolerance.[76,77] These studies are small, and it is possible that larger studies or the investigation of newer antiplatelet agents may identify a role for platelet inhibitors in

the treatment of PAH. It is worth noting, however, that many of the PAH medications, as mentioned previously, do have antiplatelet effects.[50,78]

SUMMARY

Given how heterogeneous the etiologies and pathophysiology are for each WHO group of PH, it is no surprise that the degree of hypercoagulability and benefit of anticoagulation would be variable between groups and subtypes. CTEPH is usually caused by an initial acute venous thromboembolism and has been associated with thrombophilic disorders; anticoagulation has a clear benefit in these patients. There is pathophysiological evidence that PAH is a prothrombotic state caused by the dysregulation of coagulation, fibrinolysis, and endothelial cells. These abnormalities, combined with in situ thromboses found in pulmonary arteries, argue that PAH patients are in a hypercoagulable state and may benefit from anticoagulation therapy. Studies investigating the benefit of anticoagulation in IPAH patients have yielded mixed results. Each individual subtype of APAH will need to be further investigated to assess the benefit of anticoagulation. Given that an increased bleeding risk limits the use of anticoagulation even in patients who would derive benefit, further study of DOACs and antiplatelet agents is also overdue.

ACKNOWLEDGMENTS

The authors have grateful to Ms Isabella Siegel for her artistic and creative skills in drawing the figure.

REFERENCES

1. Maron BA, Wertheim BM, Gladwin MT. Under pressure to clarify pulmonary hypertension clinical risk. Am J Respir Crit Care Med 2018;197(4):423–6.

2. Galiè N, Humbert M, Vachiery JL, et al. 2015 ESC/ERS guidelines for the diagnosis and treatment of pulmonary hypertension. The joint task force for the diagnosis and treatment of pulmonary hypertension of the European Society of Cardiology (ESC) and the European Respiratory Society (ERS) endorsed by: Association for European Paediatric and Congenital Cardiology (AEPC), International Society for Heart and Lung Transplantation (ISHLT). Eur Heart J 2015;37(1):67–119.

3. Bazan IS, Fares WH. Pulmonary hypertension: diagnostic and therapeutic challenges. Ther Clin Risk Manag 2015;11:1221–33.

4. Robinson JC, Pugliese SC, Fox DL, et al. Anticoagulation in pulmonary arterial hypertension. Curr Hypertens Rep 2016;18(6):47.

5. Humbert M, Morrell NW, Archer SL, et al. Cellular and molecular pathobiology of pulmonary arterial hypertension. J Am Coll Cardiol 2004;43(12 Suppl S):13S–24S.

6. Tuder RM, Stacher E, Robinson J, et al. Pathology of pulmonary hypertension. Clin Chest Med 2013; 34(4):639–50.

7. Tuder RM, Voelkel NF. Plexiform lesion in severe pulmonary hypertension: association with glomeruloid lesion. Am J Pathol 2001;159(1):382–3.

8. Fares WH. The other vascular beds in pulmonary arterial hypertension. Surrogates or associated? Ann Am Thorac Soc 2014;11(4):596–7.

9. Bazan IS, Fares WH. Review of the ongoing story of appetite suppressants, serotonin pathway, and pulmonary vascular disease. Am J Cardiol 2016; 117(10):1691–6.

10. Giaid A, Yanagisawa M, Langleben D, et al. Expression of endothelin-1 in the lungs of patients with pulmonary hypertension. New Engl J Med 1993; 328(24):1732–9.

11. Galie N, Manes A, Branzi A. The endothelin system in pulmonary arterial hypertension. Cardiovasc Res 2004;61(2):227–37.

12. Galie N, Olschewski H, Oudiz RJ, et al. Ambrisentan for the treatment of pulmonary arterial hypertension: results of the ambrisentan in pulmonary arterial hypertension, randomized, double-blind, placebo-controlled, multicenter, efficacy (ARIES) study 1 and 2. Circulation 2008; 117(23):3010–9.

13. Pulido T, Adzerikho I, Channick RN, et al. Macitentan and morbidity and mortality in pulmonary arterial hypertension. N Engl J Med 2013;369(9):809–18.

14. Wharton J, Strange JW, Møller GM, et al. Antiproliferative effects of phosphodiesterase type 5 inhibition in human pulmonary artery cells. Am J Respir Crit Care Med 2005;172(1):105–13.

15. Galiè N, Ghofrani HA, Torbicki A, et al. Sildenafil citrate therapy for pulmonary arterial hypertension. New Engl J Med 2005;353(20):2148–57.

16. Jones DA, Benjamin CW, Linseman DA. Activation of thromboxane and prostacyclin receptors elicits opposing effects on vascular smooth muscle cell growth and mitogen-activated protein kinase signaling cascades. Mol Pharmacol 1995;48(5): 890–6.

17. Galie N, Manes A, Branzi A. Prostanoids for pulmonary arterial hypertension. Am J Respir Med 2003; 2(2):123–37.

18. Barst RJ, Rubin LJ, Long WA, et al. A comparison of continuous intravenous epoprostenol (prostacyclin) with conventional therapy for primary pulmonary hypertension. N Engl J Med 1996;334(5):296–301.

19. Rubin LJ, Mendoza J, Hood M, et al. Treatment of primary pulmonary hypertension with continuous intravenous prostacyclin (epoprostenol). Results of a randomized trial. Ann Intern Med 1990;112(7): 485–91.

20. Badesch DB, Tapson VF, McGoon MD, et al. Continuous intravenous epoprostenol for pulmonary hypertension due to the scleroderma spectrum of disease. A randomized, controlled trial. Ann Intern Med 2000;132(6):425–34.

21. Nunes H, Humbert M, Sitbon O, et al. Prognostic factors for survival in human immunodeficiency virus-associated pulmonary arterial hypertension. Am J Respir Crit Care Med 2003;167(10):1433–9.

22. Rosenzweig EB, Kerstein D, Barst RJ. Long-term prostacyclin for pulmonary hypertension with associated congenital heart defects. Circulation 1999; 99(14):1858–65.

23. Cabrol S, Souza R, Jais X, et al. Intravenous epoprostenol in inoperable chronic thromboembolic pulmonary hypertension. J Heart Lung Transplant 2007; 26(4):357–62.

24. Stenmark KR, Gerasimovskaya E, Nemenoff RA, et al. Hypoxic activation of adventitial fibroblasts: role in vascular remodeling. Chest 2002;122(6 Suppl):326s–34s.

25. Yeager ME, Halley GR, Golpon HA, et al. Microsatellite instability of endothelial cell growth and apoptosis genes within plexiform lesions in primary pulmonary hypertension. Circ Res 2001; 88(1):E2–11.

26. Humbert M, Monti G, Fartoukh M, et al. Platelet-derived growth factor expression in primary pulmonary hypertension: comparison of HIV seropositive and HIV seronegative patients. Eur Respir J 1998; 11(3):554–9.

27. Fares WH, Ford HJ, Ghio AJ, et al. Safety and feasibility of obtaining wedged pulmonary artery samples and differential distribution of biomarkers in pulmonary hypertension. Pulm Circ 2012;2(4):477–82.

28. Marshall JD, Sauler M, Tonelli A, et al. Complexity of macrophage migration inhibitory factor (MIF) and other angiogenic biomarkers profiling in pulmonary arterial hypertension. Pulm Circ 2017;7(3):730–3.

29. Dorfmuller P, Perros F, Balabanian K, et al. Inflammation in pulmonary arterial hypertension. Eur Respir J 2003;22(2):358–63.

30. Mensah KA, Yadav R, Trow TK, et al. Lupus-associated pulmonary arterial hypertension: variable course and importance of prompt recognition. Case Rep Med 2015;2015:328435.

31. Bazan IS, Mensah KA, Rudkovskaia AA, et al. Pulmonary arterial hypertension in the setting of scleroderma is different than in the setting of lupus: a review. Respir Med 2018;134:42–6.

32. Parent F, Bachir D, Inamo J, et al. A hemodynamic study of pulmonary hypertension in sickle cell disease. N Engl J Med 2011;365(1):44–53.

33. Niu X, Nouraie M, Campbell A, et al. Angiogenic and inflammatory markers of cardiopulmonary changes

in children and adolescents with sickle cell disease. PLoS One 2009;4(11):e7956.

34. Marshall JD, Bazan I, Zhang Y, et al. Mitochondrial dysfunction and pulmonary hypertension: cause, effect, or both. Am J Physiol Lung Cell Mol Physiol 2018;314(5):L782–96.

35. Herve P, Humbert M, Sitbon O, et al. Pathobiology of pulmonary hypertension. The role of platelets and thrombosis. Clin Chest Med 2001;22(3):451–8.

36. Fuster V, Steele PM, Edwards WD, et al. Primary pulmonary hypertension: natural history and the importance of thrombosis. Circulation 1984;70(4): 580–7.

37. Wagenvoort CA, Mulder PGH. Thrombotic lesions in primary plexogenic arteriopathy. Chest 1993;103(3): 844–9.

38. Johnson SR, Granton JT, Mehta S. Thrombotic arteriopathy and anticoagulation in pulmonary hypertension. Chest 2006;130(2):545–52.

39. Inglesby TV, Singer JW, Gordon DS. Abnormal fibrinolysis in familial pulmonary hypertension. Am J Med 1973;55(1):5–14.

40. Huber K, Beckmann R, Frank H, et al. Fibrinogen, t-PA, and PAI-1 plasma levels in patients with pulmonary hypertension. Am J Respir Crit Care Med 1994; 150(4):929–33.

41. Tournier A, Wahl D, Chaouat A, et al. Calibrated automated thrombography demonstrates hypercoagulability in patients with idiopathic pulmonary arterial hypertension. Thromb Res 2010;126(6): e418–22.

42. Hoeper MM, Sosada M, Fabel H. Plasma coagulation profiles in patients with severe primary pulmonary hypertension. Eur Respir J 1998;12(6):1446–9.

43. Ruf W, Mueller BM. Tissue factor signaling. Thromb Haemost 1999;82(2):175–82.

44. Riewald M, Ruf W. Orchestration of coagulation protease signaling by tissue factor. Trends Cardiovasc Med 2002;12(4):149–54.

45. Turitto VT, Hall CL. Mechanical factors affecting hemostasis and thrombosis. Thromb Res 1998;92(6 Suppl 2):S25–31.

46. White RJ, Meoli DF, Swarthout RF, et al. Plexiform-like lesions and increased tissue factor expression in a rat model of severe pulmonary arterial hypertension. Am J Physiol Lung Cell Mol Physiol 2007; 293(3):L583–90.

47. Bakouboula B, Morel O, Faure A, et al. Procoagulant membrane microparticles correlate with the severity of pulmonary arterial hypertension. Am J Respir Crit Care Med 2008;177(5):536–43.

48. Christman BW, McPherson CD, Newman JH, et al. An imbalance between the excretion of thromboxane and prostacyclin metabolites in pulmonary hypertension. N Engl J Med 1992;327(2):70–5.

49. Lopes AA, Maeda NY, Almeida A, et al. Circulating platelet aggregates indicative of in vivo platelet activation in pulmonary hypertension. Angiology 1993;44(9):701–6.

50. Clapp LH, Gurung R. The mechanistic basis of prostacyclin and its stable analogues in pulmonary arterial hypertension: role of membrane versus nuclear receptors. Prostaglandins Other Lipid Mediat 2015; 120:56–71.

51. Friedman R, Mears JG, Barst RJ. Continuous infusion of prostacyclin normalizes plasma markers of endothelial cell injury and platelet aggregation in primary pulmonary hypertension. Circulation 1997; 96(9):2782–4.

52. Haznedaroğlu IC, Atalar E, Oztürk MA, et al. Thrombopoietin inside the pulmonary vessels in patients with and without pulmonary hypertension. Platelets 2002;13(7):395–9.

53. Tang L, Wu YY, Lip GY, et al. Heart failure and risk of venous thromboembolism: a systematic review and meta-analysis. Lancet Haematol 2016;3(1):e30–44.

54. Dartevelle P, Fadel E, Mussot S, et al. Chronic thromboembolic pulmonary hypertension. Eur Respir J 2004;23(4):637–48.

55. Dorfmuller P, Günther S, Ghigna MR, et al. Microvascular disease in chronic thromboembolic pulmonary hypertension: a role for pulmonary veins and systemic vasculature. Eur Respir J 2014;44(5):1275–88.

56. Moser KM, Bloor CM. Pulmonary vascular lesions occurring in patients with chronic major vessel thromboembolic pulmonary hypertension. Chest 1993;103(3):685–92.

57. Hoeper MM, Mayer E, Simonneau G, et al. Chronic thromboembolic pulmonary hypertension. Circulation 2006;113(16):2011–20.

58. Galie N, Kim NH. Pulmonary microvascular disease in chronic thromboembolic pulmonary hypertension. Proc Am Thorac Soc 2006;3(7):571–6.

59. Pengo V, Lensing AW, Prins MH, et al. Incidence of chronic thromboembolic pulmonary hypertension after pulmonary embolism. N Engl J Med 2004; 350(22):2257–64, 2004 Massachusetts Medical Society: United States.

60. Becattini C, Agnelli G, Pesavento R, et al. Incidence of chronic thromboembolic pulmonary hypertension after a first episode of pulmonary embolism. Chest 2006;130(1):172–5.

61. Pepke-Zaba J, Delcroix M, Lang I, et al. Chronic thromboembolic pulmonary hypertension (CTEPH): results from an international prospective registry. Circulation 2011;124(18):1973–81.

62. Galiè N, Hoeper MM, Humbert M, et al. Guidelines for the diagnosis and treatment of pulmonary hypertension: the task force for the diagnosis and treatment of pulmonary hypertension of the European Society of Cardiology (ESC) and the European Respiratory Society (ERS), endorsed by the International Society of Heart and Lung Transplantation (ISHLT). Eur Heart J 2009;30:2493–537.

63. Jamieson SW, Kapelanski DP, Sakakibara N, et al. Pulmonary endarterectomy: experience and lessons learned in 1,500 cases. Ann Thorac Surg 2003; 76(5):1457–62 [discussion: 1462–4].

64. Jenkins DP, Madani M, Mayer E, et al. Surgical treatment of chronic thromboembolic pulmonary hypertension. Eur Respir J 2013;41(3):735–42.

65. Auger WR, Kim NH. Balloon pulmonary angioplasty for chronic thrombocmbolic pulmonary hypertension: more work to be done. Circ Cardiovasc Qual Outcomes 2017;10(11) [pii:e004230].

66. Rich S, Kaufmann E, Levy PS. Levy the effect of high doses of calcium-channel blockers on survival in primary pulmonary hypertension. New Engl J Med 1992;327(2):76–81.

67. Ogata M, Ohe M, Shirato K, et al. Effects of a combination therapy of anticoagulant and vasodilator on the long-term prognosis of primary pulmonary hypertension. Jpn Circ J 1993;57(1):63–9.

68. Frank H, Mlczoch J, Huber K, et al. The effect of anticoagulant therapy in primary and anorectic drug-induced pulmonary hypertension. Chest 1997; 112(3):714–21.

69. Olsson KM, Delcroix M, Ghofrani HA, et al. Anticoagulation and survival in pulmonary arterial hypertension: results from the comparative, prospective registry of newly initiated therapies for pulmonary hypertension (COMPERA). Circulation 2014;129(1): 57–65.

70. Preston IR, Roberts KE, Miller DP, et al. Effect of warfarin treatment on survival of patients with Pulmonary Arterial Hypertension (PAH) in the Registry to Evaluate Early and Long-Term PAH Disease Management (REVEAL). Circulation 2015;132(25): 2403–11.

71. Broberg CS, Ujita M, Prasad S, et al. Pulmonary arterial thrombosis in eisenmenger syndrome is associated with biventricular dysfunction and decreased pulmonary flow velocity. J Am Coll Cardiol 2007;50(7):634–42.

72. Zylkowska J, Kurzyna M, Pietura R, et al. Recurrent hemoptysis: an emerging life-threatening complication in idiopathic pulmonary arterial hypertension. Chest 2011;139(3):690–3.

73. Patel MR, Mahaffey KW, Garg J, et al. Rivaroxaban versus warfarin in nonvalvular atrial fibrillation. New Engl J Med 2011;365(10):883–91.

74. Schulman S, Kearon C, Kakkar AK, et al. Dabigatran versus Warfarin in the treatment of acute venous thromboembolism. New Engl J Med 2009;361(24): 2342–52.

75. Delbeck M, Nickel KF, Perzborn E, et al. A role for coagulation factor Xa in experimental pulmonary arterial hypertension. Cardiovasc Res 2011;92(1): 159–68.

76. Kawut SM, Bagiella E, Lederer DJ, et al. A randomized clinical trial of aspirin and simvastatin for pulmonary arterial hypertension: ASA-STAT. Circulation 2011;123(25):2985–93.

77. Robbins IM, Kawut SM, Yung D, et al. A study of aspirin and clopidogrel in idiopathic pulmonary arterial hypertension. Eur Respir J 2006;27(3):578–84.

78. Makowski CT, Rissmiller RW, Bullington WM. Riociguat: a novel new drug for treatment of pulmonary hypertension. Pharmacotherapy 2015;35(5):502–19.

Chronic Thromboembolic Pulmonary Hypertension
An Update

Check for updates

Jean M. Elwing, MD, FCCP[a],*, Anjali Vaidya, MD[b],
William R. Auger, MD, FCCP[c]

KEYWORDS

- Chronic thromboembolic pulmonary hypertension (CTEPH)
- Chronic thromboembolic disease (CTED) • Pulmonary endarterectomy (PEA)
- Pulmonary thromboendarterectomy (PTE) • Balloon pulmonary angioplasty (BPA)
- Pulmonary hypertension (PH)

KEY POINTS

- Chronic thromboembolic pulmonary hypertension (CTEPH) is a progressive pulmonary vascular disease with significant morbidity and mortality. It occurs in approximately 4% of pulmonary embolism (PE) survivors and is a sequela of nonresolving thromboemboli with persistent arterial obstruction.
- CTEPH develops within 2 years of an acute PE. Risk for CTEPH increases with recurrent thromboembolic disease, elevated pulmonary pressures at the time of acute PE, nonresolving PE, prothrombotic conditions, hypothyroidism, malignancy, and chronic inflammatory states.
- CTEPH requires an extensive evaluation for best outcomes. Diagnostic workup includes a thorough clinical assessment of cardiopulmonary status including pulmonary hemodynamics and diagnostic imaging.
- Surgical intervention remains the optimal management strategy for CTEPH. Select inoperable patients may be candidates for catheter-based intervention with balloon pulmonary angioplasty. Patients who are not candidates for intervention or those with postintervention pulmonary hypertension are treated with medical therapy.

INTRODUCTION

Chronic thromboembolic pulmonary hypertension (CTEPH) is a rare, yet underdiagnosed pulmonary vascular disease, which is a sequela of prior pulmonary thromboemboli[1] and is classified by the World Health Organization (WHO) as group IV pulmonary hypertension (PH).[2] Although most of the pulmonary embolism (PE) survivors experience improvement over time with resolution of

Disclosure Statement: Research Support/Grants: Actelion, ARENA, Bayer, Reata, United Therapeutics, Bellerophon, Lung LLC, Eiger, Akros, Liquidia; Consulting/Advisory Committees: United Therapeutics (J.M. Elwing). Consulting: Actelion, Bayer, United Therapeutics; Speaking: Actelion, Bayer, Gilead, United Therapeutics (A. Vaidya). Research support from Bayer, co-investigator US CTEPH Registry; Consultant: Bayer (W. Auger).
^a Pulmonary Hypertension Program, Division of Pulmonary, Critical Care and Sleep Medicine, University of Cincinnati College of Medicine, 231 Albert Sabin Way, ML 0564, Cincinnati, OH 45267, USA; ^b Pulmonary Hypertension, Right Heart Failure, and Pulmonary Thromboendarterectomy Program, Advanced Heart Failure and Cardiac Transplant, Temple University School of Medicine, Temple University Hospital, 9th Floor Parkinson Pavilion, 3401 North Broad Street, Philadelphia, PA 19140, USA; ^c CTEPH Program, UC San Diego Health, University of California, San Diego, 9300 Campus Point Drive #7381, La Jolla, CA 92037, USA
* Corresponding author.
E-mail address: Jean.Elwing@UC.edu

Clin Chest Med 39 (2018) 605–620
https://doi.org/10.1016/j.ccm.2018.04.018
0272-5231/18/© 2018 Elsevier Inc. All rights reserved.

thromboembolic burden, there is a small group that develops CTEPH[3] due to an alternate natural history with limited resolution of vascular obstruction, thrombus organization, and recanalization.[1] This is associated with small pulmonary arterial vascular changes leading to increased pulmonary vascular resistance (PVR) and PH.[4] The pathophysiologic mechanisms of this condition have not been fully elucidated but seem to be a result of a complex interaction between the pulmonary arterial obstruction from prior PE and multifactorial molecular responses in the pulmonary microvasculature.[5]

EPIDEMIOLOGY AND RISK FACTORS

Conflicting data exist regarding the incidence and prevalence of CTEPH. In a recent detailed evaluation of published literature, population-based hospital databases, and surveys by Gall and colleagues,[3] it was estimated that CTEPH occurs in approximately 4% (0.1%–9.1%) of all PE survivors. These findings are similar to the results of The INFORM Study (3.8%)[6] and a prospective long-term follow-up study monitoring 223 patients after acute PE for up to 10 years (3.8%).[7] Based on this data, the annual incidence of CTEPH can be estimated at 3 to 5 cases per 100,000 in the United States and Europe with less than a third of cases (7%–29%) being diagnosed based on reviewed databases.[3] In the 2007 to 2009 International CTEPH Registry (679 newly diagnosed patients <6 months), men and women were affected equally, 75% had previous PE, and most were diagnosed in the 6th decade of life.[8] Most frequently, patients reported NYHA functional class III/IV symptoms at time of diagnosis[9] with the vast majority of CTEPH being detected within 2 years of an acute thromboembolic event.[7,10]

Several risk factors for the development of CTEPH have been identified. Pengo and colleagues[7] found in a prospective long-term follow-up study that recurrent PE, younger age, larger perfusion defects, and idiopathic presentation were all associated with increased risk of CTEPH. Several prothrombotic factors have also been associated with the development of CTEPH and include elevated factor VIII,[11] dysfibrinogenemia,[12] antiphospholipid antibodies, and lupus anticoagulant.[13] Additional factors that have been associated include splenectomy,[14,15] human leukocyte antigen (HLA) polymorphism HLA-DPB1,[16] elevated pulmonary pressures at the time of PE, lower-limb varicosities, residual obstruction on computed tomography (CT) imaging 3 months after acute PE,[10] hypothyroidism, malignancy, infected pacemaker wires, recurrent

thromboembolic disease, non-O group blood type,[15] ventriculoatrial (VA) shunts, chronic inflammation due to osteomyelitis, and inflammatory bowel disease.[17] Compression of pelvic veins has also been shown to increase the risk of venous thromboembolism (VTE) and CTEPH. Compressing uterine fibroids are associated with CTEPH, and thus a history of fibroids or menorrhagia may raise clinical suspicion for this condition. May-Thurner syndrome, where the right common iliac artery compresses the left common iliac vein, can also lead to VTE and may be evident by recurrent unprovoked left lower extremity deep vein thrombosis (DVT)[18] (**Table 1**).

PATHOPHYSIOLOGY

The pathophysiologic mechanisms involved in the development of CTEPH are not fully understood but the inciting event is nonresolving large vessel thromboembolic disease.[1] Several potential triggers for lack of thrombus resolution have been postulated, including staphylococcal infection[19] and fibrinogen aberrations.[12] The role of staphylococcus is supported by a murine model of venous thrombosis with coexisting staphylococcal infection in which there was evidence of fibrotic

Table 1 Patient characteristics and risk factors associated with the development of CTEPH	
PE History	Recurrent PE Large perfusion defect Idiopathic presentation Elevated pulmonary pressures with acute PE Residual obstruction on CT 3 mo after PE
Prothrombotic Factors	Elevated factor VIII Antiphospholipid antibodies Lupus anticoagulant Dysfibrinogenemia
Patient Characteristics	Splenectomy Malignancy Infected pacemaker wires Ventriculoatrial shunts Inflammatory bowel disease Lower extremity varicose veins Osteomyelitis Non-O blood group Hypothyroidism Uterine fibroids compressing pelvic veins May-Thurner syndrome

vascular remodeling and decreased thrombus resolution. In addition, patients with CTEPH with VA shunts for hydrocephalus and pacemaker leads who underwent pulmonary thromboendarterectomy (PTE) had staphylococcal DNA detected on pathology specimens from endarterectomy in more than 85% (6/7) of patients studied.[19] The role of dysfibrinogenemia in the development of CTEPH is supported by findings from Morris and colleagues[12] who identified several genetic variants of fibrinogen in more than than 15% (5/33) of patients with CTEPH. These variants were associated with abnormalities of fibrin polymer structure and/or lysis. Additional insights into causes of nonresolving thromboembolic disease comes from several animal models of CTEPH. These include a model of defective angiogenesis with an endothelial cell–specific conditional deletion of vascular endothelial growth factor receptor 2/kinase, which leads to paucity of vessel formation and misdirected thrombus resolution[20] as well as a model of platelet endothelial cell adhesion molecule 1 deficiency, which was associated with increased thrombus burden, decreased thrombus vascularity, and increased fibrosis.[21] Ongoing study in this area is needed to increase understanding of the pathophysiology of abnormal thrombus resolution in CTEPH and provide potential targets for future intervention.

The nonresolving large vessel obstruction from previous PE in CTEPH is associated with a subsequent complex response of the pulmonary microvascular bed.[4] This is supported by a significant pulmonary vasculopathy seen on pathology specimens from patients with CTEPH revealing the entire spectrum of small pulmonary arterial changes, some suggesting even plexiform lesions similar to those seen in pulmonary arterial hypertension (PAH).[4,22,23] The nidus for the microvascular component of this disease is uncertain; however, endothelial dysfunction and impairment of vasomodulating pathways may in part explain these small vessel changes. This is supported by decreased nitric oxide synthase in an animal model of CTEPH[24] as well as increased circulating endothelin-1 levels in patients with CTEPH, which correlated with severity of PH and poor PTE postoperative outcomes.[25]

EVALUATION OF CHRONIC THROMBOEMBOLIC PULMONARY HYPERTENSION

In the diagnostic evaluation, it remains imperative to make an accurate distinction between CTEPH and other forms of PH because the diagnosis of CTEPH bears the potential for a cure achieved by PTE.[26]

History

The clinical presentation of patients with chronic thromboembolic disease can be deceptive, because typically there are no symptoms specific to this disorder. This contributes to the delay in diagnosis, making it necessary to maintain a high index of suspicion in those patients presenting with exertional dyspnea without apparent cause. A prior history of VTE may also be elusive, the European Registry indicating that up to 25% of patients with CTEPH are not known to have had a prior PE.[8] Atypical chest pains, episodic hemoptysis, nonproductive cough, and palpitations are rarely presenting complaints. Functional limitation in the absence of overt PH seem to result from 2 physiologic abnormalities related to residual pulmonary vascular obstruction and its effect on right ventricular function—an increase in dead space ventilation and an inability to optimally augment cardiac output to sufficiently meet exercise oxygen demands. Evidence of right heart dysfunction, such as severe exercise limitation and associated chest discomfort, exertional dizziness, or syncopal episodes, can be manifest late in the disease.

Physical Examination

Typical findings of PH and right heart failure (RHF) are important indicators of the severity of disease. These include elevated jugular venous pressure, tricuspid regurgitation murmur, loud pulmonic component of the second heart sound, and peripheral edema. The presence of pulmonary bruits is particularly informative, suggesting proximal disease causing turbulent flow. This may favorably predict operable disease.

Careful examination for indwelling venous catheters, ports, or pacemakers is important as a diagnostic clue for the cause of CTEPH and in identifying a therapeutic target for removal to prevent recurrent PE.

Postthrombotic syndrome (lower extremity swelling, hyperpigmentation, skin hardening, and varicose veins) in a patient with prior lower extremity DVT may indicate recurrent VTE associated with CTEPH. Particularly if noted on the left lower extremity in a patient with no other identifiable risk for VTE, this may prompt consideration for May-Thurner syndrome.[27]

Electrocardiogram

The electrocardiogram (ECG) may range from normal to significant right-sided abnormalities depending on the degree of afterload affecting the right ventricle (RV). For example, in chronic thromboembolic disease (CTED) without the presence of PH, the ECG may be normal. In CTEPH, as in PAH, findings of right ventricular hypertrophy (RVH), right axis deviation, right atrial enlargement, and T wave inversions in the right-sided precordial and inferior leads consistent with right heart strain may be seen (**Fig. 1**).[28]

Chest Radiography

Chest radiograph findings can be nearly identical to those of PAH. A prominent main pulmonary artery (PA) with Palla's sign (enlarged descending PA along the right heart border) is often seen. Depending on the degree of RHF, chest radiograph findings can reveal an enlarged right atrium extending the cardiac silhouette laterally, and a loss of retrosternal space on a lateral film, indicating RV enlargement (**Fig. 2**).

More specific to PE and CTEPH, evidence of pulmonary infarct may be seen as a wedged or rounded opacification juxtaposing the pleura, generally in the lower lobes. An area of hypovascularity, when combined with Palla's sign, can distinguish between CTEPH and idiopathic PAH with a positive and negative predictive value of 82 and 97, respectively.[29]

Echocardiogram

The degree of echocardiographic abnormalities will vary depending on the degree of PH and afterload impact on the right side of the heart.

Although acute PE has been associated with RV enlargement and dysfunction, a more careful assessment can distinguish between acute and chronic PE. The presence of RVH (RV wall thickness >5.0 mm) gives evidence for chronic RV loading.[30] Similarly, moderate to severe PH is less likely in acute PE, and its presence may reflect the anatomically diffuse chronic changes in the pulmonary vascular bed that occur in CTEPH.[31]

Echocardiography can identify an elevated PVR even before right heart catheterization. The presence of the flying "W" on M-mode assessment of the pulmonic valve is a well-described clue to the presence of PH.[30] Assessment of the pulse wave Doppler profile in the RV outflow tract, including a reduced acceleration time and the presence of a notch in the profile shape, is highly specific and sensitive for predicting the presence of an elevated PVR.[32] Systolic interventricular septal flattening also predicts the presence of an elevated PVR.[33]

Careful assessment of RV function can be done using a variety of methods, including tricuspid annular plane systolic excursion, S′ velocity, RV fractional area change, or RV index of myocardial performance[30] (**Fig. 3**).

Cardiopulmonary Exercise Testing

Cardiopulmonary exercise testing (CPET) can be informative to further delineate physiologic contributors to a patient's dyspnea. This is particularly

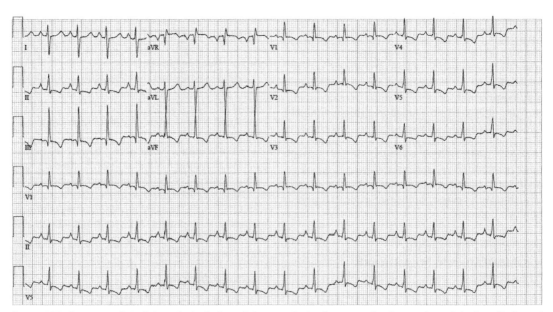

Fig. 1. ECG demonstrating right axis deviation, right ventricular hypertrophy, incomplete right bundle branch block, and right heart strain.

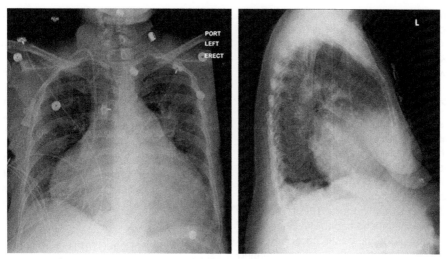

Fig. 2. Chest radiograph demonstrating right atrial enlargement, prominent pulmonary artery, and right ventricular enlargement with loss of retrosternal space.

helpful when coexisting with other cardiopulmonary diseases, obesity, deconditioning, and anemia in patients receiving anticoagulation therapy.

Findings on a CPET that represent CTEPH are those of cardiac limitation and ventilatory inefficiency. These include a reduced O_2 pulse (surrogate for stroke volume), systolic blood pressure response to exercise, ventilatory inefficiency with elevated VE/VCO_2, and reduced end-tidal CO_2 ($ETCO_2$). The degree of dead space ventilation in distal CTEPH has been shown to correlate with functional capacity and survival.[34]

Particularly in patients with CTED who do not have resting PH on echocardiography or RHC,

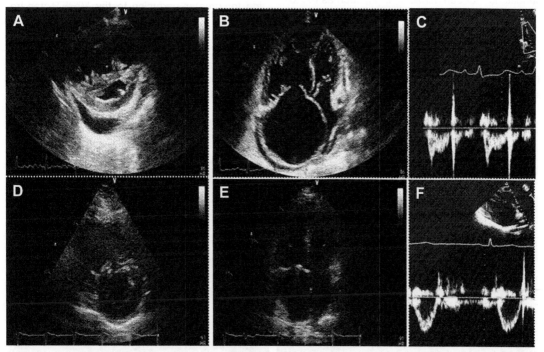

Fig. 3. Echocardiography before (*top row*) and after (*bottom row*) PTE. (*A*) Severe septal flattening with pericardial effusion. (*B*) Severe RV and RA enlargement. (*C*) RV outflow tract (RVOT) Doppler notch indicating elevated PVR. Panels (*D–F*) demonstrate resolution of these features.

but who have significant dyspnea, elevated VE/VCO$_2$, and reduced ETCO$_2$ can help secure the diagnosis of CTED.[35] This assessment can be critical in making the decision to proceed with PTE in a patient who does not have PH or RHF.

Ventilation–Perfusion (V/Q) Scintigraphy

The radioisotopic ventilation–perfusion (V/Q) scan has a sensitivity greater than 96% for detecting CTEPH. The characteristic normal ventilation with unmatched perfusion defects is highly suspicious for, but not specific for, CTEPH.[36]

Although the V/Q scan has been deemed the gold standard in screening for CTEPH, there are limitations in its diagnostic capability. Because of the partial recanalization, tracer can often pass distal to a nonobstructive clot, underestimating the thromboembolic disease burden[37] (Fig. 4).

Planar imaging depends on camera positioning and may underestimate perfusion defects on the basis of overlying lung tissue with normal perfusion. The use of single-photon emission computed tomography generates 3 dimensional images that can overcome this limitation and thus increase the sensitivity of the test in diagnosing CTEPH[38] (Fig. 5).

A perfusion defect seen on V/Q scan does not adequately distinguish between acute and chronic PE. Furthermore, unmatched perfusion defects seen on V/Q scanning can also be seen in other conditions that can mimic CTEPH, such as PA tumor emboli, fibrosing mediastinitis, or large vessel vasculitis.[39]

Computed Tomography of the Chest

The combination of high-resolution imaging with angiographic assessment using multiple cross-sectional views allows for a nearly comprehensive anatomic assessment. When PH is present, typical abnormalities of the heart are seen. This includes findings of RA enlargement, tricuspid valve annular dilatation, RV enlargement, and RV hypertrophy.[40]

Parenchymal lung abnormalities can also be distinct in CTEPH. A "mosaic" appearance results from varied perfusion leading to demarcated ground glass areas of normal perfusion with neighboring dark areas of hypoperfusion. Pulmonary infarct can be found in up to 15% of patients with PE as peripheral wedge-shaped hypovascular opacities with associated pleural thickening or fibrous, curvilinear scarring with lung volume loss[41] (Fig. 6).

Similar to PAH, in CTEPH there is vascular wall thickening and dilatation of the main pulmonary arteries. In CTEPH, however, because of heterogenous clot distribution, this may be asymmetric.[40] In contrast with acute PE, where clot is central in the lumen surrounded by contrast, CTEPH has thickening of the arterial wall with fibrous scars, webs, and vessel occlusion. Diseased areas become narrowed, accompanied by often subtle poststenotic dilatation[42] (Figs. 7 and 8).

In some cases, particularly when a disease is occlusive and proximal, arterial collaterals may be seen. These can help identify CTEPH, accounting for greater perfusion to the lungs compared with PAH. Collaterals are predominantly enlarged bronchial arteries but may also involve intercostal and internal mammary arteries. Identification requires near-simultaneous opacification of pulmonary and systemic circulations, and thus may be easily missed.[43]

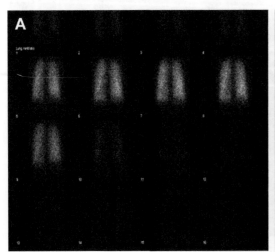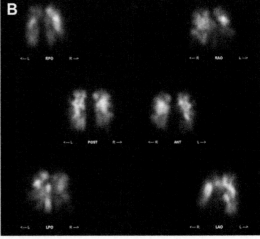

Fig. 4. V/Q scan. (*A*). Homogenous, normal ventilation. (*B*). Perfusion scan demonstrating multiple unmatched bilateral, subsegmental wedge-shaped perfusion defects.

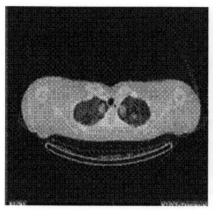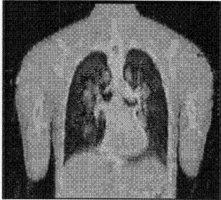

Fig. 5. Single-photon emission computed tomography demonstrating heterogenous perfusion in CTEPH.

CT angiography can distinguish between conditions that mimic CTEPH clinically and with unmatched perfusion defects on V/Q scan, but for which PTE is not indicated. Fibrosing mediastinitis is generally accompanied with calcification within the mediastinum or lining the PA walls and may be associated with pulmonary infiltrates. Systemic vasculitides (Takayasu, Behcet syndromes) have vascular aneurysms, narrowing of the main PA, systemic arterial involvement, and may be unilateral or predominantly upper lobe disease.[39,44] PA sarcoma generally involves the proximal PA, is unilateral, and may be associated with other intrapulmonary metastases.[45] Other solid tumors that have metastasized can present with pulmonary arterial tumor emboli mimicking CTEPH.[46] PA hypertension may coexist with in-situ thrombosis, particularly in the dilated vessels of systemic-to-pulmonary shunt syndromes. These clots are not flow-limiting and as such are not associated with mosaicism, collaterals, and infarction.[47]

Right Heart Catheterization

Right heart catheterization (RHC) is the gold standard for hemodynamic assessment, warranting careful attention to calibration, leveling, and measurements at end expiration. If resting hemodynamics are normal, but the suspicion for CTED remains high, exercise RHC can be performed to elicit an abnormal hemodynamic response to exercise that would support the link between CTED and functional limitation. Such abnormal findings would include an elevated RAP/PCW ratio, elevated PA pressure, a lack of reduction in PVR, or a limited cardiac output increase with exercise.

Catheter-Based Pulmonary Angiography

Invasive pulmonary angiography has been considered the most direct way to delineate the degree and anatomic location of thromboembolic burden, before consideration for PTE. Findings include vessel narrowing, poststenotic dilatation, occlusions or pouch defects, bands or webs (linear

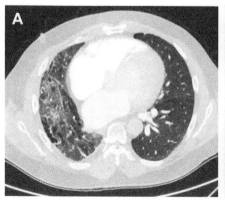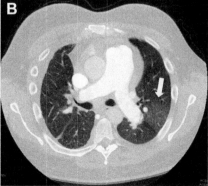

Fig. 6. CT chest (*A*). Pulmonary infarct seen as fibrous, curvilinear scarring with volume loss (*B*). Mosaic appearance with demarcated ground glass area of normal perfusion (*arrow*).

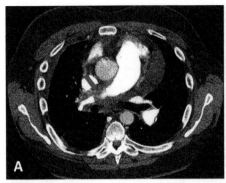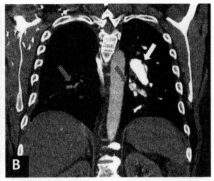

Fig. 7. CT angiography chest with arterial wall thickening and lining thrombus (*red arrow*), intravascular thrombus material (*blue arrows*), and intravascular linear web (*white arrow*) characteristic of CTEPH. (*A*) Axial plane. (*B*) Coronal plane.

lucencies within the vessel lumen), and peripheral hypovascularity in subsegmental disease.[48]

Various techniques have evolved to improve the safety and diagnostic yield of pulmonary angiography. Selective angiography of each lung ensures adequate assessment of the segmental and subsegmental branches. The use of digital subtraction angiography minimizes nonangiographic structures, simultaneously allowing for a lower volume of injected contrast.[49] Biplane angiography, or sequential anterior-posterior and lateral oblique projections, may identify filling defects otherwise obscured by normal overlying vessels (**Fig. 9**).

Venography

Recently, iliac vein abnormalities have been recognized as an important association with CTEPH. This includes compression from uterine fibroids or May-Thurner syndrome.[18] Invasive or noninvasive venography for this assessment should be considered, because it may guide further intervention toward mitigating future risk

of VTE, such as hysterectomy, myomectomy, or iliac vein stenting.

TREATMENT OF CHRONIC THROMBOEMBOLIC PULMONARY HYPERTENSION

The options for treating diagnosed chronic thromboembolic disease and CTEPH have expanded in a meaningful way over the past several years. For those selected patients with operable disease, PTE is the preferred treatment choice, given the high probability that a cure will be achieved for this form of PH. For patients with CTEPH with comorbidities precluding surgical consideration, or patients with inoperable disease, balloon pulmonary angioplasty (BPA) and PH-targeted medical therapy are currently the treatment options to consider. A recent treatment algorithm suggested in the 2015 ESC/ERS Guidelines for the Diagnosis and Treatment of Pulmonary Hypertension is presented in **Fig. 10**.[50]

With the advancements in surgical techniques and the availability of BPA, the assessment of

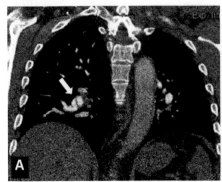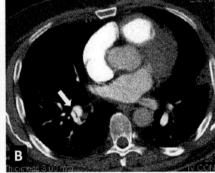

Fig. 8. CT angiography chest with intravascular linear webs characteristic of CTEPH (*arrow*). (*A*) Coronal plane. (*B*) Axial plane.

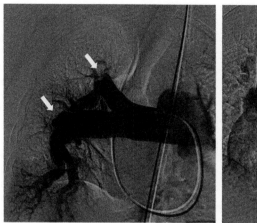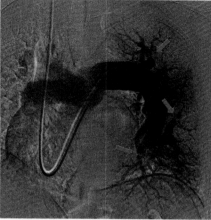

Fig. 9. Pulmonary angiography demonstrating pouch occlusions (*white arrows*), poststenotic dilatation (*red arrow*), and intravascular bands (*blue arrows*).

operability and surgical candidacy becomes increasingly important. As suggested in **Fig. 10**, every effort should be made to have patients with CTEPH evaluated at a center experienced

with performing PTE surgery. However, even at experienced CTEPH centers, operability assessment is often subjective, and a decision to proceed with a course of therapy should be accompanied

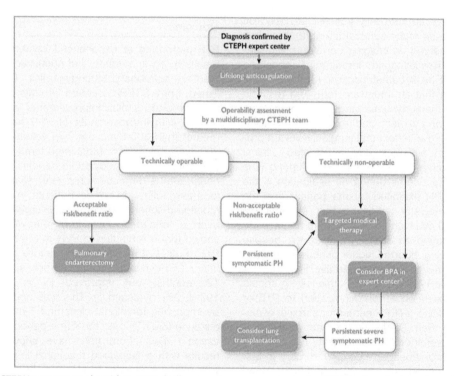

Fig. 10. CTEPH treatment algorithm. BPA, balloon pulmonary angioplasty; CTEPH, chronic thromboembolic pulmonary hypertension; PH, pulmonary hypertension. [a] Technically operable patients with nonacceptable risk/benefit ratio can be considered also for BPA. [b] In some centers medical therapy and BPA are initiated concurrently. (*Reproduced from* Galiè N, Humbert M, Vachiery JL, et al. 2015 ESC/ERS Guidelines for the diagnosis and treatment of pulmonary hypertension: The Joint Task Force for the Diagnosis and Treatment of Pulmonary Hypertension of the European Society of Cardiology (ESC) and the European Respiratory Society (ERS): Endorsed by: Association for European Paediatric and Congenital Cardiology (AEPC), International Society for Heart and Lung Transplantation (ISHLT). Eur Respir J 2015;46(4):957; doi:10.1183/13993003.01032-2015; with permission of the © 2018 European Society of Cardiology & European Respiratory Society. All rights reserved.)

by a discussion with patients weighing outcome expectations against associated risks.

PULMONARY THROMBOENDARTERECTOMY

PTE surgery has evolved significantly over the past decades, and most recently, surgical techniques have advanced to allow resection of chronic thrombotic material from the distal segmental and subsegmental vessels. However, the fundamental elements of the modern-day procedure have changed minimally since its inception. A thromboendarterectomy necessitates a median sternotomy, cardiopulmonary bypass, and deep hypothermia (for tissue protection) with circulatory arrest periods in order to provide a bloodless surgical field, allowing optimal visualization to facilitate as complete a dissection as possible. This is particularly important for an adequate distal vessel endarterectomy. Equally important to surgical success is appropriate patient selection and meticulous postoperative management.[51]

The key elements of surgical selection include the following considerations: (1) the chronic thrombotic lesions are surgically accessible based on the experience of the surgical team; (2) thrombus burden observed on imaging correlates with degree of hemodynamic impairment observed during right heart catheterization; (3) there is the anticipation that an endarterectomy will result in pulmonary hemodynamic and cardiopulmonary symptom improvement; and (4) patient comorbidities are not to an extent that surgical risks are prohibitive and outweigh any anticipated clinical benefits achieved with surgery. Among the most cited concerns during an evaluation is the degree of PH exhibited by the patient and the European Registry indicating that extreme PH (PVR >1500 dyn.s.cm^{-5}) represented an absolute contraindication to surgery.[8] However, despite centers having reported higher perioperative mortality in patients with preoperative PVR greater than 1000 to 1200 dyn.s.cm^{-5}, this finding should not be considered a contraindication to PTE or limit referral to a CTEPH center for surgical evaluation. The San Diego group has reported a declining overall operative mortality risk of 2.2% following thromboendarterectomy surgery in 500 patients operated between 2006 and 2010. However, in this same report, those patients with a preoperative PVR greater than 1000 dyn.s.cm^{-5} experienced a mortality rate of 4.1% compared with 1.6% in those patients with a PVR less than 1000 dyn.s.cm^{-5}.[26] More recently, de Perrot and colleagues[52] compared postendarterectomy outcomes in those patients with CTEPH with a preoperative total pulmonary vascular resistance of greater than (N = 26) or less than (N = 78) 1200 dyn.s.cm^{-5}. Overall in-hospital mortality after pulmonary endarterectomy was 4%, with all deaths occurring in patients with a TPR greater than 1200 dyn.s.cm^{-5} and decompensated RHF on presentation. Furthermore, advanced age by itself is not a contraindication to surgery. Over a 5-year period, Berman and colleagues[53] reported a comparable in-hospital mortality rate of 4.6% (14 of 308) for patients younger than 70 years compared with 7.8% (8 of 103) for those patients older than 70 years although total hospital days and intensive care unit days were greater in the older patient group. An elevated body mass index makes surgery and postoperative care technically more difficult but has not been shown to significantly increase mortality.[54] However, experience has established that patients with significant comorbid conditions such as severe emphysema, or those with a life-limiting malignancy, are not only at considerable perioperative risk, but are unlikely to realize the functional status benefit that might be achieved with a PTE.

Outcomes

PTE performed at experienced centers typically results in an immediate and sustained improvement in pulmonary hemodynamics. Data published from CTEPH centers around the world have reported similar improvements in hemodynamics with improvements of PVR from values greater than 800 dyn.s.cm^{-5} to values less than 400 dyn.s.cm^{-5}.[9,55,56] Most importantly, the resultant pulmonary hemodynamic benefits and functional status improvements are sustained on long-term follow-up in most patients. In a carefully monitored cohort of patients (229 surgery patients) over a decade, data from Papworth have shown that a reduction in PVR at 3 months after PTE (800 ± 494 dyn.s.cm^{-5} before surgery to 244 ± 253 dyn.s.cm^{-5}) was not only sustained at 12 months, but improved (N = 80, PVR 197 ± 289 dyn.s.cm^{-5}). This was accompanied by improving functional class and 6-minute walk distance (6MWD) over the same period of observation.[57] Data from Italy have shown similar results with a sustained functional improvement with 97% of patients NYHA III or IV before PTE and 74% improved to functional class I at 4-year follow-up.[58]

In hospital, mortality rates for PTE surgery have been reported to be 2.2%[26] and 4.2%[18] at 2 higher-volume PTE centers in the United States and 4.7% across multiple European centers.[9] Furthermore, long-term results following PTE have been excellent; representative is a report from the Netherlands demonstrating 1-, 3- and 5-year survival rates of 93.1%, 91.2%, and 88.7%, respectively.[59] A recent report from the United Kingdom examining a cohort of 880 patients undergoing long-term follow-up disclosed survival rates of 86%, 84%, 79%, and 72% at 1, 3, 5, and 10 years; the second half of the cohort exhibited a 91% and 90% at 1 and 3 years. Attributable cause of death was rarely thought to be because of RHF and CTEPH, although survivorship was adversely affected by the residual PH post-PTE as defined by a mean PA pressure greater than 38 mm Hg and a PVR greater than 425 dyn.s.cm^{-5}.[60]

Recent modifications of surgical techniques have allowed resection of chronic thromboembolic disease from the distal (segmental) pulmonary vessels. In a 2014 report from D'Armini and colleagues,[61] of 331 endarterectomies performed, 110 were classified as distal resection. Overall in-hospital mortality rate was 6.9% with no significant difference between distal versus proximal resection groups, and immediate pulmonary hemodynamic improvements were comparable (PVR 876 ± 392 to 251 + 146 dyn.s.cm^{-5} in the proximal group vs 926 ± 337 to 295 ± 161 dyne.s.cm^{-5} in the distal resection group). The sustained hemodynamic benefit at 12-month follow-up was also similar in both patient groups. This report demonstrated the possible benefits of distal vessel endarterectomy, although also emphasized that an endarterectomy performed at this level requires considerable surgical expertise.

Because perioperative mortality rates have declined, PTE surgery is now more routinely being performed in symptomatic patients with chronic thromboembolic disease (CTED) but without PH at rest. To a large extent, patients with CTED are thought to improve from PTE surgery through a reduction in dead space ventilation,[62] with the additional theoretic consideration that disease progression is abated with early surgical intervention. Recently a CTEPH center in the United Kingdom published data from 42 patients with symptomatic CTED and a baseline mean PA pressure less than 25 mm Hg who underwent PTE surgery. PTE resulted in a significant improvement in functional status and quality of life, with 95% of patients remaining NYHA class I or II at 1-year follow-up. Although there was no in-hospital mortality, postoperative complications occurred in 40% of patients.[63]

BALLOON PULMONARY ANGIOPLASTY

BPA is a percutaneous, catheter-based approach for the treatment of patients with CTEPH thought not to be candidates for endarterectomy surgery. Using selective pulmonary angiography, targeted chronic thrombotic lesions are mechanically dilated with balloons to relieve pulmonary vascular obstruction. First described in 1988[64] as a treatment option for CTEPH, there was a limited resurgence of interest in the technique in 2001.[65] With subsequent refinements reported by several Japanese groups in 2012,[66–68] BPA has now emerged as a viable treatment option for select patients with CTEPH.

Outcomes

A recent report from a multicenter registry of 7 Japanese institutions performing BPA summarizes the outcome in a total of 308 patients with CTEPH undergoing 1408 procedures (median of 4 sessions per patient) between 2004 and 2013, with the follow-up period ending in 2014. Although reflective of the early BPA experience with variation in patient selection and procedural approach, the overall results in those patients with CTEPH thought not to be candidates for PTE documented considerable efficacy. A reduction in mean PA pressure from 43.2 ± 11.0 to 24.3 ± 6.4 mm Hg after the final BPA session was observed, a result that was sustained at follow-up (196 patients undergoing follow-up catheterization at mean of 425.5 ± 280.9 days after the final BPA session). This was accompanied by an improvement in functional class and a reduction in brain-type natriuretic peptide (BNP) levels, along with a reduction in supplemental oxygen use (73.7%–21.9%) and some reduction in PH-targeted medications. Complications occurred in 36.3% of patients—lung injury observed in 17.8%, hemoptysis in 14.0%, and PA perforation in 2.9%. Overall survival during the observation period was 96.8% (1 and 2 years), and 94.5% at 3 years, with 8 of the total 12 patient deaths occurring within 30 days of BPA.[69]

Similar hemodynamic outcomes with BPA for inoperable CTEPH have been reported by other centers throughout the world.[70,71] However, with expanding experience and procedural modifications, an improved safety profile has been observed. Patient selection, accurate balloon sizing and localization of lesion types with the use of intravascular imaging modalities such as intravascular ultrasound and optical coherence tomography,[72–74] the use of intravascular pressure gradient measurements,[71,75] characterization of specific lesion types,[76] and adaptation of interventional technique to the severity of PH have variably contributed to improved safety.

To better explore the role for BPA within a practice having extensive surgical management experience, a German group reported their results with BPA in patients with CTEPH thought not to be candidates for PTE. In these 56 patients undergoing 266 BPA sessions, BPA resulted in an improvement in functional status, 6MWD, and right ventricular function. However, the observed change in pulmonary hemodynamics was more modest than that reported from other centers, with a decline in mean PA pressure of 18% and pulmonary vascular resistance of 26%. Although several possible explanations were offered, a stricter criterion for inoperability was acknowledged as potentially contributing to the difference. In this series, associated mortality rate was low at 1.8%, but the procedural complication rate of 9.4% was observed, mostly related to vascular injury and self-limited pulmonary hemorrhage.[77]

As a result of the observed efficacy of this intervention, expansion of the indications for BPA beyond inoperable CTEPH has begun to occur. Indications currently under investigation include a combined approach with endarterectomy surgery[78] for those patients with residual PH after PTE (with residual lesions amenable to angioplasty) and as a treatment option for patients with CTED.[79]

PULMONARY HYPERTENSION–TARGETED MEDICAL THERAPY

The use of PH-targeted medical therapy for treating patients with CTEPH has been reported in several different clinical settings, such as "bridging therapy" in patients with operable CTEPH and in patients with CTEPH with nonsurgical disease and as complement therapy for those patients undergoing BPA. Medications approved for use in other forms of PAH have been and continue to be used in these CTEPH patient groups, although most clinical trials have focused on those with nonsurgical disease, and very few have been randomized, controlled trials. To date, only a soluble guanylate cyclase stimulator (riociguat) has been approved by Food and Drug Administration for use in inoperable CTEPH or residual PH after PTE surgery.

Inoperable Chronic Thromboembolic Pulmonary Hypertension

Small retrospective cohort studies with prostanoids suggested efficacy in this group of patients. Cabrol and colleagues[80] retrospectively analyzed 27 patients with inoperable CTEPH treated with epoprostenol. After 3 months of therapy, there was a decrease in mean PA pressure (56 ± 9 mm Hg to 51 ± 8 mm Hg) and total pulmonary resistance (29.3 ± 7.0 U/m^2 to 23.0 ± 5.0 U/m^2). This was accompanied by an improvement in functional

status in 11 of 23 patients and an increase in 6MWD of 66 m. Similarly, in a single-center uncontrolled observational study, 28 patients with severe inoperable CTEPH were treated with subcutaneous treprostinil. Right heart catheterization was repeated in 19 patients after 19 ± 6.3 months of treatment, showing a significant reduction in PVR and an improvement in 6MWD (59 m), WHO functional class, BNP levels, and cardiac output.[81]

Early investigations of other classes of PH-targeted medical therapy for inoperable CTEPH were similarly limited in scope. Sildenafil, a phosphodiesterase-5 inhibitor, was evaluated in a single-center randomized placebo controlled trial enrolling 19 patients with inoperable CTEPH in a 12-week pilot study. Although there was no significant difference detected in the primary endpoint of the 6MWD, an improvement in WHO functional class and a pulmonary hemodynamic effect was noted during the study period (reduction in PVR of 197 dyn.sec.cm^{-5} in the treatment group). Control subjects were then transitioned to open-label sildenafil use and reassessed at 12 months. Significant improvement in 6MWD, activity and symptom scores (CAMPHOR), cardiac index, PVR, and measures of RV function were noted.[82] In a larger patient group, Reichenberger and colleagues[83] conducted an open-label study of sildenafil (50 mg 3 times a day) in 104 patients with inoperable CTEPH. After 3 months of therapy, there was a modest decrease in pulmonary vascular resistance (863 ± 38 dyn.sec.cm^{-5} to 759 ± 62 dyn.sec.cm^{-5}) and an increase in 6MWD from 310 ± 11 m to 361 ± 15 m. Further improvement in 6MWD was observed at 12 months.

The first large, randomized, controlled trial in inoperable CTEPH was conducted with the endothelin receptor antagonist, bosentan. In the BENEFiT trial, 157 patients with either inoperable CTEPH or residual PH postendarterectomy were randomized to receive either bosentan or placebo. The coprimary endpoints investigated after 16 weeks of therapy included an improvement in 6MWD and percent change from baseline in PVR. Bosentan did not improve 6MWD (+2.2 m; 95% CI: −22.5 to +26.8 m) but did reduce PVR 24% from baseline. In a subgroup analysis, the absolute reduction in PVR in the inoperable subgroup (N = 96) was to a lesser degree (−127 dyn.sec.cm^{-5}, 95% CI: −206 to −48 dyn.sec.cm^{-5}) compared with the residual PH group (N = 41; −193 dyn.sec.cm^{-5}; 95% CI: −278 to 108 dyn.sec.cm^{-5}). However, despite this hemodynamic effect, bosentan-treated patients with residual PH actually saw an 11.9 m loss in 6MWD compared with placebo-treated patients.[84]

The most recent randomized, placebo-controlled trial in patients with inoperable CTEPH examined the use of another endothelin receptor antagonist, macitentan. Merit-1 was a phase 2 trial enrolling 80 patients adjudicated as having nonsurgical disease, all patients WHO-FC II–IV with a PVR greater than 400 dyn.s.cm^{-5}. For patients more functionally compromised (WHO-FC III–IV), the concurrent use of phosphodiesterase type 5 inhibitors and oral or inhaled prostanoids were allowed (60% in the macitentan group vs 63% in the placebo group). With the primary endpoint of PVR at 16 weeks of treatment, those in the macitentan group (N = 40) demonstrated a mean PVR reduction of 73.0% of baseline compared with 87.2% decline in those receiving placebo. Six-minute walk distance at 24 weeks increased by a mean of 35.0 minutes (SD 52–52) in the macitentan group as compared with 1.0 m (SD 83–24) in those patients receiving placebo. The most common adverse effects in the macitentan group were peripheral edema (23%) and a lower hemoglobin level (15%); hemoptysis occurred in 3% of patients in both groups.[85]

Riociguat is a soluble guanylate cyclase stimulator and the first agent in this pharmaceutical class. In the CHEST-1 study, 261 patients with CTEPH (189 of whom were deemed inoperable) were randomized to 16 weeks of either riociguat (starting at 1 mg and titrated to 2.5 mg or the maximum tolerated dose) or placebo. In the riociguat-treated group, there was placebo-adjusted mean change in 6MWD of 46 m (P<.001). In addition, there were positive hemodynamic benefits in the treated group with a mean reduction in PVR of 246 dyn.sec.cm^{-5} as well as a placebo-adjusted reduction in N-terminal pro B-type natriuretic peptide of −444 pg/mL in the treated group.[86] An open-label extension phase of CHEST-1 (CHEST-2) provided riociguat for all eligible patients receiving placebo in CHEST-1. A total enrollment of 237 patients was achieved, with a cumulative treatment exposure of 378 patient years. The 6MWD improved overall by +59 (±58) m for those having received riociguat in CHEST-1 and increased to +37 (±69) m in the group previously receiving placebo. At 2 years of riociguat, survival was 93% (95% CI: 89%–96%); clinical worsening-free survival was 82% (95% CI: 84%–92%). The most common drug-related serious adverse events included syncope (2%) and hypotension (1%) in CHEST-2. In addition, 8 (3%) adverse events and 4 (2%) serious adverse events of hemoptysis and pulmonary hemorrhage occurred in the extension study.[87]

SUMMARY

CTEPH is an uncommon and underrecognized pulmonary vascular disorder that occurs in a small percentage of PE survivors.[6,7] It is a result of a complex interaction between pulmonary macrovasculature obstruction and microvascular bed's response to this.[1,4] These changes lead to a progressive pulmonary vasculopathy, which results in PH and ultimately RHF. Detection of disease requires clinical suspicion followed by a throughout evaluation including radiographic and hemodynamic assessment. Once diagnosed, consultation with a center with CTEPH expertise is recommended to formulate a management plan and to assess for operability with pulmonary endarterectomy.[26] For those deemed inoperable, catheter-based intervention[70] and medical management are considered.

In conclusion, CTEPH is a treatable and potential curable form of PH; however, its diagnosis is often delayed and frequently missed. A high index of suspicion, complete evaluation, and close collaboration with an expert center is necessary for optimal outcomes.

REFERENCES

1. Moser KM, Auger WR, Fedullo PF. Chronic major-vessel thromboembolic pulmonary hypertension. Circulation 1990;81:1735–43.
2. Simonneau G, Gatzoulis MA, Adatia I, et al. Updated clinical classification of pulmonary hypertension. J Am Coll Cardiol 2013;62:D34–41.
3. Gall H, Hoeper MM, Richter MJ, et al. An epidemiological analysis of the burden of chronic thromboembolic pulmonary hypertension in the USA, Europe and Japan. Eur Respir Rev 2017;26. https://doi.org/10.1183/16000617.0121-2016.
4. Dormüller P, Günther S, Ghigna MR, et al. Microvascular disease in chronic thromboembolic pulmonary hypertension: a role for pulmonary veins and systemic vasculature. Eur Respir J 2014;44:1275–88.
5. Quark R, Wynants M, Verbeken E, et al. Contribution of inflammation and impaired angiogenesis to the pathobiology of chronic thromboembolic pulmonary hypertension. Eur Respir J 2015;46:431–43.
6. Tapson VF, Platt DM, Xia F, et al. Monitoring for pulmonary hypertension following pulmonary embolism: the INFORM study. Am J Med 2016;129:978–85.e2.
7. Pengo V, Lensing AW, Prins MH, et al. Incidence of chronic thromboembolic pulmonary hypertension after pulmonary embolism. N Engl J Med 2004;350:2257–64.

8. Pepke-Zaba J, Delcroix M, Lang I, et al. Chronic thromboembolic pulmonary hypertension (CTEPH): results from an international prospective registry. Circulation 2011;124:1973–81.

9. Mayer E, Jenkins D, Lindner J, et al. Surgical management and outcome of patients with chronic thromboembolic pulmonary hypertension: results from an international prospective registry. J Thorac Cardiovasc Surg 2011;141:702–10.

10. Yang S, Yang Y, Zhai Z, et al. Incidence and risk factors of chronic thromboembolic pulmonary hypertension in patients after acute pulmonary embolism. J Thorac Dis 2015;7:1927–38.

11. Bonderman D, Turecek PL, Jakowitsch J, et al. High prevalence of elevated clotting factor VIII in chronic thromboembolic pulmonary hypertension. Thromb Haemost 2003;90:372–6.

12. Morris TA, Marsh JJ, Chiles PG, et al. High prevalence of dysfibrinogenemia among patients with chronic thromboembolic pulmonary hypertension. Blood 2009;114:1929–36.

13. Wolf M, Boyer-Neumann C, Parent F, et al. Thrombotic risk factors in pulmonary hypertension. Eur Respir J 2000;15:395–9.

14. Jais X, Ioos V, Jardim C, et al. Splenectomy and chronic thromboembolic pulmonary hypertension. Thorax 2005;60:1031–4.

15. Bonderman D, Wilkens H, Wakounig S, et al. Risk factors for chronic thromboembolic pulmonary hypertension. Eur Respir J 2009;33:325–31.

16. Kominami S, Tanabe N, Ota M, et al. HLA-DPB1 and NFKBIL1 may confer the susceptibility to chronic thromboembolic pulmonary hypertension in the absence of deep vein thrombosis. J Hum Genet 2009;54:108–14.

17. Bonderman D, Jakowitsch J, Adlbrecht C, et al. Medical conditions increasing the risk of chronic thromboembolic pulmonary hypertension. Thromb Haemost 2005;93:512–6.

18. Raza F, Vaidya A, Lacharite-Roberge AS, et al. Initial clinical and hemodynamic results of a regional pulmonary Thromboendarterectomy program. J Cardiovasc Surg (Torino) 2017. https://doi.org/10.23736/S0021-9509.17.10188-6.

19. Bonderman D, Jakowitsch J, Redwan B, et al. Role for staphylococci in misguided thrombus resolution of chronic thromboembolic pulmonary hypertension. Arterioscler Thromb Vasc Biol 2008;28:678–84.

20. Alias S, Redwan B, Panzenboeck A, et al. Defective angiogenesis delays thrombus resolution: a potential pathogenetic mechanism underlying chronic thromboembolic pulmonary hypertension. Arterioscler Thromb Vasc Biol 2014;34:810–9.

21. Kellermair J, Redwan B, Alias S, et al. Platelet endothelial cell adhesion molecule 1 deficiency misguides venous thrombus resolution. Blood 2013;122:3376–84.

22. Moser KM, Bloor CM. Pulmonary vascular lesions occurring in patients with chronic major vessel thromboembolic pulmonary hypertension. Chest 1993;103:685–92.

23. Yi ES, Kim H, Ahn H, et al. Distribution of obstructive intimal lesions and their cellular phenotypes in chronic pulmonary hypertension. A morphometric and immunohistochemical study. Am J Respir Crit Care Med 2000;162:1577–86.

24. Fadel E, Mazmanian GM, Baudet B, et al. Endothelial nitric oxide synthase function in pig lung after chronic pulmonary artery obstruction. Am J Respir Crit Care Med 2000;162:1429–34.

25. Reesink HJ, Meijer RC, Lutter R, et al. Hemodynamic and clinical correlates of endothelin-1 in chronic thromboembolic pulmonary hypertension. Circ J 2006;70:1058–63.

26. Madani MM, Auger WR, Pretorius V, et al. Pulmonary endarterectomy: recent changes in a single institution's experience of more than 2,700 patients. Ann Thorac Surg 2012;94:97–103.

27. Bartholomew JR. Update on the management of venous thromboembolism. Cleve Clin J Med 2017; 84(12 Suppl 3):39–46.

28. Cheng XL, He JG, Gu Q, et al. The value of the electrocardiogram for evaluating prognosis in patients with idiopathic pulmonary arterial hypertension. Lung 2017;195(1):139–46.

29. Satoh T, Kyotani S, Okano Y, et al. Descriptive patterns of severe chronic pulmonary hypertension by chest radiography. Respir Med 2005;99:329–36.

30. Vaidya A, Kirkpatrick J. Right ventricular anatomy, function, and echocardiographic evaluation. 5th edition of Otto's the practice of clinical echocardiography. Philadelphia: Elsevier Publishing; 2016.

31. Wright L, Dwyer N, Power J, et al. Right ventricular systolic function responses to acute and chronic pulmonary hypertension: assessment with myocardial deformation. J Am Soc Echocardiogr 2016; 29(3):259–66.

32. Arkles JS, Opotowsky AR, Ojeda J, et al. Shape of the right ventricular Doppler envelope predicts hemodynamics and right heart function in pulmonary hypertension. Am J Respir Crit Care Med 2011; 183(2):268–76.

33. Opotowsky AR, Ojeda J, Rogers F, et al. A simple echocardiographic prediction rule for hemodynamics in pulmonary hypertension. Circ Cardiovasc Imaging 2012;5(6):765–75.

34. Godinas L, Sattler C, Lau EM, et al. Dead-space ventilation is linked to exercise capacity and survival in distal chronic thromboembolic pulmonary hypertension. J Heart Lung Transplant 2017;36(11):1234–42.

35. Held M, Grün M, Holl R, et al. Cardiopulmonary exercise testing to detect chronic thromboembolic pulmonary hypertension in patients

with normal echocardiography. Respiration 2014; 87(5):379–87.

36. Tunariu N. Ventilation-perfusion scintigraphy is more sensitive than multidetector CTPA in detecting chronic thromboembolic pulmonary disease as a treatable cause of pulmonary hypertension. J Nucl Med 2007;48:680–4.

37. Ryan KL, Fedullo PF, Davis GB, et al. Perfusion scan findings understate the severity of angiographic and hemodynamic compromise in chronic thromboembolic pulmonary hypertension. Chest 1988;93:1180–5.

38. Soler X, Hoh CK, Test VJ, et al. Single photon emission computed tomography in chronic thromboembolic pulmonary hypertension. Respirology 2011;16:131–7.

39. Gopalan D, Blanchard D, Auger WR. Diagnostic evaluation of chronic thromboembolic pulmonary hypertension. Ann Am Thorac Soc 2016;13(3): S222–39.

40. King MA, Ysrael M, Bergin CJ. Chronic thromboembolic pulmonary hypertension: CT findings. AJR Am J Roentgenol 1998;170:955–60.

41. Frazier AA, Galvin JR, Franks TJ, et al. From the archives of the AFIP: pulmonary vasculature: hypertension and infarction. Radiographics 2000;20:491–524.

42. Hong YJ, Kim JY, Choe KO, et al. Different perfusion pattern between acute and chronic pulmonary thromboembolism: evaluation with two-phase dual-energy perfusion CT. AJR Am J Roentgenol 2013; 200:812–7.

43. Remy-Jardin M, Duhamel A, Deken V, et al. Systemic collateral supply in patients with chronic thromboembolic and primary pulmonary hypertension: assessment with multidetector row helical CT angiography. Radiology 2005;235:274–81.

44. Kerr KM, Auger WR, Fedullo PF, et al. Large vessel pulmonary arteritis mimicking chronic thromboembolic disease. Am J Respir Crit Care Med 1995;152:367–73.

45. Yi CA, Lee KS, Choe YH, et al. Computed tomography in pulmonary artery sarcoma: distinguishing features from pulmonary embolic disease. J Comput Assist Tomogr 2004;28:34–9.

46. Roberts KE, Hamele-Bena D, Saqi A, et al. Pulmonary tumor embolism: a review of the literature. Am J Med 2003;115:228.

47. Perloff JK, Hart EM, Greaves SM, et al. Proximal pulmonary arterial and intrapulmonary radiologic features of Eisenmenger syndrome and primary pulmonary hypertension. Am J Cardiol 2003;92:182–7.

48. Auger WR, Fedullo PF, Moser KM, et al. Chronic major-vessel thromboembolic pulmonary artery obstruction: appearance at angiography. Radiology 1992;182:393–8.

49. Pond GD, Ovitt TW, Capp MP. Comparison of conventional pulmonary angiography with intravenous digital subtraction angiography for pulmonary embolic disease. Radiology 1983;147(2):345–50.

50. Galie N, Humbert M, Vachiery JL, et al. 2015 ESC/ERS Guidelines for the diagnosis and treatment of pulmonary hypertension. Eur Heart J 2015;37: 67–119.

51. Madani M, Mayer E, Fadel E, et al. Pulmonary endarterectomy: patient selection, technical challenges, and outcomes. Ann Am Thorac Soc 2016;13(Suppl 3):S240–7.

52. de Perrot M, Thenganatt J, McRae K, et al. Pulmonary endarterectomy in severe chronic thromboembolic pulmonary hypertension. J Heart Lung Transplant 2015;34:369–75.

53. Berman M, Hardman G, Sharples L, et al. Pulmonary endarterectomy: outcomes in patients aged > 70. Eur J Cardiothorac Surg 2012;41:e154–60.

54. Fernandes TM, Auger WR, Fedullo PF, et al. Baseline body mass index does not significantly affect outcomes after pulmonary thromboendarterectomy. Ann Thorac Surg 2014;8:1776–81.

55. Rahnavardi M, Yan TD, Cao C, et al. Pulmonary thromboendarterectomy for chronic thromboembolic pulmonary hypertension: a systematic review. Ann Thorac Cardiovasc Surg 2011;17:435–45.

56. Condliffe R, Kiely DG, Gibbs JS, et al. Improved outcomes in medically and surgically treated chronic thromboembolic pulmonary hypertension. Am J Respir Crit Care Med 2008;177:1122–7.

57. Freed DH, Thomson BM, Berman M, et al. Functional and haemodynamic outcome 1 year after pulmonary thromboendarterectomy. Eur J Cardiothorac Surg 2008;34:525–30.

58. Corsico AG, D'Armini AM, Cerveri I, et al. Long term outcome after pulmonary thromboendarterectomy. Am J Respir Crit Care Med 2008;178: 419–24.

59. Saouti N, Morshius WJ, Heijmen RH, et al. Long-term outcome after pulmonary endarterectomy for chronic thromboembolic pulmonary hypertension: a single institution experience. Eur J Cardiothorac Surg 2009;35(6):947–52.

60. Cannon JE, Kiely DG, Page K, et al. Dynamic risk stratification of patient long-term outcome after pulmonary endarterectomy. Results from the United Kingdom National Cohort. Circulation 2016;133: 1761–71.

61. D'Armini AM, Morsolini M, Mattiucci G, et al. Pulmonary endarterectomy for distal chronic thromboembolic pulmonary hypertension. J Thorac Cardiovasc Surg 2014;148(3):1005–11.

62. van der Plas MN, Reesink HJ, Roos CM. Pulmonary endarterectomy improves dyspnea by the relief of dead space ventilation. Ann Thorac Surg 2010;89: 347–52.

63. Taboada D, Pepke-Zaba J, Jenkins DP, et al. Outcome of pulmonary endarterectomy in symptomatic chronic thromboembolic disease. Eur Respir J 2014;44(6):1635–45.

64. Voorburg JAI, Manger Cats V, Buis B, et al. Balloon angioplasty in the treatment of pulmonary hypertension caused by pulmonary embolism. Chest 1988;94:1249–53.

65. Feinstein JA, Goldhaber SZ, Lock JE, et al. Balloon pulmonary angioplasty for treatment of chronic thromboembolic pulmonary hypertension. Circulation 2001;103(1):10–3.

66. Kataoka M, Inami T, Hayashida K, et al. Percutaneous transluminal pulmonary angioplasty for the treatment of chronic thromboembolic pulmonary hypertension. Circ Cardiovasc Interv 2012;5(6):756–62.

67. Sugimura K, Fukumoto Y, Satoh K, et al. Percutaneous transluminal pulmonary angioplasty markedly improves pulmonary hemodynamics and long-term prognosis in patients with chronic thromboembolic pulmonary hypertension. Circ J 2012;76(2):485–8.

68. Mizoguchi H, Ogawa A, Munemasa M, et al. Refined balloon pulmonary angioplasty for inoperable patients with chronic thromboembolic pulmonary hypertension. Circ Cardiovasc Interv 2012;5(6):748–55.

69. Ogawa A, Satoh T, Fukuda T, et al. Balloon pulmonary angioplasty for chronic thromboembolic pulmonary hypertension: results of a multicenter registry. Circ Cardiovasc Qual Outcomes 2017;10(11) [pii: e004029].

70. Andreassen AK, Ragnarsson A, Gude E, et al. Balloon pulmonary angioplasty in patients with inoperable chronic thromboembolic pulmonary hypertension. Heart 2013;99(19):1415–20.

71. Roik M, Wretowski D, Łabyk A, et al. Refined balloon pulmonary angioplasty driven by combined assessment of intra-arterial anatomy and physiology - multimodal approach to treated lesions in patients with non-operable distal chronic thromboembolic pulmonary hypertension - technique, safety and efficacy of 50 consecutive angioplasties. Int J Cardiol 2016; 203:228–35.

72. Ikeda N, Kubota S, Okazaki T, et al. Comparison of intravascular optical frequency domain imaging versus intravascular ultrasound during balloon pulmonary angioplasty in patients with chronic thromboembolic pulmonary hypertension. Catheter Cardiovasc Interv 2016;87(7):E268–74.

73. Jorge E, Baptista R, Calisto J, et al. Optical coherence tomography of the pulmonary arteries: a systematic review. J Cardiol 2016;67(1):6–14.

74. Aoki T, Sugimura K, Tatebe S, et al. Comprehensive evaluation of the effectiveness and safety of balloon pulmonary angioplasty for inoperable chronic thromb-embolic pulmonary hypertension: long-term effects and procedure-related complications. Eur Heart J 2017;38:3152–9.

75. Inami T, Kataoka M, Shimura N, et al. Pressure-wire-guided percutaneous transluminal pulmonary angioplasty: a breakthrough in catheter-interventional therapy for chronic thromboembolic pulmonary hypertension. JACC Cardiovasc Interv 2014;7(11): 1297–306.

76. Inohara T, Kawakami T, Kataoka M, et al. Lesion morphological classification by OCT to predict therapeutic efficacy after balloon pulmonary angioplasty in CTEPH. Int J Cardiol 2015;197:23–5.

77. Olsson KM, Wiedenroth CB, Kamp JC, et al. Balloon pulmonary angioplasty for inoperable patients with chronic thromboembolic pulmonary hypertension: the intitial German experience. Eur Respir J 2017; 49:1602409.

78. Wiedenroth CB, Liebetrau C, Breithecker A, et al. Combined pulmonary endarterectomy and balloon pulmonary angioplasty in patients with chronic thromboembolic pulmonary hypertension. J Heart Lung Transplant 2016;35(5):591–6.

79. Wiedenroth CB, Olsson KM, Guth S, et al. Ballloon pulmonary angioplasty for inoperable patients with chronic thromboembolic disease. Pulm Circ 2018; 8(1):1–6.

80. Cabrol S, Souza R, Jais X, et al. Intravenous epoprostenol in inoperable chronic thromboembolic pulmonary hypertension. J Heart Lung Transplant 2007; 26(4):357–62.

81. Skoro-Sajer N, Bonderman D, Wiesbauer F, et al. Treprostinil for severe inoperable chronic thromboembolic pulmonary hypertension. J Thromb Haemost 2007;5(3):483–9.

82. Suntharalingam J, Treacy CM, Doughty NJ, et al. Long-term use of sildenafil in inoperable chronic thromboembolic pulmonary hypertension. Chest 2008;134:229–36.

83. Reichenberger F, Voswinckel R, Enke B, et al. Long-term treatment with sildenafil in chronic thromboembolic pulmonary hypertension. Eur Respir J 2007;30: 922–7.

84. Jais X, D'Armini AM, Jansa P, et al. Bosentan for treatment of inoperable chronic thromboembolic pulmonary hypertension: BENEFiT (bosentan effects in iNopErable forms of chronic thromboembolic pulmonary hypertension), a randomized, placebo-controlled trial. J Am Coll Cardiol 2008;52:2127–34.

85. Ghofrani HA, Simmoneau G, D'Armini AM, et al. Macitentan for the treatment of inoperable chronic thromboembolic pulmonary hypertension (MERIT-1): results from the multicentre, pahse2, randomised, double-blind, placebo-controlled study. Lancet Respir Med 2017;10:785–94.

86. Ghofrani HA, D'Armini AM, Grimminger F, et al. Riociguat for the treatment of chronic thromboembolic pulmonary hypertension. N Engl J Med 2013;369:319–29.

87. Simonneau G, D'Armini AM, Ghofrani HA, et al. Predictors of long-term outcomes in patients treated with riociguat for chronic thromboembolic pulmonary hypertension: data from the CHEST-2 open-label, randomised, long-term extension trial. Lancet Respir Med 2016;4:372–80.

Pulmonary Embolism Response Team
Inpatient Structure, Outpatient Follow-up, and Is It the Current Standard of Care?

Rachel Rosovsky, MD, MPH[a],*, Jorge Borges, MD[b],
Christopher Kabrhel, MD, MPH[c], Kenneth Rosenfield, MD[b]

KEYWORDS

- Pulmonary embolism (PE) • Pulmonary embolism response team (PERT) • Multidisciplinary care
- Follow-up clinic • Anticoagulation management • Direct oral anticoagulants (DOACs)

KEY POINTS

- Pulmonary embolism (PE) is a major cause of morbidity and mortality in the United States; although many novel strategies and tools have emerged to advance the treatment of patients with high-risk PE, the mortality rate for these patients remains high.
- To address this crisis, pulmonary embolism response teams (PERTs) are developing around the United States and internationally to provide rapid, individualized, and evidenced-based care for patients with acute PE. The creation of PERTs may reflect a paradigm shift in the treatment of PE.
- The infrastructure of each PERT will depend on the needs and resources of each institution, and a key component to any PERT program is the development of an outpatient follow-up clinic.
- PERTs have come together to establish the PERT Consortium with the vision to guide and influence the care of PE worldwide.

INTRODUCTION

Pulmonary embolism (PE) is a major cause of morbidity and mortality in the United States.[1] Venous thromboembolism (VTE) has an incidence of 1 to 2 per 1000 adults per year, is the third most common cause of cardiovascular death, and the number one cause of preventable in-hospital deaths in the United States.[2] The diagnosis of PE can be complex, and the severity ranges from an incidentally identified PE of minimal clinical significance to a massive PE that causes hemodynamic collapse. Many novel strategies and tools have emerged recently to advance the treatment of

Disclosures: R. Rosovsky discloses the following relationships: research support from Janssen Pharmaceuticals and Bristol Meyer Squibb; consultant to Bayer. J. Borges has no disclosures. C. Kabrhel discloses the following relationships: consultant to Diagnostica Stago, Janssen Pharmaceuticals, Siemens, Pfizer, and Portola Pharmaceuticals; grant recipient from Diagnostica Stago, Siemens Healthcare, Janssen Pharmaceuticals, and Boehringer Ingelheim. K. Rosenfield discloses the following relationships: consultant to Cardinal Health and SurModics; grants/contracts with Abbott Vascular, Atrium, Lutonix/BARD, and The Medicines Company; equity with Access Closure, Inc and AngioDynamics/Vortex; personal compensation from Cook, HCRI, and The Medicines Company; board member with VIVA Physicians.
[a] Division of Hematology and Oncology, Department of Medicine, Massachusetts Hospital, 55 Fruit Street, Boston, MA 02114, USA; [b] Division of Cardiology, Section of Vascular Medicine and Intervention, Department of Medicine, Massachusetts Hospital, 55 Fruit Street, Boston, MA 02114, USA; [c] Department of Emergency Medicine, Center for Vascular Emergencies, Massachusetts General Hospital, 55 Fruit Street, Boston, MA 02114, USA
* Corresponding author.
E-mail address: rprosovsky@partners.org

Clin Chest Med 39 (2018) 621–630
https://doi.org/10.1016/j.ccm.2018.04.019
0272-5231/18/© 2018 Elsevier Inc. All rights reserved.

patients with high-risk PEs. Despite these advances, the mortality rate for patients who present with massive PEs remains as high as 50%.[3,4] Furthermore, rigorously vetted guidelines and robust data comparing various strategies are lacking, so clinical decisions vary depending on which specialist is evaluating the patients. As a result, treatment approaches may be inconsistent and uncoordinated with no single centralized location of care or systematic way to evaluate the response to therapy. To address this, in 2012, the Massachusetts General Hospital (MGH) created a multidisciplinary rapid-response team to assess and provide clinical recommendations for patients with PE in real time.[5,6] Since then, many institutions around the world have developed pulmonary embolism response teams (PERTs) to expeditiously bring together a multidisciplinary team of experts to coordinate the care of patients with PE and provide the most appropriate therapeutic option for each patient. These teams have recently formed the PERT Consortium whose mission is to advance the diagnosis, treatment, and outcomes of patients with life-threatening PEs. The purpose of this article is to describe the concept and purpose of a PERT as well as the different ways to build an inpatient structure and outpatient follow-up clinic. The authors discuss whether the PERT approach is becoming the new standard of care for patients who present with PE.

CASE PRESENTATION

A 48-year-old man with a history of Guillain-Barré syndrome (unknown cause) for the prior 3 years presented to a local hospital with acute shortness of breath and lightheadedness while taking a shower. A computed tomography pulmonary angiogram (CTPA) showed extensive bilateral PEs and right ventricular to left ventricular (RV/LV) ratio greater than 1 (**Fig. 1**). The patient received one dose of enoxaparin and was sent to MGH for further evaluation and management. On arrival, he had pulse oximetry reading of 87% on room air and required 15 L of nasal cannula, heart rate of 150 beats per minute, respiratory rate of 28 breaths per minute, and blood pressure of 140/79 mm Hg. He was unable to speak in full sentences. An echocardiogram demonstrated a dilated and hypokinetic RV with septal flattening and RV systolic pressure (RVSP) of 54 mm Hg. He had a troponin-T of 0.28 ng/mL (normal <0.03). Ultrasound of his legs demonstrated a right lower extremity deep venous thrombosis (DVT), partially occlusive in the right popliteal vein and occlusive in the right posterior tibial vein. PERT was activated on the patient's arrival to the emergency department. An immediate multidisciplinary consultation ensued whereby PERT members reviewed the history, vital signs, imaging, and laboratory values. The team thought he had all the characteristics of a high-risk submassive PE. Given his extreme tachycardia, shortness of breath, oxygen dependence, right heart strain, and clot in his main pulmonary arteries, all members of PERT agreed that an advanced therapy (beyond anticoagulation alone) was warranted. The team discussed all available options. Because of his Guillain-Barré and concern for respiratory recovery, the team thought that surgical intervention would be too dangerous and catheter-directed thrombolysis alone may not be adequate given the location of his PEs. The team then discussed systemic intravenous thrombolysis versus percutaneous clot extraction with catheter-directed thrombolysis and decided on the latter. Even though the patient had a DVT, the team did not recommend an inferior vena cava filter, as he could be fully anticoagulated. These decisions were discussed with the patient and his family and they

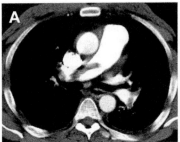 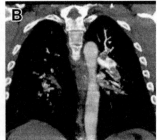 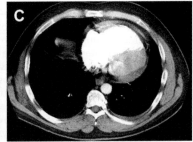

Fig. 1. CTPA findings of PE from case presentation. (*A*) Main pulmonary artery is enlarged measuring 3.5 cm. Acute occlusive and nonocclusive pulmonary artery emboli involving the main pulmonary artery, the right main pulmonary artery extending into the lobar arteries of the right upper, lower, and middle lobes. (*B*) Pulmonary artery emboli involving the left main pulmonary artery extending to the lobar arteries of the upper, lower, and lingular lobes. (*C*) Enlargement of the RV with an RV/LV ratio greater than 1 indicating evidence for right heart strain.

agreed to proceed. He was immediately taken to the cardiac catheterization laboratory, where percutaneous embolectomy was followed by placement of bilateral pulmonary artery catheters for catheter-directed thrombolysis. Both procedures were successfully performed. Hemodynamics and symptoms improved overnight with a decrease in his heart rate, respiratory rate, and oxygen requirement. He was discharged home from the intensive care unit 2 days later on a direct oral anticoagulant.

PURPOSE OF PULMONARY EMBOLISM RESPONSE TEAM

This case illustrates the complexity and urgency with which patients with acute PE present. Over the past decade, a myriad of promising and novel therapeutic tools has been developed to treat these patients. However, few guidelines exist on how to determine which patients are most appropriate for which therapy, so decisions are often left to the expert opinion of a single specialist. As demonstrated in this case, PERT provides an infrastructure that immediately and simultaneously brings together multiple experts to rapidly assess patients and initiate and implement a thoughtful treatment plan. PERT provides a platform for specialists to discuss a case in real time, generate and vet what is thought to be the best treatment plan, communicate the plan to all providers, and quickly assemble the appropriate resources to carry out the plan.

Although there are preliminary reports from a few institutions detailing the potential value of PERT,[5,7,8] the benefits and effectiveness in regard to patient outcomes, quality of life, and cost need to be further investigated. Fortunately, a venue exists to perform such evaluations. Institutions throughout the United States and internationally recently came together to form the PERT Consortium to define what is needed to have a PERT (**Box 1**) and to guide PE care around the world. The formation of this consortium will allow institutions to share experiences and data and collaborate on much needed research projects.

INPATIENT STRUCTURE OF PULMONARY EMBOLISM RESPONSE TEAM

There are many ways to develop a PERT, and there are several issues to consider when thinking about starting one. The structure of each PERT will depend on the local clinical demands, available resources, and infrastructure of the institution, so these factors must be assessed first. Determining which specialties are available and interested in

---

Box 1
Definition of a pulmonary embolism response team, according to the bylaws of the Pulmonary Embolism Response Team Consortium

PERT is an institutionally based multidisciplinary team that

- Has the ability to rapidly assess and provide treatment for patients with acute PE
- Has a formal mechanism to exercise a full range of medical, surgical, and endovascular therapies
- Can provide appropriate multidisciplinary follow-up of patients
- When feasible, collects, evaluates, and shares data regarding the effectiveness of the treatment rendered

---

joining the team is the next step. A recent survey illustrating the diversity of PERTs around the country found that the specialties most commonly engaged in PERTs were pulmonary/critical care, interventional cardiology, and emergency medicine followed by cardiac surgery, interventional radiology, noninterventional cardiology, hematology, and vascular medicine.[9] The organizational structure of each PERT may also vary.[10] Teams may choose to have one physician in charge of managing the team or a steering committee that runs the team together. The size of the teams may differ as well, ranging from a small intimate group to a large inclusive group. The PERT Consortium Research Committee recently surveyed 31 PERT programs and found that a variety of types and sizes of hospitals were successful in establishing PERT programs. Although most of the PERTs surveyed were in academic hospitals (71%), one-quarter of the programs were in community hospitals.

The structure of the PERT will depend on the availability of specific interventions and the specialists who can perform each procedure. Often, there may be different specialists who can perform the same procedure, so determining who will take the lead on each case will be important to establish upfront. Moreover, PERT programs may need to be modified if certain interventions are not available at all times.

Operationally, each PERT will need to create a system to identify appropriate patients, activate the team, mobilize resources, and develop a comprehensive follow-up program. Establishing a set of guidelines about which cases are appropriate for a PERT activation upfront will help eliminate excessive calls about patients with uncomplicated or low-risk PE. There are several different ways to activate a PERT. The two main approaches are engaging the entire multidisciplinary team upfront or using a tiered approach whereby a single physician responds initially and engages a multidisciplinary team for more complex cases. A recent PERT consortium survey found that in most institutions, a full multidisciplinary team responded to the initial PERT (63%), whereas a tiered approach was used less often (32%).[9]

Teams may communicate in a variety of ways as well, via a phone call, conference call, or virtual meeting. As an example, to activate PERT at MGH, a provider calls a 24-hour hotline. Most PERT activations at MGH come from the emergency department (50%–60%), followed by intensive care units (20%–25%), and inpatient/ward services (15%–20%).[11,12] A call to the hotline triggers a rapid response, whereby a page is sent to the on-call PERT fellow who performs the initial evaluation of patients and assesses the severity of the case. Although patients are categorized according to accepted risk stratification systems, the multidisciplinary team is also able to consider individual patient factors (eg, the presence of syncope, the chronicity of symptoms, or evidence of chronic pulmonary hypertension on echocardiogram) that are not included in most guidelines for risk stratification.

Once patients are risk stratified, the PERT fellow and attending decide if the case warrants activation of the entire team (**Fig. 2**). If so, a page and e-mail are sent to each specialist on the team with basic information about the patient. The e-mail provides instructions on how to access commercially available online meeting software

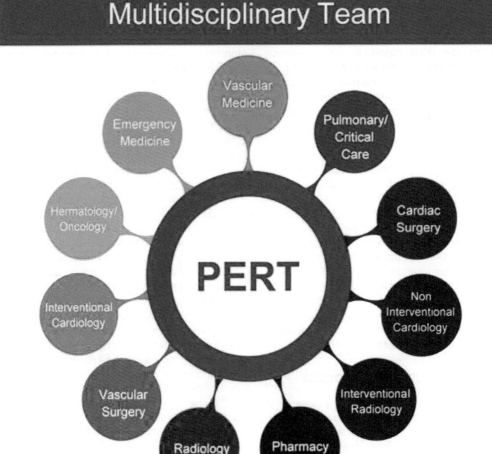

Fig. 2. The composition of a PERT.

that physicians can open on any device, including desktop or laptop computers, tablets, or even their smartphone. A Web-based meeting ensues that allows the group to converse and view the laboratory tests and radiographic images in real time. The team reviews the case, weighs the pros and cons of each therapeutic option, generates further diagnostic and treatment recommendations, and assembles the appropriate resources if advanced interventions are necessary (**Fig. 3**). Occasionally, the patients themselves or a family member will join the call. A fundamental aspect of a PERT program is the inclusion of many specialists; some cases require the input of nontraditional PERT clinicians, such as the need for an obstetrician and neonatal specialist in the case of pregnant patients with PE. Establishing an infrastructure that allows other specialists to engage in the discussion is, therefore, essential.[13]

CONTINUATION OF CASE PRESENTATION

The 48-year-old man who underwent percutaneous embolectomy and catheter-directed thrombolysis for his acute high-risk submassive PE came to the MGH multidisciplinary PERT follow-up clinic 1 month after discharge. He reported feeling "Great", the best he had felt in years. He denied dyspnea on exertion, and his repeat echocardiogram showed no signs of right heart strain. He reported no problems with anticoagulation compliance. However, on review of his records, he was noted to have a hematocrit of 26% (normal for adult men is 41%–53%) during his hospitalization. This test was repeated and again returned at 26%. A workup followed and revealed a 4.31 g/dL immunoglobulin G kappa M component on his serum protein electrophoresis concerning for multiple myeloma. Bone marrow biopsy confirmed this diagnosis, and he is currently undergoing treatment.

OUTPATIENT FOLLOW-UP CLINIC

The continuation of this case illustrates the importance of having a follow-up clinic for PERT patients, which can bridge the gap between their inpatient hospital stay and their outpatient long-term follow-up care. During follow-up, many issues can be addressed, including additional inquiry into the cause of the PE, screening for long-term complications of PE and DVT, and decisions surrounding anticoagulation management (**Box 2**).

While in the hospital, patients are often overwhelmed or too sick to comprehend what happened to them. Reviewing their clinical course

in the outpatient setting can be helpful for their understanding and recovery. Often patients want to know why they developed a PE and what their risk of recurrence is. Determining if their PE was provoked or unprovoked may also help guide long-term management.

Occult Malignancy Screening

The follow-up clinic provides further opportunities to evaluate patients for the cause of their PE. VTE may be a forewarning of occult malignancy in as high as 10% in patients with unprovoked DVT or PE. Thus, screening for occult cancers in these patients is often considered. Studies have demonstrated that although an extensive screening strategy may detect more cancer cases initially, or cancers at an earlier stage of disease than limited screening, it is unknown whether this translates into improved patient-important outcomes.[14–16] Therefore, current guidelines recommend age-appropriate cancer-related screening. For women, this may include mammogram, Papanicolaou test and colonoscopy. For men, this may include prostate-specific antigen and colonoscopy. Although there is no role for performing an exhaustive search for malignancy, it is important to pursue any abnormalities identified after performing a comprehensive history and physical examination or on routine blood work, as the aforementioned case illustrates.

Thrombophilia Testing

Inherited and acquired thrombophilias are recognized to increase the risk of a first VTE. However, recommendations for routine hypercoagulable testing are controversial; no validated testing guidelines have been published. For patients with a first VTE provoked by strong triggers, routine thrombophilia testing is not recommended,[17–20] though for patients who present with weak triggers, unprovoked or recurrent VTEs, VTE in unusual sites, or a strong family history, thrombophilia testing may be considered.[18] Providers should carefully review the limitations of the testing and know how to use the results before ordering any tests. Other studies to consider during the follow-up clinic in patients with an unprovoked left-sided DVT may include assessing for the presence of May-Thurner syndrome, a rare condition in which the right common iliac artery overlies and compresses the left common iliac vein.

Anticoagulation Management

Another important element in the follow-up care of every patient with PE is determining the type and

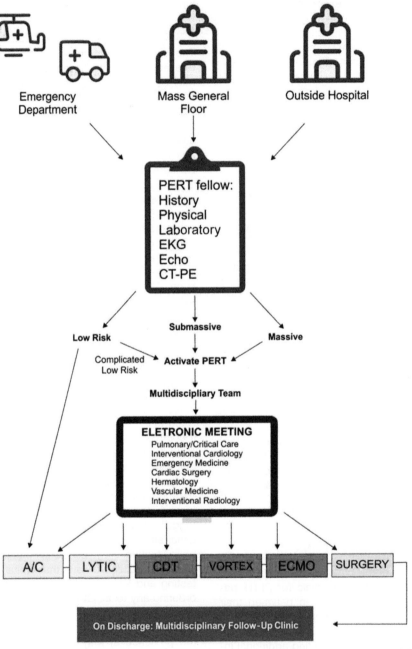

Fig. 3. The model and process of a PERT activation. When a PE is diagnosed at MGH, the PERT fellow is paged, gathers pertinent clinical information, and assesses the severity of the case. If necessary, the entire multidisciplinary team convenes and attends an electronic meeting. Diagnostic and treatment options are discussed, recommendations are generated, and appropriate resources are mobilized. On discharge, patients follow up in a multidisciplinary follow-up clinic. A/C, anticoagulation; CDT, catheter-directed therapy; ECMO, extracorporeal membrane oxygenation; EKG, electrocardiogram; LYTIC, systemic lytic therapy. (*Adapted from* Rosenfeld K, Rosovosky RP. Multidisciplinary care for pulmonary embolism. Advances in Motion. 2017. Available at: https://advances.massgeneral.org/cardiovascular/article.aspx?id=1007.)

Box 2
Outpatient follow-up clinic provides an opportunity to improve care

1. Further exploration into the cause of PE

    a. Ensure age-specific cancer-related screening and investigation into any abnormal history, physical examination, or laboratory findings

    b. Consider thrombophilia testing only in patients who present with weak triggers, unprovoked or recurrent VTEs, VTE in unusual sites, or strong family history

    c. Look for May-Thurner in the appropriate context

2. Long-term anticoagulation management

    a. Determine the type and length of anticoagulation

    b. Encourage adherence

3. Evaluation and management of complications

    a. Investigate signs and symptoms suggestive of pulmonary hypertension and chronic PEs

length of anticoagulation. Over the past decade, 4 new direct oral anticoagulants (DOACs) have gained approval from the US Food and Drug Administration after demonstrating noninferiority to warfarin in the prevention and treatment of VTE. Rivaroxaban, apixaban, and edoxaban are factor Xa inhibitors, whereas dabigatran is a factor II inhibitor. These agents are attractive and convenient for many patients, as they are oral, do not require monitoring for safety and efficacy, and have few food and drug interactions. Indeed, according to the American College of Chest Physicians' most recent guidelines, for most patients without cancer, DOACs are recommended as the first-line therapy.[20] However, deciding which agent to use is not always straightforward and depends on a variety of factors, including patient-related factors (comorbidities, bleeding risk, adherence behaviors, preferences, and weight), medication-related factors (properties of the drugs and potential drug-drug interactions), and if any intervention or procedures are planned.[21] An additional deciding factor, and one that is often the most influential, is whether a medication is covered by the patients' insurance. Having PERT patients present to an outpatient follow-up clinic allows providers to discuss the different anticoagulant options and determine the most reasonable one for each patient.

Although there are no head-to-head trials comparing the 4 DOACs with each other, there are a few key differences that may help guide the optimal choice of treatment.[22] Rivaroxaban and edoxaban are once-daily medications, whereas apixaban and dabigatran are twice-daily medications. Rivaroxaban and apixaban require a higher dose initially, whereas edoxaban and dabigatran require a parenteral anticoagulant for the first 5 to 10 days. Rivaroxaban must be taken with food, and dabigatran should be avoided in patients with dyspepsia and coronary artery disease. Dabigatran has an approved reversal agent, idarucizumab, whereas the reversal agent for the factor Xa inhibitor, andexanet alpha, is currently in clinical trials. Given the complexities associated with the DOACs, especially with respect to their different dosing regimens, having PERT patients present to a follow-up clinic may help minimize medication errors and maximize compliance. The outpatient clinic also provides an opportunity to determine the length of anticoagulation for each patient. For patients in whom a transient risk has resolved, short-term (eg, 3 month) therapy may be reasonable. Alternatively, for patients with an unprovoked VTE or a provoked VTE with ongoing risk factors, indefinite anticoagulation may be warranted.[20,23]

Chronic Thromboembolic Pulmonary Hypertension Evaluation

The outpatient follow-up clinic also allows providers to evaluate their patients for potential long-term consequences of VTE, such as post-thrombotic syndrome (in patients with DVT), post-PE syndrome, and chronic thrombotic pulmonary hypertension (CTEPH).[24,25] Although CTEPH is fortunately rare (incidence: 1%–9% of patients with PE), engaging pulmonary specialists in a follow-up clinic may help identify cases more accurately and earlier.[26,27] Patients who experience persistent dyspnea on exertion or impaired exercise tolerance after their PE should be evaluated for possible CTEPH.[28] In these patients, a repeat echocardiogram should be performed; if there is evidence of chronic PE, persistent right heart dysfunction, or pulmonary hypertension, a ventilation/perfusion (V/Q) scan is warranted. If the V/Q scan suggests CTEPH, patients should be referred to a center that specializes in this complication. Subsequently, pulmonary angiography with right heart catheterization may be performed to establish the diagnosis. Patients with persistent symptoms and evidence of chronic PE but without CTEPH may benefit from a cardiopulmonary exercise test. Results from these tests will dictate which treatments are most appropriate for patients with chronic PEs, such as indefinite anticoagulation, adjunctive medications, balloon pulmonary angioplasty, or pulmonary thromboendarterectomy.

Inferior Vena Cava Filter Retrieval

A recent study found that 21% of retrievable inferior vena cava filters (IVCFs) were not retrieved because of loss to follow-up, discontinued care, or physician oversight.[29] An outpatient follow-up clinic can ensure that patients who required an IVCF during their acute illness have it retrieved when it is no longer indicated.

SUMMARY

Establishing a comprehensive outpatient follow-up program for PERT patients is a way not only to continue the collaborative care they received as an inpatient but also to provide optimal long-term care and to facilitate the recognition and management of complications associated with PE.

IS PULMONARY EMBOLISM RESPONSE TEAM THE NEW STANDARD OF CARE?

The pervasive nature and diverse circumstances under which PE occurs, in community and hospital settings and on any service or floor within the hospital, makes it "any-person's disease." Furthermore, the broad array of treatment options, coupled with the absence of reliable comparative effectiveness studies to define the real benefit for one type of treatment over others, makes selection of therapy challenging. This dilemma, combined with the broad array of specialists who treat PE, each with different backgrounds and biases, leads to enormous variations in therapy. Many clinicians who are actively treating patients with PE think PERTs may become a new standard of care for patients with this life-threatening and common disease. That said, given the novelty of the PERT concept, data have yet to be accumulated to confirm the value of PERT as a mechanism to improve outcomes for patients with PE.

In the absence of a PERT, vulnerable patients with PE would receive the care plan outlined by an individual clinician. This plan might be completely different depending on the clinician or specialty who happened to see the patients or receive the referral. Importantly, patients themselves are unaware that different clinicians within the same institution would offer different treatment plans. PE is not the only disease state for which there are many different treatment options and the potential for variations in approach. For example, many oncologic conditions may be approached surgically, medically, with radiation, or combinations of these. In such situations in medicine, whereby multiple options are available and none is clearly the winner, the team-based approach has proven time and time again to be the preferred strategy for both clinicians and patients. Recently, the team-based approach has proven to be highly successful and satisfying in other areas, such as the heart team approach to transcutaneous aortic valve replacement and complex coronary artery disease. For these diseases, reimbursement has been tied to this multidisciplinary deliberation.

Expanding this approach into the treatment of PE seems logical. As described in detail earlier, key to the success of any PERT is the ability to address the needs of patients with PE in a rapid-response fashion, good communication between specialties, access to the full range of treatment modalities, and ongoing follow-up care. These elements of PERT, more than the actual treatment rendered, are what define a new standard of care for PE management. Actual treatments for PE vary because of physician and patient preferences and the paucity of comparative data and definitive guidelines. However, group discussion, rather than an individual decision-making, may reduce this variation.

Establishment of a PERT can improve care for PE in other, less obvious, ways. For example, institutions with PERTs may have an increased awareness of PE. PE can be a challenging diagnosis to make, and the influence of the PERT education and getting clinicians to think of PE as a possible diagnosis can make a great impact. Other institutional benefits include increasing interdisciplinary communication and collaboration and eliminating silos of care. These partnerships may enhance safety and peer-to-peer oversight in a positive manner. Lastly, co-locating and consolidating the care of very ill patients with PE may lead to more consistent management in sites where protocols can be applied, and the dosing of drugs and the use of technology could become more standardized.

In summary, while it is too early to state definitively that PERTs create a new standard of care, a team-based PERT approach facilitates the rapid delivery of care, provides built-in checks and balances, may reduce unnecessary treatment variation while increasing awareness and diagnostic acumen, and seems likely to improve the overall care of PE patients. By participating in the PERT Consortium, member institutions and their PERT professionals have access to the numerous educational resources and a community of like-minded, clinicians interested in improving the care of patients with PE.

Finally, as the PERT model is adopted by more institutions around the world, a large body of data will be generated by entry into a central registry. These data will enable sites to better evaluate quality of PE care and to benchmark their performance against other sites around the country and internationally. When carefully analyzed, these data will also provide the evidence base needed to enhance care, define best practices, and optimize outcomes for patients with PE.

REFERENCES

1. Heit JA. Venous thromboembolism: disease burden, outcomes and risk factors. J Thromb Haemost 2005; 3:1611–7.
2. Deitelzweig SB, Johnson BH, Lin J, et al. Prevalence of clinical venous thromboembolism in the USA: current trends and future projections. Am J Hematol 2011;86:217–20.
3. Kucher N, Rossi E, De Rosa M, et al. Massive pulmonary embolism. Circulation 2006;113:577–82.
4. Jimenez D, de Miguel-Diez J, Guijarro R, et al. Trends in the management and outcomes of acute pulmonary embolism: analysis from the RIETE registry. J Am Coll Cardiol 2016;67:162–70.
5. Kabrhel C, Rosovsky R, Channick R, et al. A multidisciplinary pulmonary embolism response team: initial 30-month experience with a novel approach to delivery of care to patients with submassive and massive pulmonary embolism. Chest 2016;150:384–93.
6. Provias T, Dudzinski DM, Jaff MR, et al. The Massachusetts General Hospital Pulmonary Embolism Response Team (MGH PERT): creation of a multidisciplinary program to improve care of patients with massive and submassive pulmonary embolism. Hosp Pract 1995;2014(42):31–7.
7. Carroll BJ, Pemberton H, Bauer KA, et al. Initiation of a multidisciplinary, rapid response team to massive and submassive pulmonary embolism. Am J Cardiol 2017;120:1393–8.
8. Serhal M, Haddadin IS, Heresi GA, et al. Pulmonary embolism response teams. J Thromb Thrombolysis 2017;44:19–29.
9. Barnes GD, Kabrhel C, Courtney DM, et al. Diversity in the pulmonary embolism response team model: an organizational survey of the national PERT consortium members. Chest 2016;150:1414–7.
10. Barnes G, Giri J, Courtney DM, et al. Nuts and bolts of running a pulmonary embolism response team: results from an organizational survey of the National PERT Consortium members. Hosp Pract 1995; 2017(45):76–80.
11. Deadmon EK, Giordano NJ, Rosenfield K, et al. Comparison of emergency department patients to inpatients receiving a pulmonary embolism response team (PERT) activation. Acad Emerg Med 2017;24:814–21.
12. Kabrhel C, Rosovsky R, Baugh C, et al. The creation and implementation of an outpatient pulmonary embolism treatment protocol. Hosp Pract 1995; 2017(45):123–9.
13. Monteleone PP, Rosenfield K, Rosovsky RP. Multidisciplinary pulmonary embolism response teams and systems. Cardiovasc Diagn Ther 2016;6:662–7.
14. Delluc A, Antic D, Lecumberri R, et al. Occult cancer screening in patients with venous thromboembolism: guidance from the SSC of the ISTH. J Thromb Haemost 2017;15:2076–9.
15. Carrier M, Lazo-Langner A, Shivakumar S, et al. Screening for occult cancer in unprovoked venous thromboembolism. N Engl J Med 2015; 373:697–704.
16. Robertson L, Yeoh SE, Stansby G, et al. Effect of testing for cancer on cancer- and venous thromboembolism (VTE)-related mortality and morbidity in people with unprovoked VTE. Cochrane Database Syst Rev 2017;(8):CD010837.
17. Baglin T, Gray E, Greaves M, et al. Clinical guidelines for testing for heritable thrombophilia. Br J Haematol 2010;149:209–20.
18. Connors JM. Thrombophilia testing and venous thrombosis. N Engl J Med 2017;377:1177–87.
19. Hicks LK, Bering H, Carson KR, et al. The ASH choosing wisely(R) campaign: five hematologic tests and treatments to question. Blood 2013;122: 3879–83.
20. Kearon C, Akl EA, Ornelas J, et al. Antithrombotic therapy for VTE disease: CHEST guideline and expert panel report. Chest 2016;149:315–52.
21. Streiff MB, Agnelli G, Connors JM, et al. Guidance for the treatment of deep vein thrombosis and pulmonary embolism. J Thromb Thrombolysis 2016; 41:32–67.
22. Rosovsky R, Merli G. Anticoagulation in pulmonary embolism: update in the age of direct oral anticoagulants. Tech Vasc Interv Radiol 2017;20: 141–51.
23. Kearon C, Akl EA, Comerota AJ, et al. Antithrombotic therapy for VTE disease: antithrombotic therapy and prevention of thrombosis, 9th ed: American College of Chest Physicians evidence-based clinical practice guidelines. Chest 2012;141: e419S–96S.
24. Sista AK, Klok FA. Late outcomes of pulmonary embolism: the post-PE syndrome. Thromb Res 2018; 164:157–62.
25. Ende-Verhaar YM, Cannegieter SC, Vonk Noordegraaf A, et al. Incidence of chronic thromboembolic pulmonary hypertension after acute pulmonary embolism: a contemporary view of the published literature. Eur Respir J 2017;49 [pii: 1601792].

26. Becattini C, Agnelli G, Pesavento R, et al. Incidence of chronic thromboembolic pulmonary hypertension after a first episode of pulmonary embolism. Chest 2006;130:172–5.

27. Pengo V, Lensing AW, Prins MH, et al. Incidence of chronic thromboembolic pulmonary hypertension after pulmonary embolism. N Engl J Med 2004;350: 2257–64.

28. Task Force for Diagnosis and Treatment of Pulmonary Hypertension of European Society of Cardiology (ESC), European Respiratory Society (ERS), International Society of Heart and Lung Transplantation (ISHLT), et al. Guidelines for the diagnosis and treatment of pulmonary hypertension. Eur Respir J 2009;34:1219–63.

29. Jia Z, Fuller TA, McKinney JM, et al. Utility of retrievable inferior vena cava filters: a systematic literature review and analysis of the reasons for nonretrieval of filters with temporary indications. Cardiovasc Intervent Radiol 2018;41(5):675–82.

Endovascular and Open Surgery for Deep Vein Thrombosis

Cassius Iyad Ochoa Chaar, MD, MS*, Afsha Aurshina, MBBS

KEYWORDS

- Deep vein thrombosis • Postthrombotic syndrome • Thrombolysis • Thrombectomy
- Angioplasty and stenting

KEY POINTS

- Catheter-directed thrombolysis is a safe and effective modality for treatment of extensive, typically iliofemoral deep vein thrombosis (DVT) in selected patients.
- Early removal of thrombus restores venous patency, preserves valve function, and can lead to faster relief of symptoms and decrease the long-term risk of severe postthrombotic syndrome.
- Chronic venous obstruction is commonly a late manifestation of DVT and can lead to severe postthrombotic syndrome and venous ulceration. Endovascular recanalization with balloon angioplasty and stenting can relieve symptoms and promote ulcer healing.
- Open venous surgery in the form of thrombectomy for acute DVT and venous bypass for chronic venous obstruction is an effective treatment modality that is typically reserved for patients who fail endovascular therapy.

INTRODUCTION

Deep vein thrombosis (DVT) is the third most common cause of cardiovascular morbidity with acute life-threatening complications, including pulmonary embolism and rarely limb-threatening complications such as phlegmasia cerulea dolens.[1,2] Chronic sequelae of DVT, popularly known as postthrombotic syndrome (PTS) occurs in 20% to 50% of the patients. PTS usually occurs within 2 years of onset of DVT despite anticoagulation and compression and is associated with significant morbidity and health care costs.[3–5]

Although traditional conservative measures such as anticoagulation and compression stockings remain the primary treatment of acute DVT, percutaneous endovascular surgical therapy can lead to rapid relief of symptoms with low complications and low subsequent incidence of PTS.[6–9] In chronic DVT, endovenous recanalization and stenting of venous obstruction is an effective and durable treatment for patients with moderate to severe PTS. Open thrombectomy and venous bypass are traditional surgical options used in limb threatening conditions such as phlegmasia and in cases where endovascular interventions fail or are not possible. This article reviews the current options for treatment of DVT in the acute and chronic settings.

ACUTE DEEP VEIN THROMBOSIS
Rationale for Thrombus Removal

Early removal of thrombus can prevent a high sustained venous pressure, restore venous patency, and preserve valve function by limiting damage to venous valves, thus preserving the physiology of veins.[7,10] Studies have reported that poor

No conflicts of interest.

Section of Vascular Surgery, Department of Surgery, Yale University School of Medicine, 330 Cedar street, Boardman 204, New Haven, CT 06510, USA

* Corresponding author.

E-mail address: cassius.chaar@yale.edu

Clin Chest Med 39 (2018) 631–644

https://doi.org/10.1016/j.ccm.2018.04.014

0272-5231/18/Published by Elsevier Inc.

thrombus clearance can lead to valve dysfunction and recurrent thrombosis and is associated with development of PTS.[8,11] This led to the "open vein hypothesis," which has been used as the rationale of early thrombus removal using endovascular techniques.[8,12,13]

Catheter-Directed Thrombolysis

Indications

Catheter-directed thrombolysis (CDT) for acute DVT is still controversial, despite its wide adoption, because of the lack of level I evidence. This dilemma is probably best illustrated by the guidelines of the American College of Chest Physicians that initially favored lysis for treatment of iliofemoral DVT in the 8th edition (2008) but subsequently changed to favor anticoagulation alone in the following editions.[14,15] The Society of Vascular Surgery, Society of Interventional Radiology, and American Heart Association favor CDT for acute iliofemoral DVT presenting within 2 weeks of onset of symptoms in patients who have good life expectancy and are at low risk for bleeding and complications.[16–18] The ATTRACT trial was completed recently and was designed to compare CDT with anticoagulation alone in patients with proximal DVT and help vascular specialists to identify patients who could benefit most from this therapy.[12] The results of the trial have just been released and will be reviewed separately.

The use of systemic thrombolysis for acute iliofemoral DVT has been abandoned because of the high rate of incomplete thrombolysis and bleeding complications associated with it.[9] CDT involves local delivery of thrombolytic agent directly into the thrombus, which minimizes the total amount of thrombolytic agent required, treatment time, and risk of bleeding. The indication for performing CDT can be emergent, urgent, or elective as described in **Table 1**.[19]

Technique

The first step for performing CDT is to determine the access site in order to maximize the infusion of thrombolytic agents within the thrombus. An ultrasound-guided venous puncture is performed typically in the popliteal vein. Other access options include the common femoral vein, the internal jugular, or the posterior tibial vein. An angiogram is performed to assess the extent of the thrombus (**Fig. 1**). Using fluoroscopic guidance, a combination of a catheter and a wire are advanced through the vein to traverse all the thrombus. An attempt should be made to cross all of the thrombus and confirm the location of the vein free of clot with an angiogram. The angiographic catheter is then exchanged for a

Table 1		
Indication for catheter-directed thrombolysis		
Indication	**Diagnosis**	**Treatment Goal**
Emergent	Phlegmasia cerulea dolens	Limb salvage
Urgent	Inferior vena cava thrombosis (risk of renal failure and Budd–Chiari syndrome)	Prevent pulmonary embolism, preserve visceral organ drainage, relieve pelvic congestion
Elective	Acute iliofemoral DVT, with moderate to severe symptoms Severe symptomatic acute femoropopliteal DVT worsening despite anticoagulation	Immediate symptom relief, prevent PTS

multiside-hole catheter with infusion length that ideally matches the length of the thrombosed segment of the vein. The thrombolytic agent is then delivered directly into the thrombus through the infusion catheter. The thrombolytic agent commonly used is recombinant tissue plasminogen activator at a dose of 1 mg/h. A venogram is performed 12 to 24 hours after initiation of lysis to assess the degree of thrombus and the response to lytic therapy (**Fig. 2**). After 24 to 48 hours of thrombolytic therapy, all acute thrombus in the vein should be dissolved. Frequently, stenotic lesions especially in the iliac veins are uncovered that contribute to stasis and to the occurrence of DVT. These lesions are commonly related to arterial compression of the veins at the iliac arterial bifurcations.[20] They usually respond poorly to balloon angioplasty alone and require stenting (**Fig. 3**). Iliac lesions can sometimes be very subtle to detect on plane angiography, and the introduction of intravascular ultrasound (IVUS) has become the standard of care and is the best method to uncover hidden lesions.[21]

Adjunctive therapy

Since the introduction of CDT, several devices and techniques have been developed to enhance and accelerate intravascular thrombus removal. In addition to treating stenotic lesions that potentially

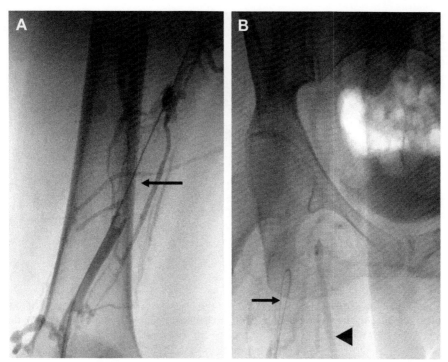

Fig. 1. Initial angiogram of left leg catheter-directed thrombolysis for extensive DVT. (*A*) Filling defect and large thrombus demonstrated in the femoral vein (*arrow*) with prominent collaterals. (*B*) No visualization of the common femoral vein or iliac veins because of extensive thrombosis. A wire (*arrow*) is advanced into the proximal femoral vein but no contrast is seen in the vein because of the thrombus. The only vein visualized is the profunda femoral vein (*arrow head*).

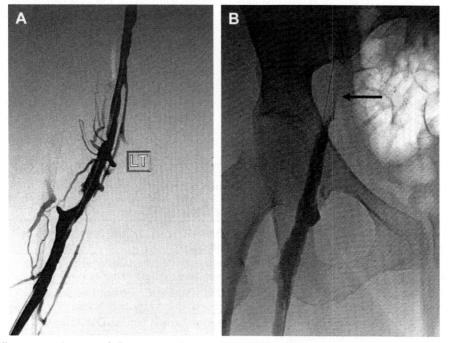

Fig. 2. Follow-up angiogram of the same patient demonstrating resolution of thrombus in the femoral vein distally (*A*) and more proximally including the common femoral vein (*B*). There is still poor filling of the iliac veins because of persistent thrombus and venous obstruction (*arrow*).

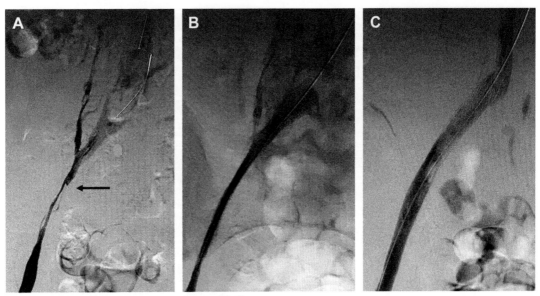

Fig. 3. Pelvic angiogram demonstrating stenotic lesion of the iliac vein (*arrow*) after 48 hours of lysis and resolution of acute thrombus (*A*). The lesion responds poorly to balloon angioplasty alone (*B*). Stenting the iliac veins works best to restore flow (*C*).

precipitate thrombosis, balloon angioplasty is used to macerate large clots and enhance the penetration of lytic agent into them. Large-bore catheters are used for aspiration of thrombus. Pharmacomechanical thrombectomy (PMT) uses catheter-based mechanical devices to combine thrombus fragmentation/maceration with distribution of thrombolytic agents and thrombus aspiration. The major advantage of using PMTs is rapid thrombus dissolution and clearance in a single session sometimes and overall decrease in the overall duration of thrombolysis. In case of contraindication to thrombolysis, mechanical thrombectomy alone can be used for endovascular management of DVT. PMTs include rotational,

rheolytic and ultrasound-accelerated devices, which have been summarized in **Table 2**.[22]

Outcomes

The technical success of CDT for acute extensive DVT is 80% to 90%. In fact, focusing on more recent literature of the 21st century, the success rate is consistently greater than 90% and is likely related to refinement of the techniques and advances in PMT technology (**Table 3**). Bleeding remains the most feared complication during CDT. It is often related to the access site and can be treated conservatively with transfusions, local pressure, and placement of additional sutures at the access site. Rarely, it has been noted to be

Table 2
Available pharmacomechanical thrombectomy adjuncts

Device (Company)	Principle	Mode of Action
Arrow-Trerotola (Teleflex)	Rotational thrombectomy	Rotational helix used to break the thrombus by a rotating wire or cage
AngioJet (Boston Scientific)	Rheolytic thrombectomy	Pressure gradient created using Bernoulli effect to fragment and aspirate thrombus
EKOS (BTG Interventional)	Ultrasound-accelerated	Ultrasound waves into thrombus help fragmentation of thrombus and increase penetration of lytic agent
Indigo (Penumbra)	Suction thrombectomy	High-velocity vacuum suction with catheter
AngioVac (AngioDynamics)	Cannula and circuit thrombectomy	Large-caliber suction cannula and filter in extracorporeal venovenous bypass circuit

Table 3
Technical success and patency of CDT for treatment of DVT

Author, Year	n	Design	Technical Success (%)	Patency (%)	Mean Follow-up (mo)
Semba et al,[26] 1994	21	RS	85	85	3
Bjarnason et al,[27] 1997	77	PS	79	63	12
Mewissen et al,[23] 1999	287	RS	83	60	12
Razavi et al,[28] 2002	31	PS	89	83.3	20
Grunwald et al,[29] 2004	74	RS	98	n/a	1
Vedantham et al,[30] 2004	18	RS	100	96	1
Protack et al,[31] 2007	69	RS	97	77	25
Baekgaard et al,[32] 2010	101	PS	95	82	72
Warner et al,[33] 2013	32	RS	92	75	29
Engelberger et al,[34] 2014	87	PS	98	87	12
Fiengo et al,[35] 2015	24	PS	91	83	24
Du et al,[36] 2015	427	RS	97.5	87	24

Abbreviations: PS, prospective study; RS, retrospective study.

fatal or leads to devastating consequences especially when it occurs in the central nervous system. Among 473 patients in a multicenter National Venous Registry study with CDT, complications included bleeding in 54 (11%), neurologic in 2 (0.4%), PE in 6 (1%), and death in 2 (0.4%). Bleeding complications were most common at the venous insertion site (4%) or in the retroperitoneum (1%). Major neurologic complications, including one fatal intracranial hemorrhage and one subdural hematoma, occurred in only 2 patients (0.4%).[23] More recently, in a meta-analysis, Wang and colleagues[24] compared complications posttreatment between CDT versus anticoagulation alone. They reported that a significant increase in complication rate (odds ratio [OR] = 4.36; 95% confidence interval [CI]: 2.94–6.47; $P<.001$) was noted with CDT. There was an increased risk of bleeding (OR = 3.19; 95% CI: 0.76–13.42; $P = .114$) as well as higher risk of PE (OR = 1.57; 95% CI: 1.37–1.79; $P<.001$). In a database study of the Nationwide Inpatient Sample, there was no difference in mortality of patients admitted with DVT and treated with CDT compared with anticoagulation alone. However, CDT was associated with increased transfusions, PE, and intracranial hemorrhage.[25] The long-term patency of the veins treated with CDT is 60% to 80% in studies with follow-up between 12 and up to 72 months (see **Table 3**). Several comparative studies have correlated patency of the venous system with a decrease in PTS when CDT was compared with anticoagulation alone.

The catheter-directed venous thrombolysis (CaVenT) study is a randomized multicenter trial comparing CDT and anticoagulation alone for treatment of DVT. It demonstrated an increase in the vein patency from 36% to 64% and a relative risk reduction of 26% in PTS over 2 years of follow-up (41.1% vs 55.6%, $P = .04$) with CDT compared with anticoagulation alone.[37] Also, technical success after CDT was high, with a mean complete thrombus removal of 82% ± 25%. Removal of more than 50% thrombus was achieved in 90% patients. However, the CaVenT study had a few limitations because of use of CDT alone without PMT and limited use of stents compared with that of other studies. Similar clinical outcomes were noted within the Thrombus Obliteration by Rapid Percutaneous Endovenous Intervention in Deep Venous Occlusion (TORPEDO) study. In a single-centered study, Sharifi and colleagues[38,39] reported a significantly lower recurrence of DVT (4.5% vs 16%, $P = .002$) and incidence of PTS (6.8% vs 29.6%, $P<.001$) with CDT compared with anticoagulation at 2.5-year follow-up. The Acute Venous Thrombosis: Thrombus Removal with Adjunctive Catheter Directed Thrombolysis (ATTRACT) study randomized 692 patients to CDT or anticoagulation alone. There was no statistically significant difference in the incidence of PTS (CDT = 47% vs A = 48%, $P = .56$) or recurrent venous thromboembolism (VTE) (CDT = 12% vs A = 8%, $P = .09$) at 24-months follow-up. CDT was associated with a significantly increased risk of major bleeding in the first 10 days (CDT = 1.7% vs A = 0.3%, $P = .049$) (**Table 4**). Even though the ATTRACT trial failed to prove the hypothesis that CDT prevents the incidence of PTS, it demonstrated a significant decrease in moderate to severe PTS after 24 months (18% CDT vs 24% A,

Table 4
Studies comparing CDT versus anticoagulation alone

Author, Year	Design	Patients (n)	CDT + A vs A	Outcomes	F/U (mo)
AbuRahma et al,[40] 2001	PS	51	18 vs 33	Patency (83% CDT vs 3% A at 30 d, $P<.001$) Primary patency at 1, 3, and 5 y: CDT: 83%,69%,69% vs A: 24%,18%,18%	60
Elsharawy et al,[41] 2002	RCT	35	18 vs 17	Patency (72% CDT vs 12% A, $P<.001$) Reflux (41% A vs 11% CDT, $P = .04$)	6
Enden et al,[37] 2009 (CaVenT)	RCT	103	50 vs 53	Patency (64% CDT vs 35.8% A, $P = .004$) Obstruction (20% CDT vs 49% A, $P = .004$)	6
Enden et al,[8] 2012 (CaVenT)	RCT	189	90 vs 99	Patency (65.9% CDT vs 47.4% A, $P = .012$) PTS (41% CDT vs 55.6% A, $P = .047$)	24
Sharifi et al,[38] 2012 (TORPEDO)	RCT	183	91 vs 92	Recurrent VTE (4.5% CDT vs 16%A, $P = .02$) PTS (6.8% CDT vs 29.6% A, $P<.001$)	30
Lee et al,[42] 2013	RS	53	27 vs 26	Patency (69.2% CDT vs 38.5% A, $P<.05$) PTS (19.2% CDT vs 50% A, $P = .04$)	12
Haig et al,[10] 2016	RCT	176	87 VS. 89	PTS (43% CDT vs71% A, $P<.0001$) Patency (79.1% CDT vs 70.9% A, $P = .218$)	60
Vedantham et al,[43] 2017 (ATTRACT)	RCT	692	336 vs 355	PTS (48.7% CDT vs 48.2% A, $P = .56$) Moderate to Severe PTS (18% CDT vs 24% A, $P = .04$) Recurrent VTE (12.5% CDT;8.5% A, $P = .08$)	24

Abbreviations: A, anticoagulation; F/U, follow-up; PS, prospective study; PTA, percutaneous transluminal angioplasty; RCT, randomized control trial; RS, retrospective study.

$P = .04$). It also showed a significant improvement in symptoms of leg pain and swelling at 10 and 30 days when compared with anticoagulation. With no procedural mortality and a major bleeding rate of 1.7%, ATTRACT proved again that CDT is a safe procedure in experienced centers. We typically offer CDT for patients with extensive acute iliofemoral DVT who have moderate to severe symptoms. Patients are admitted to the hospital, receive heparin drip and compression stockings and are monitored for 24 to 48 hours. If the symptoms and ability to ambulate do not improve, we proceed with CDT only in patients at low risk of bleeding and with good life expectancy.

Open Surgical Thrombectomy

Open surgical thrombectomy is used selectively for patients with acute severe DVT, especially patients presenting with phlegmasia and arterial compromise that require rapid decompression of the venous outflow. It is typically achieved via a groin incision to perform a femoral venotomy and thrombectomy using Fogarty balloons. A counter-incision is frequently needed with a distal venotomy to facilitate passage of the thrombectomy catheter in the direction of the valves. Although the use of lysis has significantly increased over the past decade, the use of thrombectomy has remained stable.[44]

Plate and colleagues[45] demonstrated the superiority of thrombectomy over anticoagulation alone in a prospective randomized study at follow-up after 10 years. After treatment, persistent venous symptoms were noted in 62% in the thrombectomy group and 88% in the anticoagulation group. Casey and colleagues[9] in a meta-analysis compared 3 available treatment strategies: CDT, anticoagulation alone, and open surgical thrombectomy. The meta-analysis included 15 studies that fulfilled the eligibility criteria. They reported that a significant reduction in risk of both PTS (RR: 0.19, 95% CI: 0.07–0.48) and venous obstruction (RR: 0.38, 95% CI: 0.18–0.37) was noted with CDT over anticoagulation alone. Also, when surgical thrombectomy was compared with anticoagulation, a similar risk reduction in PTS (RR: 0.67, 95% CI: 0.52–0.87) and venous obstruction (RR: 0.68, 95% CI: 0.46–0.99) was reported. There was, however, insufficient data to compare CDT with thrombectomy. The study also demonstrated no significant effects of surgical thrombectomy on the outcomes of death (RR, 0.80; 95% CI: 0.10–6.22), PE (RR: 0.56; 95% CI, 0.08–4.18), or recurrent VTE (RR: 0.69; 95% CI: 0.24–2.01).

CHRONIC DEEP VEIN THROMBOSIS
Defining Chronic Deep Vein Thrombosis

Patients with "chronic DVT" present with venous insufficiency as a result of venous obstruction and deep valvular reflux.[46,47] Both pathophysiologic processes (venous obstruction and reflux) are known late sequelae of acute DVT and define the basic mechanism behind PTS. "Chronic DVT" has no thrombus unlike in the acute phase. In fact, the residual thrombus in the vein is totally replaced by fibrotic scar tissue characterized by collagen and calcifications. These changes have been noted in surgical specimens as early as 7 months and up to 25 years after acute DVT.[48] There is no current effective surgical therapy for deep venous reflux and the recommendation is to use compression therapy for symptomatic

relief. Recent advances with IVUS and high-resolution imaging have enhanced our ability to recognize the obstructive component and the major role it plays in the pathophysiology of PTS.[49]

Endovascular therapy with angioplasty and stenting under IVUS guidance is the treatment of choice for those lesions. Open surgical bypass or phlebectomy is usually reserved for patients who fail endovascular therapy. The correction of venous obstruction alone using stenting usually allows a significant relief in patients despite uncorrected reflux.[50]

Venous Stenting

Indications
Patients presenting with moderate to severe PTS symptoms despite compression therapy undergo evaluation for venous obstruction typically in the iliac veins and the inferior vena cava. Patients with venous ulcers typically in the malleolar area should be treated with compression therapy and local wound care. Even though local wound care alone improves patient symptoms and can promote healing of a venous ulcer, patients should get an evaluation for venous outflow obstruction especially if they have a history of DVT (**Fig. 4**). We typically obtain a magnetic resonance angiography (MRA) of the pelvis to assess the iliac veins in patients with unilateral symptoms and MRA of the abdomen and pelvis when the bilateral lower extremities are affected. In our experience, MRA gives excellent definition of the contour of the veins and allows to uncover short focal areas of stenosis or occlusion. It also allows the visualization of large collateral vessels (**Fig. 5**). Treatment

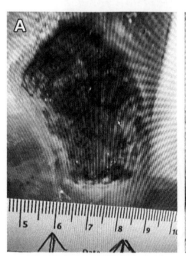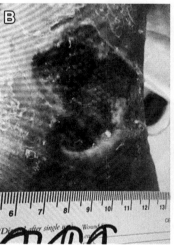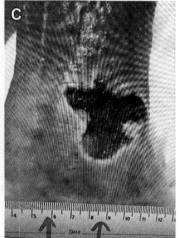

Fig. 4. Patient with history of extensive DVT presenting for evaluation of a right medial malleolar ulcer. The ulcer was debrided and was 3 × 4 cm in size (*A*). With local wound care the size decreased to 3 × 3 cm after 1 month (*B*) and to 2.5 × 2 cm after 3 months (*C*) and stayed stable at that size for 2 months.

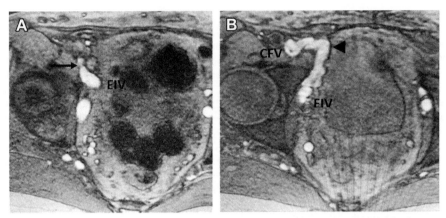

Fig. 5. Cross-sectional MRA of the pelvis demonstrates severe stenosis of the right external iliac vein (EIV) tapering down into complete occlusion (*arrow*) (*A*). Another level demonstrates a large collateral (*arrowhead*) connecting the right common femoral vein (CFV) to the EIV (*B*).

of severe areas of stenosis or occlusion of the iliac veins by stenting can enhance venous return and decrease venous hypertension promoting wound healing (**Fig. 6**).

Technique

The popliteal vein is typically accessed for treatment of postthrombotic venous outflow obstruction. This enables treatment of the common femoral vein or the distal external iliac vein, if affected. In selected cases where the obstruction is confined to the common iliac vein or inferior vena cava, femoral vein access is adequate if the femoral vein is patent on ultrasound. Another alternative access is the internal jugular vein. Recent literature by Ye and colleagues[51] suggested high technical safety and feasibility in using a transpopliteal approach for stent placement in iliofemoral vein. Venous access is obtained under ultrasound guidance. A 6-Fr sheath is placed and angiography of the lower extremity and pelvis is performed (**Fig. 7**). A hydrophilic wire is directed toward the iliofemoral obstruction using an angled tip catheter. The lesion is crossed into the iliac veins using a combination of soft and stiff hydrophilic wires and a low-profile

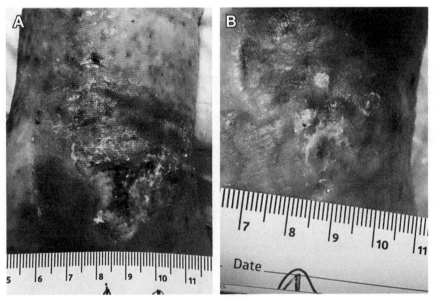

Fig. 6. The same patient's medial malleolar ulcer stopped improving for 2 months. He underwent iliac vein stenting for focal postthrombotic lesion of the right EIV. The size of the ulcer subsequently decreased to 2 × 1.5 cm 1 month after intervention (*A*) and healed 3 months later (*B*).

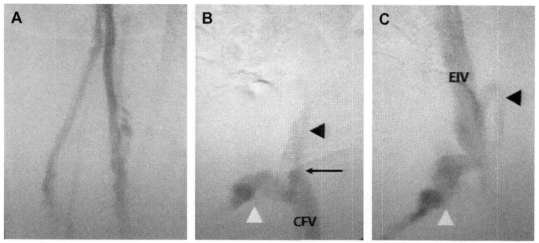

Fig. 7. Initial angiogram of the right lower extremity after popliteal vein access. The femoral veins show some collaterals and likely a duplicated femoral vein (A). There is a focal occlusion of the most distal right external iliac vein (EIV) (arrow) The common femoral vein (CFV) is filled with contrast and there is filling of transpelvic collaterals (white arrowhead) and collaterals around the occlusion (black arrowhead) (B). The EIV has delayed filling via the collateral (black arrowhead) (C).

crossing catheter. After crossing the lesion, the patient is anticoagulated. IVUS is performed to assess the degree of stenosis and get measurements for sizing of the stent (**Fig. 8**A). Balloon dilatation and stenting is subsequently performed to treat the lesion (**Fig. 9**A). An oversized self-expanding stent is then deployed. The lesions need to be stented without any skip areas to avoid residual symptoms and intra-stent stenosis. Completion angiography is performed to assess flow and resolution of filling of collaterals (**Fig. 9**B). Repeat IVUS is also performed to document the increase in the stented area and to rule out any residual subtle areas of stenosis (**Fig. 8**B).

Outcomes
The role of endovascular angioplasty and stenting to maintain long-term venous patency and provide symptomatic relief is well established (**Table 5**).

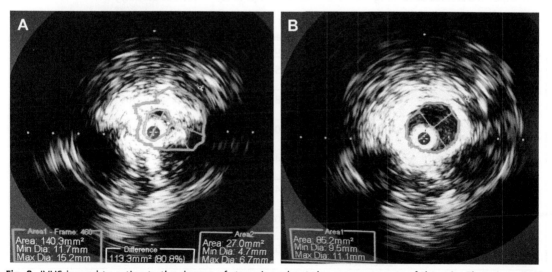

Fig. 8. IVUS is used to estimate the degree of stenosis and get size measurements of the vein. There is an 80% area reduction (blue) when compared with a reference adjacent vein (green) and the average size of the normal vein is 14 mm (A). IVUS after placement of 16-mm self-expanding stent and balloon angioplasty demonstrates expansion of the area of stenosis from 27 mm^2 to 85.2 mm^2 (B).

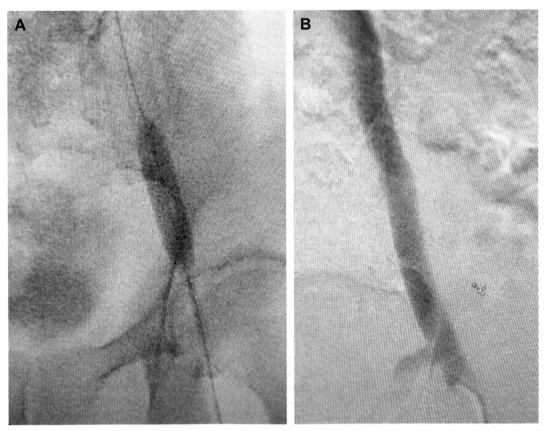

Fig. 9. Balloon angioplasty and stenting of the right external iliac vein (A). Completion angiogram shows excellent flow in the iliac with minimal filling of collateral vessels (B).

Table 5
Retrospective studies describing technical success and patency of venous stenting

Author	Patients (n)	Stent	Technical Success	Primary Patency	Assisted Primary Patency	Secondary Patency	Mean Follow-up (mo)
Blanch Alerany et al,[54] 2014	36	Wallstent Zilver Vena	95%	74%	87%	89%	21
de wolf et al,[55] 2015	63	Wallstent, Sinus-XL Zilver Vena	88%	74%	81%	96%	12
Kurklinsky et al,[56] 2012	89	Wallstent, SMART, Protégé, Luminexx	100%	81%	94%	95%	11
Neglen et al,[52] 2007	982	Wallstent, Nitinol	94%	57%	80%	86%	30
Sang et al,[57] 2014	67	Wallstent, SMART, Luminexx	94%	70.7%	N/A	82.8%	36
Stanley et al,[58] 2013	27	Wallstent	100%	82%	N/A	N/A	46
Titus et al,[59] 2011	23	Nitinol, Stainless steel stent	95.6%	78.3%	82.7%	95%	10.5
Ye et al,[51] 2014	110	Wallstent, Lifestent, EverFlex	95%	70%	90%	94%	25

Abbreviation: N/A, not available in study.

Neglen and Raju, in a large retrospective study, reported cumulative rates of complete pain and swelling resolution of 62% and 32% at 5-year follow-up.[52] The rate of ulcer healing has also been improved with use of endovenous stenting and has been reported as high as 78% and 58% at 2- and 5-year follow-up.[51,52] In a recent meta-analysis by Razavi and colleagues[53], the technical success rate of endovascular therapy for acute thrombotic and chronic postthrombotic disease was 94.2% and 94.1%, respectively. The meta-analysis also reported that the rate of complete pain resolution, relief of edema, and complete ulcer healing as derived from 14 chronic DVT studies were 69.3%, 63.6%, and 70.8%, respectively.

Despite the high clinical and technical success with endovenous stenting, approximately 20% of stented limbs require reinterventions over time because of either in-stent restenosis (ISR) or stent compression.[49] Neglen and colleagues[60] reported only 23% limbs (n = 324 limbs) with no ISR at long-term follow-up (42 months). They also reported a diameter reduction of greater than 20% and greater than 50% in 61% and 15% patients, respectively. The investigators thus reported 3 major risk factors associated with ISR, which included presence of thrombotic disease, history of thrombophilia, and long stents. Similar results were suggested by Ye and colleagues,[51] which described that in patients with long stents (extending below the inguinal ligament) and visible collateral circulation after stenting, there was a higher rate of ISR (HR = 1.77–6.5, P = .014; 22.5% vs 6%, P = .007, respectively). Few studies have reported bleeding complication following intervention in the form of retroperitoneal bleed or arterial injury requiring blood transfusion.[55,58] The rate of various complications as summarized in a meta-analysis of 25 studies (13 acute DVT, 12 chronic DVT) have been illustrated in **Table 6**.[53]

Table 6
Complications after venous stenting

Complication		Rate (%)	95% CI
Early thrombosis	Acute DVT	6.5	3.2–11
	Chronic DVT	6.8	3.8–10.6
Major bleeding	Acute DVT	1.1	0.3–2.6
	Chronic DVT	0.9	0.3–1.9
Pulmonary embolism	Acute DVT	0.9	0.1–2.3
	Chronic DVT	0.6	0.1–1.4
Periprocedural mortality	Acute DVT	0.7	0.1–1.8
	Chronic DVT	0.3	0.1–0.7

Open Surgery for Venous Obstruction

Open venous surgery typically is reserved for fit patients who have debilitating symptoms or ulceration and fail endovascular therapy. A variety of configurations and conduits have been described.[61–64] Most commonly, a large-caliber prosthetic bypass is used in conjunction with a temporary arteriovenous fistula to enhance flow and prevent thrombosis.

Even though open surgery in selected patients can be done with no mortality or pulmonary embolization, approximately one-third of patients develop perioperative complications. Early morbidity is due to thrombosis, bleeding, and wound infections. Despite a 5-year primary patency of 42%, 60% of patients had resolution of symptoms. Repeat intervention with CDT or open revision is effective for graft salvage and increases secondary patency to 59% at 5 years.[62] The patency of the bypass varies depending on the conduit and anatomic location, with Palma cross femoral bypasses having highest reported patency of 70% after 5 years.[62,63,65,66]

SUMMARY

Surgical therapy for DVT is primarily endovascular in the acute and chronic settings. It is safe and effective in providing relief for patients with moderate to severe symptoms. Open surgery is reserved for patients who fail endovascular therapy.

REFERENCES

1. Perkins JM, Magee TR, Galland RB. Phlegmasia caerulea dolens and venous gangrene. Br J Surg 1996;83(1):19–23.
2. Hirsh J, Hoak J. Management of deep vein thrombosis and pulmonary embolism. A statement for healthcare professionals. Council on thrombosis (in consultation with the council on cardiovascular radiology), American Heart Association. Circulation 1996;93(12):2212–45.
3. Kahn SR, Shbaklo H, Lamping DL, et al. Determinants of health-related quality of life during the 2 years following deep vein thrombosis. J Thromb Haemost 2008;6(7):1105–12.
4. Porter JM, Moneta GL. Reporting standards in venous disease: an update. International Consensus Committee on chronic venous disease. J Vasc Surg 1995;21(4):635–45.
5. Guanella R, Ducruet T, Johri M, et al. Economic burden and cost determinants of deep vein thrombosis during 2 years following diagnosis: a prospective evaluation. J Thromb Haemost 2011;9(12):2397–405.

6. Enden T, Resch S, White C, et al. Cost-effectiveness of additional catheter-directed thrombolysis for deep vein thrombosis. J Thromb Haemost 2013;11(6): 1032–42.

7. Watson L, Broderick C, Armon MP. Thrombolysis for acute deep vein thrombosis. Cochrane Database Syst Rev 2016;(11):CD002783.

8. Enden T, Haig Y, Kløw NE, et al. Long-term outcome after additional catheter-directed thrombolysis versus standard treatment for acute iliofemoral deep vein thrombosis (the CaVenT study): a randomised controlled trial. Lancet 2012;379(9810):31–8.

9. Casey ET, Murad MH, Zumaeta-Garcia M, et al. Treatment of acute iliofemoral deep vein thrombosis. J Vasc Surg 2012;55(5):1463–73.

10. Haig Y, Enden T, Grotta O, et al. Post-thrombotic syndrome after catheter-directed thrombolysis for deep vein thrombosis (CaVenT): 5-year follow-up results of an open-label, randomised controlled trial. Lancet Haematol 2016;3(2):e64–71.

11. Comerota AJ. The ATTRACT trial: rationale for early intervention for iliofemoral DVT. Perspect Vasc Surg Endovasc Ther 2009;21(4):221–4 [quiz: 224–5].

12. Vedantham S, Goldhaber SZ, Kahn SR, et al. Rationale and design of the ATTRACT study: a multicenter randomized trial to evaluate pharmacomechanical catheter-directed thrombolysis for the prevention of postthrombotic syndrome in patients with proximal deep vein thrombosis. Am Heart J 2013;165(4): 523–530 e3.

13. Vedantham S, Piazza G, Sista AK, et al. Guidance for the use of thrombolytic therapy for the treatment of venous thromboembolism. J Thromb Thrombolysis 2016;41(1):68–80.

14. Kearon C, Akl EA, Comerota AJ, et al. Antithrombotic therapy for VTE disease: antithrombotic therapy and prevention of thrombosis, 9th ed: American college of chest physicians evidence-based clinical practice guidelines. Chest 2012; 141(2 Suppl):e419S–96S.

15. Kearon C, Kahn SR, Agnelli G, et al. Antithrombotic therapy for venous thromboembolic disease: American college of chest physicians evidence-based clinical practice guidelines (8th edition). Chest 2008;133(6 Suppl):454S–545S.

16. Meissner MH, Gloviczki P, Comerota AJ, et al. Early thrombus removal strategies for acute deep venous thrombosis: clinical practice guidelines of the society for vascular surgery and the American Venous Forum. J Vasc Surg 2012;55(5):1449–62.

17. Vedantham S, Millward SF, Cardella JF, et al. Society of interventional radiology position statement: treatment of acute iliofemoral deep vein thrombosis with use of adjunctive catheter-directed intrathrombus thrombolysis. J Vasc Interv Radiol 2009;20(7 Suppl):S332–5.

18. Jaff MR, McMurtry MS, Archer SL, et al. Management of massive and submassive pulmonary embolism, iliofemoral deep vein thrombosis, and chronic thromboembolic pulmonary hypertension: a scientific statement from the American Heart Association. Circulation 2011;123(16):1788–830.

19. Vedantham S, Thorpe PE, Cardella JF, et al. Quality improvement guidelines for the treatment of lower extremity deep vein thrombosis with use of endovascular thrombus removal. J Vasc Interv Radiol 2006; 17(3):435–47 [quiz: 48].

20. Raju S, Neglen P. High prevalence of nonthrombotic iliac vein lesions in chronic venous disease: a permissive role in pathogenicity. J Vasc Surg 2006; 44(1):136–44.

21. Lee AI, Ochoa Chaar CI. CLINICAL PROBLEM-SOLVING. The hidden lesion. N Engl J Med 2016; 374(22):2160–5.

22. Kohi MP, Kohlbrenner R, Kolli KP, et al. Catheter directed interventions for acute deep vein thrombosis. Cardiovasc Diagn Ther 2016;6(6):599–611.

23. Mewissen MW, Seabrook GR, Meissner MH, et al. Catheter-directed thrombolysis for lower extremity deep venous thrombosis: report of a national multicenter registry. Radiology 1999; 211(1):39–49.

24. Wang L, Zhang C, Mu S, et al. Safety of catheter-directed thrombolysis for the treatment of acute lower extremity deep vein thrombosis: a systematic review and meta-analysis. Medicine 2017;96(35): e7922.

25. Bashir R, Zack CJ, Zhao H, et al. Comparative outcomes of catheter-directed thrombolysis plus anticoagulation vs anticoagulation alone to treat lower-extremity proximal deep vein thrombosis. JAMA Intern Med 2014;174(9):1494–501.

26. Semba CP, Dake MD. Iliofemoral deep venous thrombosis: aggressive therapy with catheter-directed thrombolysis. Radiology 1994;191(2): 487–94.

27. Bjarnason H, Kruse JR, Asinger DA, et al. Iliofemoral deep venous thrombosis: safety and efficacy outcome during 5 years of catheter-directed thrombolytic therapy. J Vasc Interv Radiol 1997;8(3): 405–18.

28. Razavi MK, Wong H, Kee ST, et al. Initial clinical results of tenecteplase (TNK) in catheter-directed thrombolytic therapy. J Endovasc Ther 2002;9(5): 593–8.

29. Grunwald MR, Hofmann LV. Comparison of urokinase, alteplase, and reteplase for catheter-directed thrombolysis of deep venous thrombosis. J Vasc Interv Radiol 2004;15(4):347–52.

30. Vedantham S, Vesely TM, Sicard GA, et al. Pharmacomechanical thrombolysis and early stent placement for iliofemoral deep vein thrombosis. J Vasc Interv Radiol 2004;15(6):565–74.

31. Protack CD, Bakken AM, Patel N, et al. Long-term outcomes of catheter directed thrombolysis for lower extremity deep venous thrombosis without prophylactic inferior vena cava filter placement. J Vasc Surg 2007;45(5):992–7 [discussion: 997].

32. Baekgaard N, Broholm R, Just S, et al. Long-term results using catheter-directed thrombolysis in 103 lower limbs with acute iliofemoral venous thrombosis. Eur J Vasc Endovasc Surg 2010;39(1):112–7.

33. Warner CJ, Goodney PP, Wallaert JB, et al. Functional outcomes following catheter-based iliac vein stent placement. Vasc Endovascular Surg 2013; 47(5):331–4.

34. Engelberger RP, Fahrni J, Willenberg T, et al. Fixed low-dose ultrasound-assisted catheter-directed thrombolysis followed by routine stenting of residual stenosis for acute ilio-femoral deep-vein thrombosis. Thromb Haemost 2014;111(6):1153–60.

35. Fiengo L, Bucci F, Khalil E, et al. Original approach for thrombolytic therapy in patients with Ilio-femoral deep vein thrombosis: 2 years follow-up. Thromb J 2015;13:40.

36. Du X-L, Kong L-S, Meng Q-Y, et al. Safety and efficacy of low dosage of urokinase for catheter-directed thrombolysis of deep venous thrombosis. Chin Med J 2015;128(13):1787–92.

37. Enden T, Klow NE, Sandvik L, et al. Catheter-directed thrombolysis vs. anticoagulant therapy alone in deep vein thrombosis: results of an open randomized, controlled trial reporting on short-term patency. J Thromb Haemost 2009;7(8):1268–75.

38. Sharifi M, Bay C, Mehdipour M, et al. Thrombus obliteration by rapid percutaneous endovenous intervention in deep venous occlusion (TORPEDO) trial: midterm results. J Endovasc Ther 2012;19(2): 273–80.

39. Sharifi M, Mehdipour M, Bay C, et al. Endovenous therapy for deep venous thrombosis: the TORPEDO trial. Catheter Cardiovasc Interv 2010;76(3):316–25.

40. AbuRahma AF, Perkins SE, Wulu JT, et al. Iliofemoral deep vein thrombosis: conventional therapy versus lysis and percutaneous transluminal angioplasty and stenting. Ann Surg 2001;233(6):752–60.

41. Elsharawy M, Elzayat E. Early results of thrombolysis vs anticoagulation in iliofemoral venous thrombosis. A randomised clinical trial. Eur J Vasc Endovasc Surg 2002;24(3):209–14.

42. Lee CY, Lai ST, Shih CC, et al. Short-term results of catheter-directed intrathrombus thrombolysis versus anticoagulation in acute proximal deep vein thrombosis. J Chin Med Assoc 2013;76(5):265–70.

43. Vedantham S, Goldhaber SZ, Julian JA, et al. Pharmacomechanical catheter-directed thrombolysis for deep-vein thrombosis. N Engl J Med 2017;377(23): 2240–52.

44. Brahmandam A, Abougergi MS, Ochoa Chaar CI. National trends in hospitalizations for venous thromboembolism. J Vasc Surg Venous Lymphat Disord 2017;5(5):621–629 e2.

45. Plate G, Eklof B, Norgren L, et al. Venous thrombectomy for iliofemoral vein thrombosis–10-year results of a prospective randomised study. Eur J Vasc Endovasc Surg 1997;14(5):367–74.

46. Labropoulos N, Volteas N, Leon M, et al. The role of venous outflow obstruction in patients with chronic venous dysfunction. Arch Surg 1997;132(1):46–51.

47. Johnson BF, Manzo RA, Bergelin RO, et al. Relationship between changes in the deep venous system and the development of the postthrombotic syndrome after an acute episode of lower limb deep vein thrombosis: a one- to six-year follow-up. J Vasc Surg 1995;21(2):307–13.

48. Comerota AJ, Oostra C, Fayad Z, et al. A histological and functional description of the tissue causing chronic postthrombotic venous obstruction. Thromb Res 2015;135(5):882–7.

49. Raju S. Treatment of iliac-caval outflow obstruction. Semin Vasc Surg 2015;28(1):47–53.

50. Raju S, Kirk O, Davis M, et al. Hemodynamics of "critical" venous stenosis and stent treatment. J Vasc Surg Venous Lymphat Disord 2014;2(1): 52–9.

51. Ye K, Lu X, Jiang M, et al. Technical details and clinical outcomes of transpopliteal venous stent placement for postthrombotic chronic total occlusion of the iliofemoral vein. J Vasc Interv Radiol 2014; 25(6):925–32.

52. Neglen P, Hollis KC, Olivier J, et al. Stenting of the venous outflow in chronic venous disease: long-term stent-related outcome, clinical, and hemodynamic result. J Vasc Surg 2007;46(5):979–90.

53. Razavi MK, Jaff MR, Miller LE. Safety and effectiveness of stent placement for iliofemoral venous outflow obstruction: systematic review and meta-analysis. Circ Cardiovasc Interv 2015;8(10): e002772.

54. Blanch Alerany M, Izquierdo Lamoca LM, Ramirez Ortega M, et al. Endovascular treatment of iliofemoral chronic post-thrombotic venous flow obstruction. J Vasc Surg Venous Lymphat Disord 2014;2(1): 2–7.

55. de Wolf MA, de Graaf R, Kurstjens RL, et al. Short-term clinical experience with a dedicated venous nitinol stent: initial results with the sinus-venous stent. Eur J Vasc Endovasc Surg 2015; 50(4):518–26.

56. Kurklinsky AK, Bjarnason H, Friese JL, et al. Outcomes of venoplasty with stent placement for chronic thrombosis of the iliac and femoral veins: single-center experience. J Vasc Interv Radiol 2012;23(8):1009–15.

57. Sang H, Li X, Qian A, et al. Outcome of endovascular treatment in postthrombotic syndrome. Ann Vasc Surg 2014;28(6):1493–500.

58. Stanley GA, Murphy EH, Plummer MM, et al. Midterm results of percutaneous endovascular treatment for acute and chronic deep venous thrombosis. J Vasc Surg Venous Lymphat Disord 2013; 1(1):52–8.

59. Titus JM, Moise MA, Bena J, et al. Iliofemoral stenting for venous occlusive disease. J Vasc Surg 2011; 53(3):706–12.

60. Neglen P, Raju S. In-stent recurrent stenosis in stents placed in the lower extremity venous outflow tract. J Vasc Surg 2004;39(1):181–7.

61. Husni E. Clinical experience with femoropopliteal venous reconstruction. In: Berganand JJ, Yao JST, editors. Venous problems. Chicago: Yearbook Medical Publishers; 1978. p. 485–91.

62. Garg N, Gloviczki P, Karimi KM, et al. Factors affecting outcome of open and hybrid reconstructions for nonmalignant obstruction of iliofemoral veins and inferior vena cava. J Vasc Surg 2011; 53(2):383–93.

63. Jost CJ, Gloviczki P, Cherry KJ Jr, et al. Surgical reconstruction of iliofemoral veins and the inferior vena cava for nonmalignant occlusive disease. J Vasc Surg 2001;33(2):320–7 [discussion: 327–8].

64. Palma EC, Esperon R. Vein transplants and grafts in the surgical treatment of the postphlebitic syndrome. J Cardiovasc Surg 1960;1:94–107.

65. Harris JP, Kidd J, Burnett A, et al. Patency of femorofemoral venous crossover grafts assessed by duplex scanning and phlebography. J Vasc Surg 1988;8(6):679–82.

66. Mendes BC, Gloviczki P, Akhtar N. Patency and clinical success 22 years after the Palma procedure. J Vasc Surg Venous Lymphat Disord 2016; 4(1):95–6.

Inferior Vena Cava Filters
Why, Who, and for How Long?

Brian P. Holly, MD[a],*, Brian Funaki, MD[b], Mark L. Lessne, MD[c]

KEYWORDS

- Vena cava • Filter • Venous thromboembolism

KEY POINTS

- Vena cava filters are indicated for the prevention of pulmonary emboli (PE) in patients who are unable to receive anticoagulation.
- Retrievable vena cava filters should be removed once the indication for PE prevention is no longer present.
- Patients with inferior vena cava (IVC) filters in place require close follow-up to ensure timely removal.

INTRODUCTION

The mainstay of treatment of patients with venous thromboembolic (VTE) disease is anticoagulation. Patients on anticoagulation have low rates of recurrent VTE, and patients with deep venous thrombosis (DVT) have low rates of subsequently developing pulmonary embolism (PE).[1,2] Before current practice of anticoagulation, primary PE prophylaxis often consisted of surgical ligation or interruption of the inferior vena cava (IVC) as means of disrupting the route for PE to develop. These surgical procedures paved the way for IVC filters, which are used today. IVC filters are implantable devices designed to intercept thrombus that has broken free from the lower extremities or pelvis and prevent its migration to the lungs. The purpose of this article is to review IVC filters and their impact on VTE treatment.

TYPES OF INFERIOR VENA CAVA FILTERS

IVC filters are divided into 2 main categories: *permanent and retrievable*. *Permanent* IVC filters are designed to remain within the patient for the duration of their lifetime and have no engineering considerations to facilitate removal. *Retrievable* (also known as *optional* or *removable*) IVC filters are specifically designed to allow for retrieval once the high-risk period for VTE has passed; however, these filters are also US Food and Drug Administration (FDA) approved to remain permanently. A novel category of IVC filters, the *temporary* IVC filter, are filters that are tethered to a cord or other device, such as a central venous catheter. These filters can be left in place for a very short amount of time while the patient is in the hospital and must be removed. Preliminary data suggest these temporary IVC filters may safely prevent PE in patients with transient indications for IVC filtration, such as trauma.[3,4]

There is no consensus on any one filter design or type being superior to another. To date, no comparative studies of permanent versus retrievable filters have been conducted nor have there been any head-to-head studies of different filters within either category. Nonetheless, current

---

Disclosure Statement: M.L. Lessne is a paid speaker for Cook Medical.
The remaining authors of this article have no financial or commercial interests relevant to this article.
[a] Vascular and Interventional Radiology, Johns Hopkins Hospital, Interventional Radiology Center, Sheikh Zayed Tower, Suite 7203, 1800 Orleans Street, Baltimore, MD 21287, USA; [b] Vascular and Interventional Radiology, Department of Radiology, University of Chicago Medicine, 5840 South Maryland, MC 2026, Chicago, IL 60637, USA; [c] Vascular & Interventional Specialists, Charlotte Radiology, 700 East Morehead Street, Charlotte, NC 28202, USA
* Corresponding author.
E-mail address: bholly3@jhmi.edu

Clin Chest Med 39 (2018) 645–650
https://doi.org/10.1016/j.ccm.2018.04.015
0272-5231/18/© 2018 Elsevier Inc. All rights reserved.

practice patterns have led to a significant increase in the use of retrievable IVC filters, which are now placed much more commonly than permanent filters.[5] Physicians should consider the length of time IVC filtration is necessary because there are some data to suggest that permanent IVC filters have fewer long-term complications than retrievable filters, and they are more cost-effective.[6–8] However, if the indication for filtration is likely to be temporary (ie, the patient may be able to resume anticoagulation in the future), then a retrievable filter would be favored.

INDICATIONS/CONTRAINDICATIONS FOR INFERIOR VENA CAVA FILTER PLACEMENT

In the late 1990s, the PREPIC study was conducted to determine the safety and efficacy of IVC filters in the setting of proximal DVT.[9] The landmark study found initial benefit of IVC filters in preventing PE, but this was offset by an increase in recurrent DVT in patients with an IVC filter. This study remains one of the few randomized controlled trials (RCT) that has been performed evaluating IVC filters, and the results play a major role in how IVC

filters are currently used. In today's practice, the most widely accepted indication for placement of an IVC filter is the prevention of PE in a patient with VTE and a contraindication to anticoagulation: this is the only unanimously agreed upon indication. Findings from a more recent RCT ("PREPIC II"), which included patients with a diagnosis of PE and DVT, confirmed that there was no reduction in the risk of recurrent, symptomatic PE at 3 months in anticoagulated patients who received an IVC filter versus patients on anticoagulation alone.[10] Other accepted indications for placement of an IVC filter include a complication of anticoagulation, worsening of VTE despite adequate anticoagulation, VTE with poor cardiopulmonary reserve, high-risk or massive PE, and free-floating caval or iliac DVT. The most updated societal guidelines regarding the indications for placement of an IVC filter are highlighted in **Table 1**.

There are no absolute contraindications to IVC filter placement. The most updated recommendations from the American College of Chest Physicians (ACCP) state, "In patients with acute DVT or PE who are treated with anticoagulants, we recommend against the use of an inferior vena

Table 1
Societal guidelines for the placement of inferior vena cava filters

Guideline	Recommendations
CHEST/ACCP Guidelines[1,2]	• In patients with acute VTE and contraindication to anticoagulation (AC), recommend the use of an IVC filter • In patients with high-risk/massive PE, consider IVC filter in addition to anticoagulation • In patients with recurrent VTE despite adequate AC, IVC filter is an option of last resort
SIR Guidelines[31]	IVC filters are indicated in patients with PE or IVC, iliac, femoral, or popliteal DVT and one or more of the following: • Contraindication to AC • Complication of AC • Failure of AC • Inability to achieve/maintain adequate AC • Thrombus progression despite adequate AC • High-risk/massive PE with residual DVT • Free-floating caval or iliac DVT • Severe cardiopulmonary disease and DVT Prophylactic IVC filters (no documented DVT/PE) are indicated in the following settings: • Severe trauma, closed head injury, spinal cord injury, multiple long-bone or pelvic fractures • Patients at high risk for VTE (immobilized, ICU patient, and so forth)
AHA Guidelines[39]	• Adult patients with any confirmed acute PE (or proximal DVT) with contraindications to anticoagulation or with active bleeding complication should receive an IVC filter • For patients with recurrent acute PE despite therapeutic anticoagulation, it is reasonable to place an IVC filter • Placement of an IVC filter may be considered for patients with acute PE and very poor cardiopulmonary reserve, including those with high-risk/massive PE

cava (IVC) filter."[2] Although this is not a true contraindication, it bears mention because a recent RCT failed to show any benefit from placing an IVC filter in patients who are receiving anticoagulation.[10] There have been reports of patients with a nickel allergy having a reaction to the IVC filter, but these are rare and routine screening is not necessary.[11] Anatomic issues may preclude IVC filter placement (ie, caval thrombosis, anatomic variants, invasion or compression by tumor), but these are also rare. Bacteremia should prompt the physician to weigh the risks of infection versus the benefit of filter placement; although infection of an IVC filter is exceedingly unusual, several cases have been reported.[12]

INFERIOR VENA CAVA FILTER PLACEMENT

Before IVC filter placement, patients should have all relevant laboratory work up-to-date, including a complete blood count, basic metabolic panel, and prothrombin time/international normalized ratio if indicated. Typically, iodinated contrast is used for the filter placement procedure, and therefore, renal function should be within acceptable limits; patients need to be evaluated for a contrast allergy. For patients unable to receive iodinated contrast, intravascular ultrasound, carbon dioxide, and gadolinium-based contrasts are alternatives.

IVC filters are typically placed in an angiography suite using fluoroscopic guidance. Either the jugular or the femoral vein is accessed; the ideal filter position is determined using fluoroscopic guidance, and the filter is typically deployed in the infrarenal IVC. Ideally, the filter is placed so that the apex is centered within the cava, just below the level of the most inferior renal vein. Physicians placing IVC filters need to be aware of anatomic variants that could limit the filter's effectiveness or make placement challenging. For example, if the caval diameter is greater than 30 to 40 mm, so called, megacava, many filters are not approved for use at that caval size, and the patient may require placement of 2 filters, one in each of the bilateral iliac veins. Duplicated IVC, circumaortic and retroaortic renal veins, and caval interruption likewise require attention and technical modifications during filter placement.

COMPLICATIONS OF INFERIOR VENA CAVA FILTERS

When performed in an angiography suite, procedural complications during IVC filter placement are infrequent and typically of little clinical significance. One study detailing a single-center experience with IVC filters reported a 0.3% major complication rate.[13] Rarely, there can be a problem with filter deployment (ie, filter placement at an unintentional location within the IVC or in an unintentional vessel), which may prompt immediate retrieval and replacement.

On the other hand, the long-term complications of indwelling IVC filters are far more common and have led to increased scrutiny of IVC filters in recent years. In 2010, the FDA issued a safety communication urging physicians placing retrievable IVC filters to consider removal once the indication for their placement has resolved. The safety communication was in response to more than 900 reports of adverse events involving IVC filters. Complications such as filter fracture, embolization, migration, caval wall penetration, and thrombosis are the most worrisome.

Filter fracture occurs when one of the struts or filter components becomes discontinuous with the main filter element. A fracture increases the risk of embolization of the fractured fragment or migration of the filter itself. Fracture is the most common major complication of retrievable IVC filters.[14] Although the overall incidence of filter fracture is hard to discern, recent reports cite fracture rates of 10% to 15%, with the risk of fracture increasing with increasing dwell times.[15,16] Typically, fractured filter fragments are of little clinical significance; however, filter fracture can be symptomatic if embolization occurs or if the component perforates adjacent retroperitoneal structures or other organs along the downstream blood flow from the filter (ie, kidneys, liver, heart, or lungs).

Filter migration occurs when the entire filter moves from its original deployment location and, although rare, extreme migration to an intracardiac location has been reported.[17]

Caval wall penetration involves the struts of the filter protruding beyond the limits of the caval wall while remaining attached to the filter. Multiple reports exist describing complications involving penetration of adjacent structures.[18,19]

Caval thrombosis can occur as a result of the filter trapping a large thrombus and failing to recanalize or because of recurrent thrombus forming inside the filter and propagating to the point of caval stenosis or occlusion. Caval thrombosis is also rare, with a recent systematic review reporting a frequency of caval thrombosis or stenosis for patients receiving a retrievable IVC filter of 2.8%.[17] In vitro models suggest that normal caval flow dynamics are impaired by the presence of an IVC filter, especially in the setting of trapped thrombus or a tilted filter.[20,21] This increased turbulence may help explain the increased rate of recurrent DVT. There is currently no consensus on the recommendations for anticoagulation following IVC filter placement. There is some evidence to suggest that patients with an IVC filter who remain on anticoagulation have lower rates of recurrent VTE and are less likely to form thrombus within the filter.[22,23]

INFERIOR VENA CAVA FILTER RETRIEVAL

As previously mentioned, most of the IVC filters placed today are designed to be retrieved. Current retrievable filter designs (**Fig. 1**) commonly include a hook at the cranial or caudal filter apex, which is used to retrieve the filter once it is no longer needed. The procedure to retrieve the filter typically entails obtaining jugular venous access, as most filters are designed to be removed from a jugular vein approach. After performing a venogram, the physician then engages the hook with a snare device, and the filter is collapsed into a vascular sheath and removed. Technical success of IVC filter retrieval is generally very high (>95%) and depends on several factors (dwell time of filter, degree of filter tilt, and so forth).[24–26] If the filter is tilted or embedded in the wall of the IVC, more advance techniques may be required to remove the filter. In addition, there is no absolute cutoff time after which IVC filter retrieval should not be attempted. In cases of prolonged IVC filter dwell time, extreme tilt, caval penetration, caval ingrowth or filter migration, filter removal may require referral to centers specifically experienced in complex filter removals.

Although against their indications for use, permanent IVC filters can be safely removed from patients if the indication to do so is sufficiently strong.

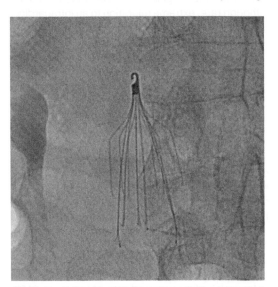

Fig. 1. A retrievable IVC filter (Denali; Bard Medical, Covington, GA, USA). Note the hook at the filter apex to facilitate retrieval.

Findings from prior studies show that chronically indwelling IVC filters put these patients at risk for future VTE.[9] Unfortunately, many patients receive permanent IVC filters even though they may only have a temporary indication for IVC filtration. In these instances, it may be prudent to remove a permanent filter; however, this often entails advanced techniques that increase the risk of the retrieval procedure.[27,28] Consultation with a physician who is experienced in complex filter removals is recommended.

In 2010, and again in 2014, the FDA issued a safety communication urging all physicians who place IVC filters to take an active role in ensuring proper follow-up for patients who have received an IVC filter. The goal is to ensure that patients who no longer have an indication for IVC filtration have their filters evaluated for removal in a timely manner. Many IVC filter practices have now adopted dedicated IVC filter clinics to follow these patients. Recent studies have shown that when physicians follow their IVC filter patients in a formal IVC filter clinic, retrieval rates are significantly improved. One study reported an improvement in retrieval rate from 29% in the preclinic period to 60% in the postclinic period.[29] Another study reported an increase in retrieval rate from 8% to 52% after implementation of a system of mailing the patient and referring physician a follow-up letter as well as automatically scheduling patients for a follow-up clinic visit at the time of filter placement.[30] Similarly, an additional IVC filter practice was able to achieve a follow-up rate of 83.5% in all patients by creating an IVC filter patient database and periodically mailing the patient a letter regarding their IVC filter.

ADDITIONAL TOPICS

Prophylactic IVC filters: Certain patients, such as critically ill patients in an intensive care unit or polytrauma patients, are at a higher risk for VTE. If a DVT were to develop, these patients often have a contraindication to anticoagulation because of their injuries or the potential need for multiple surgical procedures. Although level I data are lacking, The Society of Interventional Radiology and the Eastern Association for the Surgery of Trauma advocate the placement of an IVC filter, even if no DVT is present, in these high-risk patients.[31–33]

Superior vena cava (SVC) filters: The incidence of PE resulting from an upper extremity DVT is small, approximately 2%.[34] Although it is possible that thrombus located in an upper extremity vein could break free and embolize to the pulmonary arterial system, the available data suggest this is less likely to be clinically significant compared with thrombus embolizing from the lower extremity.[35] Although the ACCP guidelines do recommend anticoagulation for upper extremity DVT, SVC filters are not routinely used in these patients. Placement of IVC filters in the SVC is considered an off-label use, and data on safety and efficacy are limited. Moreover, retrieval of SVC filters may prove higher risk than those in the IVC secondary to the risk of cardiac injury.[36]

Novel filter designs: Since the advent of the retrievable IVC filter, the general design concept of the IVC filter has not significantly changed. However, research and development of novel filter designs are ongoing. Future directions include devices that are composed of biocompatible materials that allow all or part of the filter to dissolve.[37,38] If this technology provides a viable filter model, it could potentially alleviate the issue of patients being lost to follow-up with an IVC filter in place.

SUMMARY

IVC filters, when used appropriately, have been proven safe and effective. Societal guidelines vary in the indications for IVC filter placement; however, most agree that IVC filters are indicated to prevent PE in patients with active lower-extremity DVT who cannot receive anticoagulation. It is imperative that patients with retrievable IVC filters are followed closely and that their IVC filters are removed once no longer indicated.

REFERENCES

1. Kearon C, Akl EA, Comerota AJ, et al. Antithrombotic therapy for VTE disease: antithrombotic therapy and prevention of thrombosis, 9th ed: American College of Chest Physicians evidence-based clinical practice guidelines. Chest 2012; 141(2 Suppl):e419S–496.

2. Kearon C, Akl EA, Ornelas J, et al. Antithrombotic therapy for VTE disease: CHEST guideline and expert panel report. Chest 2016;149(2):315–52.

3. Tapson VF, Hazelton JP, Myers J, et al. Evaluation of a device combining an inferior vena cava filter and a central venous catheter for preventing pulmonary embolism among critically ill trauma patients. J Vasc Interv Radiol 2017;28(9):1248–54.

4. Jia W, Liu J, Tian X, et al. Tempofilter II implantation in patients with lower extremity fractures and proximal deep vein thrombosis. Diagn Interv Radiol 2014;20(3):245–50.

5. Smouse BJA. Is market growth of vena cava filters justified. Endovascular Today 2010;74–7.

6. Eifler AC, Lewandowski RJ, Gupta R, et al. Optional or permanent: clinical factors that optimize inferior vena cava filter utilization. J Vasc Interv Radiol 2013;24(1):35–40.

7. Janne d'Othee B, Faintuch S, Reedy AW, et al. Retrievable versus permanent caval filter procedures: when are they cost-effective for interventional radiology? J Vasc Interv Radiol 2008;19(3):384–92.

8. Desai TR, Morcos OC, Lind BB, et al. Complications of indwelling retrievable versus permanent inferior vena cava filters. J Vasc Surg Venous Lymphat Disord 2014;2(2):166–73.

9. Decousus H, Leizorovicz A, Parent F, et al. A clinical trial of vena caval filters in the prevention of pulmonary embolism in patients with proximal deep-vein thrombosis. N Engl J Med 1998;338(7):409–15.

10. Mismetti P, Laporte S, Pellerin O, et al. Effect of a retrievable inferior vena cava filter plus anticoagulation vs anticoagulation alone on risk of recurrent pulmonary embolism: a randomized clinical trial. JAMA 2015;313(16):1627–35.

11. Morshedi MM, Kinney TB. Nickel hypersensitivity in patients with inferior vena cava filters: case report and literature and MAUDE database review. J Vasc Interv Radiol 2014;25(8):1187–91.

12. Rottenstreich A, Bar-Shalom R, Bloom AI, et al. Endovascular infection following inferior vena cava (IVC) filter insertion. J Thromb Thrombolysis 2015; 40(4):452–7.

13. Athanasoulis CA, Kaufman JA, Halpern EF, et al. Inferior vena caval filters: review of a 26-year single-center clinical experience. Radiology 2000; 216(1):54–66.

14. Andreoli JM, Lewandowski RJ, Vogelzang RL, et al. Comparison of complication rates associated with permanent and retrievable inferior vena cava filters: a review of the MAUDE database. J Vasc Interv Radiol 2014;25(8):1181–5.

15. Vijay K, Hughes JA, Burdette AS, et al. Fractured bard recovery, G2, and G2 express inferior vena cava filters: incidence, clinical consequences, and outcomes of removal attempts. J Vasc Interv Radiol 2012;23(2):188–94.

16. Nicholson W, Nicholson WJ, Tolerico P, et al. Prevalence of fracture and fragment embolization of Bard retrievable vena cava filters and clinical implications including cardiac perforation and tamponade. Arch Intern Med 2010;170(20):1827–31.

17. Angel LF, Tapson V, Galgon RE, et al. Systematic review of the use of retrievable inferior vena cava filters. J Vasc Interv Radiol 2011;22(11):1522–30.e3.

18. Jia Z, Wu A, Tam M, et al. Caval penetration by inferior vena cava filters: a systematic literature review of clinical significance and management. Circulation 2015;132(10):944–52.

19. Bos A, Van Ha T, van Beek D, et al. Strut penetration: local complications, breakthrough pulmonary embolism, and retrieval failure in patients with Celect vena cava filters. J Vasc Interv Radiol 2015;26(1):101–6.

20. Leask RL, Johnston KW, Ojha M. Hemodynamic effects of clot entrapment in the TrapEase inferior vena cava filter. J Vasc Interv Radiol 2004;15(5):485–90.

21. Singer MA, Wang SL. Modeling blood flow in a tilted inferior vena cava filter: does tilt adversely affect hemodynamics? J Vasc Interv Radiol 2011;22(2):229–35.

22. Ray CE Jr, Prochazka A. The need for anticoagulation following inferior vena cava filter placement: systematic review. Cardiovasc Intervent Radiol 2008;31(2):316–24.

23. Hajduk B, Tomkowski WZ, Malek G, et al. Vena cava filter occlusion and venous thromboembolism risk in persistently anticoagulated patients: a prospective, observational cohort study. Chest 2010;137(4):877–82.

24. Lynch FC. A method for following patients with retrievable inferior vena cava filters: results and lessons learned from the first 1,100 patients. J Vasc Interv Radiol 2011;22(11):1507–12.

25. Binkert CA, Drooz AT, Caridi JG, et al. Technical success and safety of retrieval of the G2 filter in a prospective, multicenter study. J Vasc Interv Radiol 2009;20(11):1449–53.

26. Dinglasan L, Oh J, Schmitt J, et al. Complicated inferior vena cava filter retrievals: associated factors identified at preretrieval CT. Radiology 2013;266(2):347–54.

27. Tamrazi A, Wadhwa V, Holly B, et al. Percutaneous retrieval of permanent inferior vena cava filters. CardioVascular Intervent Radiol 2016;39(4):538–46.

28. Kuo WT, Odegaard JI, Rosenberg JK, et al. Excimer laser-assisted removal of embedded inferior vena cava filters: a single-center prospective study. Circ Cardiovasc Interv 2013;6(5):560–6.

29. Minocha J, Idakoji I, Riaz A, et al. Improving inferior vena cava filter retrieval rates: impact of a dedicated inferior vena cava filter clinic. J Vasc Interv Radiol 2010;21(12):1847–51.

30. Sutphin PD, Reis SP, McKune A, et al. Improving inferior vena cava filter retrieval rates with the define, measure, analyze, improve, control methodology. J Vasc Interv Radiol 2015;26(4):491–8.e1.

31. Caplin DM, Nikolic B, Kalva SP, et al. Quality improvement guidelines for the performance of inferior vena cava filter placement for the prevention of pulmonary embolism. J Vasc Interv Radiol 2011;22(11):1499–506.

32. Haut ER, Garcia LJ, Shihab HM, et al. The effectiveness of prophylactic inferior vena cava filters in trauma patients: a systematic review and meta-analysis. JAMA Surg 2014;149(2):194–202.

33. Rogers FB, Cipolle MD, Velmahos G, et al. Practice management guidelines for the prevention of venous thromboembolism in trauma patients: the EAST practice management guidelines work group. J Trauma 2002;53(1):142–64.

34. Levy MM, Albuquerque F, Pfeifer JD. Low incidence of pulmonary embolism associated with upper-extremity deep venous thrombosis. Ann Vasc Surg 2012;26(7):964–72.

35. Munoz FJ, Mismetti P, Poggio R, et al. Clinical outcome of patients with upper-extremity deep vein thrombosis: results from the RIETE registry. Chest 2008;133(1):143–8.

36. Nguyen ML, Yevich SM, Black JH, et al. Endovascular removal of an embedded superior vena cava filter after 6 years. J Vasc Interv Radiol 2015;26(1):131–3.

37. Eggers MD, McArthur MJ, Figueira TA, et al. Pilot in vivo study of an absorbable polydioxanone vena cava filter. J Vasc Surg Venous Lymphat Disord 2015;3(4):409–20.

38. Hohenwalter EJ, Stone JR, O'Moore PV, et al. Multicenter trial of the VenaTech convertible vena cava filter. J Vasc Interv Radiol 2017;28(10):1353–62.

39. Jaff MR, McMurtry MS, Archer SL, et al. Management of massive and submassive pulmonary embolism, iliofemoral deep vein thrombosis, and chronic thromboembolic pulmonary hypertension: a scientific statement from the American Heart Association. Circulation 2011;123(16):1788–830.

Catheter-Based Therapies for Pulmonary Emboli

Jeffrey S. Pollak, MD

KEYWORDS

- Catheter-directed therapy • Catheter-directed thrombolysis • Percutaneous intervention
- Pulmonary embolism • Thrombolysis • Transcatheter embolectomy • Transcatheter thrombectomy

KEY POINTS

- Acute pulmonary embolism remains a significant cause of mortality and morbidity, prompting care beyond anticoagulation for patients with massive and possibly submassive disease.
- Transcatheter therapies for acute pulmonary embolism consist of catheter-based thrombolysis directly into the clot, catheter-based thrombus debulking, and combinations of these.
- Evidence suggests that catheter-based thrombolysis at lower doses than standard systemic thrombolysis achieves an outcome including mortality that is variably the same or better at a lower bleeding risk.
- Catheter-based thrombus debulking consists of fragmentation and/or clot removal. This holds the promise of even faster hemodynamic improvement and can be used in patients with contraindications to thrombolysis, but no adequate or proved method or device is currently available.

INTRODUCTION

Although anticoagulation remains the mainstay of treatment of acute pulmonary embolism (PE), this disease still carries an estimated 30-day mortality of 9% to 11% and 3 month rate of 9% to 17%, with 100,000 to 200,000 deaths annually in the United States, concentrated in those with massive (high-risk) and less so in those with submassive (intermediate-risk) involvement.[1,2] Acute PE is believed the third most common cause of death in hospitalized patients and limited data suggest the possibility of long-term cardiopulmonary sequela even short of actual chronic thromboembolic pulmonary hypertension, which itself occurs in perhaps 1% to 4%.[3] Consequently, more advanced therapy should be considered in patients with massive and submassive involvement given their higher risk for these complications as long as the risks of such therapy are acceptable.

The acute goals of any therapy more aggressive than anticoagulation are to provide rapid relief of pulmonary arterial obstruction and restore pulmonary and systemic perfusion, reduce pulmonary artery pressure, reduce right ventricular compromise, and improve oxygenation. Options consist of systemic thrombolysis, catheter-based or catheter-directed therapies (CDT), surgical embolectomy, and extracorporeal membrane oxygenation.

TYPES OF TRANSCATHETER THERAPIES

Catheter-based therapies can be divided into catheter-directed thrombolysis, transcatheter mechanical thrombus debulking, and combinations of these. The rationale is to achieve clot reduction and clinical improvement with a lower bleeding risk than systemic thrombolysis and perhaps greater efficacy. Major limitations are the size and volume of clots, their age because older

Disclosure statements: No financial interest in the subject matter or materials discussed in this article or with a company making a competing product (J.S. Pollak).
Department of Radiology and Biomedical Imaging, Section of Vascular and Interventional Radiology, Yale University School of Medicine, PO Box 208042, 333 Cedar Street, New Haven, CT 06520-8042, USA
E-mail address: jeffrey.pollak@yale.edu

Clin Chest Med 39 (2018) 651–658
https://doi.org/10.1016/j.ccm.2018.04.016

thromboemboli have started to organize and adhere to the vessel wall and be more resistant to pharmacologic or mechanical treatment, and the status of patients—considering individual risks for pharmacologic thrombolysis, level of cardiopulmonary instability, and the time available for any intervention.

General Concepts

Once a decision has been made to proceed with a transcatheter intervention, pulmonary artery catheterization becomes the first procedural step. Access usually is through a femoral or internal jugular vein and less commonly an upper extremity vein and should be done under ultrasound guidance to minimize punctures or inadvertent entry into a nearby artery, which increases the risk for access site bleeding. Two sheaths can be placed in one vein adjacent to each other if more than 1 catheter is needed for treatment. Right heart and pulmonary artery pressures should be obtained; at least the pulmonary artery value can be followed to determine patient response. Pulmonary angiography is usually done to visualize the emboli, but some proceduralists may skip this when a prior CT angiogram (CTA) permits confident guidance for thrombolysis. After the procedure, patients are followed in an intensive care setting, monitoring hemodynamics, respiratory status, and for possible complications related to the procedure, such as bleeding. An echocardiogram within 2 days is helpful in assessing response.

Catheter-Directed Thrombolysis

Systemic thrombolysis has been shown to accelerate dissolution of acute PE with more rapid lowering of pulmonary artery pressure and more rapid imaging response than anticoagulation along with reduced early mortality but at a cost of a higher risk of bleeding, most worrisomely, intracranially.[4,5] Furthermore, 30-day mortality is not always found reduced. Multiple contraindications exist for systemic thrombolysis, which are based on factors placing patients at higher risk for bleeding.[6] Absolute contraindications include past intracranial hemorrhage; recent ischemic stroke within the past 3 months; a central nervous system structural lesion; such as a tumor, major trauma or surgery within several weeks to months; and active bleeding. Relative contraindications include an ischemic stroke older than 3 months, oral anticoagulation, uncontrolled more severe hypertension, recent internal bleeding, pregnancy, advanced liver disease, and advanced age (variably >65–75 years). Depending on the patient, even absolute contraindications can become relative. A meta-analysis comparing systemic thrombolysis plus anticoagulation to just anticoagulation showed risks of major bleeding of 9.24% to 3.42% and of intracranial hemorrhage of 1.46% to 0.19%.[4]

Transcatheter thrombolysis directly into pulmonary thromboemboli has the theoretic advantages of supplying a high local concentration of the agent to a greater surface area of the clot yet at a lower dose than systemic administration and with lower systemic exposure. This should translate to greater efficacy with a lower risk of bleeding. Still, the 2016 guidelines for antithrombotic therapy for VTE disease by the American College of Chest Physicians recommend systemic thrombolysis over catheter-directed thrombolysis, reserving the latter as an option in patients at higher risk of bleeding or as a possible adjunct to catheter-assisted thrombus removal in patients with hypotension who have a high bleeding risk, have failed systemic thrombolysis, or have shock that is likely to cause death before systemic thrombolysis can take effect.[7] Typically, a multi-sidehole catheter is advanced into the clot in one lung or two catheters are used, one for each pulmonary artery (**Fig. 1**) and a fibrinolytic agent is infused, such as tissue plasminogen activator (TPA) at rates of 0.5-1 mg/hour per catheter when two catheters are used and 0.5-2 mg/hour if just one catheter is used. The duration of the infusion is usually 12-24 hours, giving average total doses of 20 to 28 mg.[8,9] Note that administering the thrombolytic agent proximal to the PE is believed to provide no benefit over systemic administration as the drug will preferentially course into unobstructed branches.[10] Systemic heparin is generally delivered at a subtherapeutic dose of 500-600 units/hour during the fibrinolytic instillation given concern over a greater potential for bleeding if fully anticoagulated.

In an attempt to further enhance the effectiveness and speed of clot dissolution, intrathrombotic fibrinolytic instillation can be combined with high-frequency, low intensity ultrasound waves delivered simultaneously with the drug through a multi-sidehole EkoSonic Endovascular System Infusion Catheter (EKOS Corp, Bothell, WA), which is called ultrasound-assisted or ultrasound-accelerated thrombolysis. The ultrasound disrupts and thins fibrin strands, increasing permeability and exposure to plasminogen activator sites deep in the clot (**Fig. 2**). This system has received an FDA indication for the treatment of pulmonary embolism.

The ULTIMA study randomized the use of ultrasound-assisted thrombolysis for acute intermediate

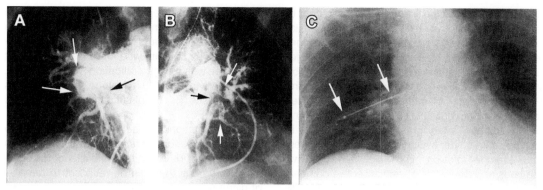

Fig. 1. An 84-year-old woman with left lower extremity cellulitis who became unresponsive with hypoxia requiring intubation and ventilatory support. Bilateral pulmonary angiography showed large bilateral emboli, occlusive in the right middle lobe and occlusive and nonocclusive in several lower lobe segments (*arrows [A]*) and near-occlusive in left lobar and segmental arteries (*arrows [B]*). Multi–side-hole catheters were placed into each pulmonary artery for thrombolytic infusions. The right catheter had its side holes extending from the inter-lobar artery into the occluded right middle lobe artery (*arrows [C]*). The infusions were continued for 12 hours. The patient's clinical status improved and she was extubated on day 3.

risk PE to anticoagulation alone and found hemody-namic improvement based on a lower right to left ventricular ratio with no major bleeding in the thrombolytic group, although no significant differ-ence in 90 day mortality.[11] In a prospective sin-gle-arm study, the SEATTLE II trial, found lower right to left ventricular ratios, pulmonary artery pressures, and clot burden with a 10% major bleeding rate but none intracranial of fatal.[12] In an effort to determine the optimal dose and duration of ultrasound-assisted thrombolysis, the OPTA-LYSE PE study looked at four infusion regimens from 1 to 2 mg of TPA per catheter and 2, 4, or 6 hour infusions.[13] Even at these short infusion times,

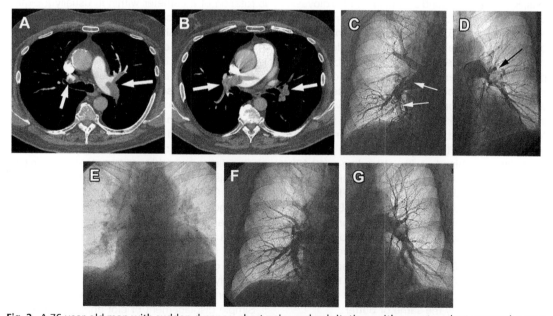

Fig. 2. A 76-year-old man with sudden dyspnea, chest pain, and palpitations with no antecedent event who now had submassive PE. Echocardiography revealed severely increased right ventricular cavity size with moderately decreased systolic function and a right ventricular systolic pressure of 56 mm Hg. A chest CTA showed bilateral PE (*A, B*). Bilateral pulmonary angiography confirmed extensive PE (*arrows [C, D]*). Ultrasound-assisted thrombo-lytic catheters were placed into the clot in each pulmonary artery with TPA infusing at 1 mg/h through each (*E*). Repeat pulmonary angiography the next day showed marked reduction in emboli (*F, G*) and pulmonary artery pressure was 44/11 with a mean of 22 mm Hg. An echocardiogram at 2 months was normal, with insufficient tricuspid regurgitation to permit estimation of the right ventricular systolic pressure.

all four groups had significant decreases in right to left ventricular ratios at 48 hours, which were similar between them, with three major bleeds. Nevertheless, at the current time, proof does not exist for an advantage of ultrasound-accelerated thrombolysis over plain catheter directed thrombolysis. The PERFECT registry of catheter-directed therapies for PE found no significant differences in pre and post pulmonary artery pressures and changes in the pressures, the average thrombolytic doses, and average infusion times between the two methods and Graif et al in a retrospective comparison of 60 patients with mostly submassive PE found no significant difference in complications or 30 day mortality with significantly greater procedure and fluoroscopy times for ultrasound-assisted thrombolysis compared to use of a pigtail catheter in the pulmonary artery.[8,14]

While no randomized comparisons of catheter-directed thrombolysis to systemic thrombolysis exist, several larger analyses have looked at the risks and efficacy. In a multicenter registry and meta-analysis of patients treated with CDT, Bloomer et al found intracranial hemorrhage to be 1.5% and 0.35% and major complications of 9.5% and 4.65% (generally just transfusions) for massive and submassive PE.[15] In another meta-analysis looking at ultrasound-assisted thrombolysis, Kaymaz et al found all cause and cardiovascular mortalities of 3.2% and 2.2% with major and minor bleeding 5.5% and 6.9%, and when compared to three randomized systemic thrombolytic trials, the death rate was similar but major bleeding was lower.[16] In a more direct comparison, Aurora et al looked at 3107 patients treated with systemic thrombolysis and 1319 with CDT in the National Readmission Database for 2013 to 2014 and found that the systemic group had higher mortality (14.9% compared to 6.12%), mortality combined with bleeding (18.1% compared to 8.4%), and readmission rates (10.6% compared to 7.6%) than the CDT group.[17] In looking at the National Inpatient Database, Liang et al did not find improved mortality but did find lower risk of hemorrhage stroke in the nonshock group, which would correspond to intermediate risk PE.[18] Therefore, evidence is suggestive that CDT carries a lower risk than systemic thrombolysis while outcome including mortality is variably the same or better.

Transcatheter Mechanical Thrombus Debulking

Catheter based mechanical methods to treat pulmonary embolism can be divided into fragmentation and thromboembolectomy (removal). These can provide more rapid reduction in clot burden and improvement in hemodynamic parameters than thrombolysis and may be appropriate in more tenuous patients who need faster treatment or in those with a contraindication to thrombolysis. In addition to being used alone, such methods may be used in combination with a fibrinolytic agent.

Major limitations for debulking techniques are the large volume of clot relative to the limited sizes and effects of devices; the coexistence of organized thrombus that can be resistant to removal of disruption; multiple pulmonary artery branches that can be problematic to catheterize; and risks, including access site bleeding or thrombosis, pulmonary artery injury with bleeding or occlusion, distal embolization with occlusion of pulmonary artery branches resulting in worsened obstruction and pulmonary hypertension, cardiac injury, and blood loss, particularly with aspiration systems. No optimal or even adequate device or method currently exists and there is no device specifically having US Food and Drug Administration approval to use for PE.

Pure fragmentation and clot displacement

The simplest and probably most commonly used method to fragment clot in the pulmonary artery is rotation of a catheter within it, usually a pigtail catheter. This is facilitated by advancing the catheter over a wire using a distal side hole for entry. The pigtail of the catheter is now alongside the wire, and rotation of the shaft results in rotation of pigtail in a large arc within the pulmonary artery (**Fig. 3**). Other described methods are use of a balloon and wire to macerate thrombus. Two specific fragmentation devices are the Helix Clot Buster (Ev3 Covidien, Plymouth, Minnesota), a rotational mechanical thrombectomy device with an impeller powered by compressed air or nitrogen that is no longer available in the United States, and the Cleaner Rotational Thrombectomy System (Argon Medical Devices, Frisco, Texas), a sinusoidal-shaped motorized wire housed in a 6-French or 7-French catheter approved for mechanical declotting and controlled and selective infusion of physician specified fluids, including thrombolytics, in the peripheral vasculature and arteriovenous dialysis fistulae/grafts (see **Fig. 3**).

Simple displacement of clot against the vessel wall may be accomplished by balloon dilatation or stenting. This is less effective for fresh thrombus that can more readily recoil or prolapse back into the lumen than for older organized thrombus. These methods rely on a patent distal vessel and are reserved for situations not responsive to other treatments.

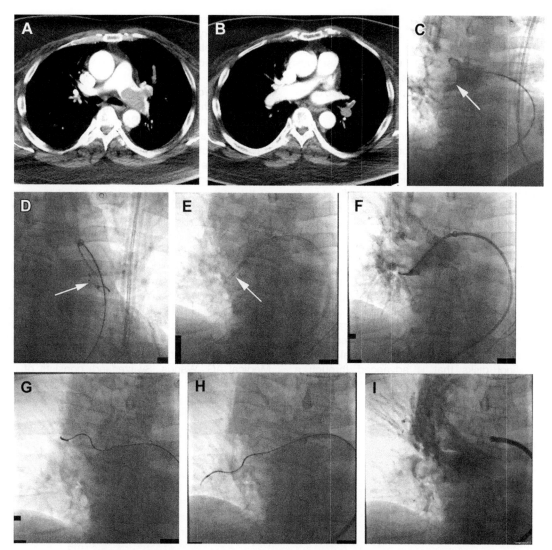

Fig. 3. A 60-year-old man with past repeated venous thromboembolic disease who developed massive PE 5 days after resection of a meningioma when anticoagulation was temporarily held for a fall, with persistent hypotension and hypoxemia into the 40s despite intravenous TPA. (*A, B*) Chest CTA 5 days before the current event in which a large near-occlusive left main PE was present but the right pulmonary artery was patent. Segmental emboli were present in the right lung on other images. Pulmonary angiography now showed a near-occlusive right main pulmonary artery embolism (*arrow* [*C*]). A rotating pigtail catheter was employed for fragmentation, as depicted in the left pulmonary artery (*arrow* [*D*]) and a large caliber guide catheter for suction, as depicted in the right pulmonary artery (*arrow* [*E*]) but with no improvement (*F*). The Cleaner Rotational Thrombectomy System was then used in the right main, upper, interlobar, and middle lobe pulmonary arteries (*G, H*) with moderate angiographic improvement (*I*), consisting of better flow into the right upper and middle lobes. Dramatic clinical improvement occurred over the next 30 minutes, with normalization of hemodynamics and oxygenation.

Pure aspiration-removal

Large-caliber guide catheters and sheaths may be introduced into the pulmonary arteries to permit manual suction of embolic material (see **Fig. 3**E). Specialty catheters, such as the Pronto thrombectomy catheter (Vascular Solutions, Minneapolis, Minnesota) have also been designed for manual aspiration. The sizes of these catheters remain a limitation compared with the large size and volume of the clot present in patients with major PE. Alternatively, several devices providing mechanical aspiration have been devised.

The AngioVac Venous Drainage System (AngioDynamics, Latham, New York) consists of a 22-French coil-reinforced cannula with a balloon-expandable funnel-shaped tip through which blood, including clot, is suctioned into an extracorporeal circuit using a pump, passes through a filter to trap the clot, and then returned through a large reinfusion cannula. This requires a perfusionist. Use of this device in the pulmonary arteries has had limited technical success and serious complications attributed to its size and lack of flexibility and steerability, with reports of cardiac damage with perforation and clot fragmentation with embolization.[19,20]

The Indigo Mechanical Thrombectomy System (Penumbra, Alameda, California) consists of an 8-French aspiration catheter that connects to a suction pump through aspiration tubing and a separator wire with an expanded distal end to help macerate clot and facilitate more easy passage through the catheter. The system is approved for removal of thrombus in the peripheral arterial and venous systems. Preliminary experience in a limited number of patients having submassive or massive PE has been favorable, with stabilization of hemodynamics and survival to discharge in 83% (**Fig. 4**).[21]

The FlowTriever System (Inari Medical, Irvine, California) is an investigational device consisting of a flow restoration catheter with 3 distal expanding nitinol disks that is advanced through a 20-French aspiration guide catheter within the pulmonary artery. Manual aspiration and withdrawal of the disks through the guide catheter results in partial thrombus removal.[22]

Fragmentation-aspiration

Rheolytic thrombectomy AngioJet Peripheral Thrombectomy System (Boston Scientific, Marlborough, Massachusetts) relies on a saline jet traveling backward across openings in the distal aspect of the catheter to create a lower pressure zone causing a vacuum effect, with maceration of the clot and at least partial removal through the return lumen. A modification to powerfully inject pulses of a thrombolytic agent directly into the clot (power-pulse) can enhance its effectiveness; this is a form of pharmacomechanical thrombolysis. Concern exists over the use of this in the pulmonary arterial system given reports of bradycardia, heart block, hemoglobinuria, renal insufficiency, hemoptysis, and death, although technical modifications may reduce these risks.[23,24]

The Aspirex thrombectomy catheter (Straub Medical AG, Wangs, Switzerland) consists of a

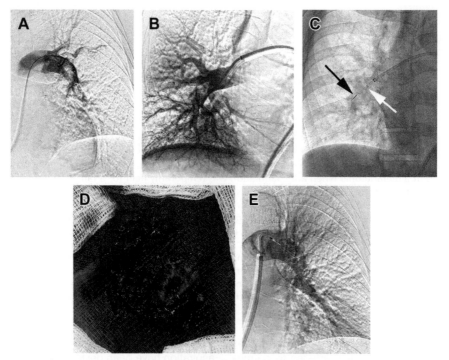

Fig. 4. A 60-year-old man who developed acute hypoxemia and transient hypotension 3 weeks to 4 weeks after resection of a brain tumor who had submassive PE, with evidence of right ventricular strain based on imaging and biomarkers. He was approved for anticoagulation but not thrombolytic therapy. Pulmonary angiography showed extensive bilateral PE (A, B). The 8-French Penumbra Indigo catheter was used for suction embolectomy bilaterally, showing the catheter (*white arrow*) and the separator (*black arrow*) in the right pulmonary artery (C). A moderate amount of clot was retrieved (D) and angiography showed reduction in the filling defects and improved flow, as shown on a postinterventional angiogram of the left side (E).

rapidly rotating spiral inside a catheter generating negative pressure to draw in clot through a side window and macerate and aspirate it.[25] This system is not available in the United States.

Combinations of Catheter-Directed Therapies

Catheter-based treatments can be combined together or occasionally with systemic thrombolysis to achieve better results. For massive PE, Kuo and colleagues[24] looked at 35 uncontrolled trials from 1990 to 2008 in which 594 patients were treated with CDT in whom the vast majority had insufficient time or a contraindication to full-dose systemic thrombolysis, whereas the 4% who had prior systemic thrombolysis had persistent hemodynamic abnormalities. Mechanical methods alone were used in one-third and mechanical combined with local thrombolysis in the remainder. A majority of mechanical methods involved rotation of a pigtail catheter either as the sole method or in combination with another technique, whereas the remainder was a variety of other methods. Clinical success, as defined by stability of hemodynamics, resolution of hypoxia, and survival, was achieved in 86.5%, and it was higher in studies in which at least 80% of patients also received local thrombolysis, particularly for an extended time. Major complications occurred in 2.4%, most commonly groin hematomas or other hemorrhage requiring transfusion, and minor complications in 7.9%, most commonly hemorrhage not requiring transfusion. Patients exposed to the AngioJet device had the highest complication rates, 28% major and 27% minor. For submassive PE, a meta-analysis by Lou and colleagues[9] looked at 422 patients in which the vast majority had CDT (ultrasound-assisted twice as common as simple catheter infusion) infrequently in conjunction with mechanical methods and 26 were treated with mechanical methods alone. They concluded that these techniques provided therapeutic efficacy based on a decrease in pulmonary artery pressure and right-to-left ventricular ratio with a low rate of adverse events. In-hospital and 30-day mortalities were 1.29% and 1.6%, respectively; major hemorrhage 2.1% with intracranial hemorrhage 0.45%; and recurrent PE in only 0.79%. The PERFECT (Pulmonary embolism response to fragmentation, embolectomy, and catheter thrombolysis) registry looked at CDT in 101 patients in whom 28 had massive PE and were treated with mechanical or pharmacomechanical methods (fragmentation, intraclot fibrinolytic injection, and/or aspiration embolectomy), with possibly subsequent direct thrombolysis, and 73 had submassive PE, who were all treated

with catheter-directed thrombolysis using either standard or ultrasound-assisted infusions of TPA or urokinase.[8] Clinical success was achieved in 86% of patients with massive PE and 97% of those with submassive PE, as defined by stabilization of hemodynamics, improvement in right ventricular strain and/or pulmonary hypertension (seen in at least 85%), and survival to hospital discharge—4 patients with massive PE and 2 with submassive PE died. Average drug doses were 28 mg for TPA and 2.7 million units for urokinase, and no major bleeding occurred, including none intracranially. Self-limited minor bleeding occurred in 13%, not requiring transfusion.

SUMMARY

Transcatheter treatment of major acute PE is an evolving field. Current evidence indicates that catheter-directed thrombolysis improves cardiovascular status (pulmonary artery pressure, right ventricular strain, and systemic hemodynamics) at least similar to systemic thrombolysis and with correspondingly similar improvements in mortality and variably lower mortality. A major advantage over systemic thrombolysis is that catheter-directed thrombolysis using lower doses locally administered into the clot seems to result in a lower rate of major bleeding. This may favor more liberal use in those with submassive PE, a group in which therapy beyond just anticoagulation is more controversial, especially if they seem at higher risk for deterioration. Although catheter-directed mechanical methods may permit more rapid clot reduction or redistribution and so faster hemodynamic improvement in more unstable patients and those at higher risk for any form of thrombolysis, the methods and devices available remain suboptimal considering the large volume of clot typically present in an extensive vascular bed. The major role for such techniques is currently for massive PE and the best results are generally seen when combined with pharmacologic thrombolysis.

More work is needed to identify those patients who would benefit acutely from transcatheter therapies, what the best therapy is for any particular patient, and whether long-term advantages may exist.

REFERENCES

1. Konstantinides SV, Torbicki A, Agnelli G, et al. 2014 ESC guidelines on the diagnosis and management of acute pulmonary embolism. Eur Heart J 2014; 35(43):3033–69, 3069a–k.
2. Park B, Messina L, Dargon P, et al. Recent trends in clinical outcomes and resource utilization for

pulmonary embolism in the United States: findings from the nationwide inpatient sample. Chest 2009; 136(4):983–90.

3. Kahn SR, Houweling AH, Granton J, et al. Long-term outcomes after pulmonary embolism: current knowledge and future research. Blood Coagul Fibrinolysis 2014;25(5):407–15.

4. Chatterjee S, Chakraborty A, Weinberg I, et al. Thrombolysis for pulmonary embolism and risk of all-cause mortality, major bleeding, and intracranial hemorrhage: a meta-analysis. JAMA 2014;311(23):2414–21.

5. Meyer G, Vicaut E, Danays T, et al. Fibrinolysis for patients with intermediate-risk pulmonary embolism. N Engl J Med 2014;370(15):1402–11.

6. Virk HUH, Chatterjee S, Sardar P, et al. Systemic thrombolysis for pulmonary embolism: evidence, patient selection, and protocols for management. Interv Cardiol Clin 2018;7(1):71–80.

7. Kearon C, Akl EA, Ornelas J, et al. Antithrombotic therapy for VTE disease: CHEST guideline and expert panel report. Chest 2016;149(2):315–52.

8. Kuo WT, Banerjee A, Kim PS, et al. Pulmonary embolism response to fragmentation, embolectomy, and catheter thrombolysis (PERFECT): initial results from a prospective multicenter registry. Chest 2015;148(3):667–73.

9. Lou BH, Wang LH, Chen Y. A meta-analysis of efficacy and safety of catheter-directed interventions in submassive pulmonary embolism. Eur Rev Med Pharmacol Sci 2017;21(1):184–98.

10. Schmitz-Rode T, Kilbinger M, Gunther RW. Simulated flow pattern in massive pulmonary embolism: significance for selective intrapulmonary thrombolysis. Cardiovasc Intervent Radiol 1998;21(3):199–204.

11. Kucher N, Boekstegers P, Muller OJ, et al. Randomized, controlled trial of ultrasound-assisted catheter-directed thrombolysis for acute intermediate-risk pulmonary embolism. Circulation 2014;129(4):479–86.

12. Piazza G, Hohlfelder B, Jaff MR, et al. A prospective, single-arm, multicenter trial of ultrasound-facilitated, catheter-directed, low-dose fibrinolysis for acute massive and submassive pulmonary embolism: the SEATTLE II study. JACC Cardiovasc Interv 2015; 8(10):1382–92.

13. Tapson VF, Piazza G, Goldhaber SZ, et al. Optimum duration and dose of R-TPA with the acoustic pulse thrombolysis procedure for intermediate-risk (submassive) pulmonary embolism: optalyse PE. Am J Respir Crit Care Med 2017;195:A2835.

14. Graif A, Grilli CJ, Kimbiris G, et al. Comparison of ultrasound-accelerated versus pigtail catheter-directed thrombolysis for the treatment of acute massive and submassive pulmonary embolism. J Vasc Interv Radiol 2017;28(10):1339–47.

15. Bloomer TL, El-Hayek GE, McDaniel MC, et al. Safety of catheter-directed thrombolysis for massive and submassive pulmonary embolism: results of a multicenter registry and meta-analysis. Catheter Cardiovasc Interv 2017;89(4):754–60.

16. Kaymaz C, Akbal OY, Tanboga IH, et al. Ultrasound-assisted catheter-directed thrombolysis in high-risk and intermediate-high-risk pulmonary embolism: a meta-analysis. Curr Vasc Pharmacol 2017;16(2): 179–89.

17. Arora S, Panaich SS, Ainani N, et al. Comparison of in-hospital outcomes and readmission rates in acute pulmonary embolism between systemic and catheter-directed thrombolysis (from the national readmission database). Am J Cardiol 2017;120(9): 1653–61.

18. Liang NL, Avgerinos ED, Singh MJ, et al. Systemic thrombolysis increases hemorrhagic stroke risk without survival benefit compared with catheter-directed intervention for the treatment of acute pulmonary embolism. J Vasc Surg Venous Lymphat Disord 2017;5(2):171–6.e1.

19. Al-Hakim R, Park J, Bansal A, et al. Early experience with angiovac aspiration in the pulmonary arteries. J Vasc Interv Radiol 2016;27(5):730–4.

20. Del Rosario T, Basta M, Agarwal S. Angiovac suction thrombectomy complicated by thrombus fragmentation and distal embolization leading to hemodynamic collapse: a case report. A A case Rep 2017;8(8):206–9.

21. Ciampi-Dopazo JJ, Romeu-Prieto JM, Sanchez-Casado M, et al. Aspiration thrombectomy for treatment of acute massive and submassive pulmonary embolism: initial single-center prospective experience. J Vasc Interv Radiol 2018;29(1):101–6.

22. Tukaye DN, McDaniel M, Liberman H, et al. Percutaneous pulmonary embolus mechanical thrombectomy. JACC Cardiovasc Interv 2017; 10(1):94–5.

23. Das S, Das N, Serota H, et al. A retrospective review of patients with massive and submassive pulmonary embolism treated with AngioJet rheolytic thrombectomy with decreased complications due to changes in thrombolytic use and procedural modifications. Vascular 2018;26(2):163–8.

24. Kuo WT, Gould MK, Louie JD, et al. Catheter-directed therapy for the treatment of massive pulmonary embolism: systematic review and meta-analysis of modern techniques. J Vasc Interv Radiol 2009;20(11):1431–40.

25. Bayiz H, Dumantepe M, Teymen B, et al. Percutaneous aspiration thrombectomy in treatment of massive pulmonary embolism. Heart Lung Circ 2015;24(1):46–54.

Surgical Management of Acute and Chronic Pulmonary Embolism

Barbara L. LeVarge, MD[a],*, Cameron D. Wright, MD[b],
Josanna M. Rodriguez-Lopez, MD[c]

KEYWORDS

- Pulmonary embolism • Chronic thromboembolic pulmonary hypertension
- Surgical pulmonary embolectomy • Pulmonary thromboendarterectomy

KEY POINTS

- Patients with proximal pulmonary embolism (PE) who are at increased risk for mortality are potential candidates for surgical pulmonary embolectomy (SPE), a procedure now seeing renewed interest as an option for PE management.
- Outcomes of SPE vary greatly depending on the studied population; survival has improved over time and currently rivals that of systemic thrombolysis based on observational data.
- For patients with chronic PE and associated pulmonary hypertension, pulmonary thromboendarterectomy (PTE) has benefitted from much evolution over the past several decades and is now associated with low morbidity and mortality in experienced centers.
- PTE remains a highly technical surgery requiring multidisciplinary input and planning; with advancements in technique, marked improvements in hemodynamics can be achieved in a greater number of patients.

INTRODUCTION

Acute pulmonary embolism (PE) is a common clinical condition that results in at least 100,000 deaths yearly in the United States.[1] Acute PE is described as high risk (massive) when otherwise unexplained hypotension is present; these patients have particularly high mortality risk from right ventricular (RV) failure and cardiovascular collapse. Those without hemodynamic instability are labeled as having intermediate-risk (submassive) PE if there is evidence of RV strain or dysfunction. Patients without these features have low-risk PE and are typically managed with anticoagulation alone with good outcomes.

Patients with high-risk and intermediate-risk PE may be considered for interventions beyond anticoagulation in efforts to decrease short-term mortality risk. This is particularly true of high-risk PE, because associated mortality can be greater than 50%.[2] Available management options vary by center but include systemic thrombolysis, catheter-based thrombolysis or embolectomy, extracorporeal membrane oxygenation (ECMO) support, and surgical embolectomy. In past years, surgical treatment has been reserved for very ill

Disclosure Statement: The authors attest that they have no relationships to disclose.
[a] Division of Pulmonary Diseases and Critical Care Medicine, Department of Medicine, University of North Carolina, 130 Mason Farm Road CB 7020, Chapel Hill, NC 27599, USA; [b] Division of Thoracic Surgery, Department of Surgery, Massachusetts General Hospital, 55 Fruit Street, Boston, MA 02114, USA; [c] Division of Pulmonary and Critical Care Medicine, Department of Medicine, Massachusetts General Hospital, 55 Fruit Street, Boston, MA 02114, USA
* Corresponding author.
E-mail address: barbara_levarge@med.unc.edu

Clin Chest Med 39 (2018) 659–667
https://doi.org/10.1016/j.ccm.2018.04.017
0272-5231/18/© 2018 Elsevier Inc. All rights reserved.

patients, usually with either contraindication to or failure of systemic thrombolysis.

After an episode of acute PE, endogenous thrombolysis progressively reduces the embolic burden, with minimal residual thrombus expected in most patients. In some individuals, however, these mechanisms fail and chronic PE develops. After an episode of acute PE, 1% to 4% of patients further develop chronic thromboembolic pulmonary hypertension (CTEPH) from these vascular obstructions with associated impact on RV function.[3,4] When this occurs, time and anticoagulation are insufficient to normalize the vasculature. These patients, however, are candidates for meticulous surgical removal of the obstructive material with endarterectomy.

Surgery can be highly effective in management of appropriate patients with acute and chronic PE. Despite similarity in name, surgical pulmonary embolectomy (SPE) and pulmonary thromboendarterectomy (PTE) are different procedures. Both typically require sternotomy and cardiopulmonary bypass, but removal of the luminal thrombotic material is more straightforward in SPE. PTE requires careful dissection of affected arteries with removal of vascular intima along with thrombus. PTE remains the gold standard for management of CTEPH, although other medical and interventional approaches are also gaining popularity. In contrast, SPE had long been regarded as salvage therapy for acute PE but now sees increasing interest in evolving the technique and indications. This review focuses on the role of SPE and PTE in the management of patients with acute and chronic PE.

SURGICAL PULMONARY EMBOLECTOMY FOR ACUTE PULMONARY EMBOLISM
History

A surgical approach to acute PE was first developed by Friedrich Trendelenburg in the early 1900s. In 1908 he presented his technique at the annual Congress of the German Surgical Association, reporting on the first unsuccessful use of SPE. The Trendelenburg SPE involved exposure of the pulmonary artery (PA) and aorta via 2 perpendicular incisions over the left sternal border and second rib followed by encircling the vessels with rubber tubing. Tension was placed on the tubing to occlude both vessels, and the PA was rapidly incised with subsequent clot extraction using blunt tipped forceps. The arteriotomy incision was then held together with forceps and a clamp while flow through the great vessels was restored; the incision was then sutured. Arteriotomy and embolectomy were completed in less than 1 minute.[5]

Trendelenburg's 3 reported SPE procedures in humans resulted in removal of thrombus, but death occurred in the operative or early postoperative period. In 1924, Trendelenburg's trainee, Martin Kirschner, performed SPE on a 38-year-old woman who had sudden collapse after hernia surgery. Large thrombi were removed, and the patient fully recovered, marking the first truly successful procedure of its kind.[5]

The development of cardiopulmonary bypass (CPB) was a major advance to successful SPE, although ability to mobilize CPB urgently took some time. SPE on bypass was first achieved by Sharp in 1961[6]; subsequently, performance of SPE significantly increased.[7–9]

Indications for Surgery

Patients with confirmed, life-threatening acute PE affecting the central vasculature are potential candidates for SPE. In these patients with high-risk or intermediate-risk PE, mortality risk with anticoagulation alone is often unacceptably high. SPE should be strongly considered in such patients with contraindication to thrombolysis (although importantly they must be able to tolerate heparinization for CPB), which is supported by clinical practice guidelines from the American College of Chest Physicians,[10] American Heart Association,[11] and European Society of Cardiology.[12] SPE should also be considered in those deemed to have insufficient time to allow thrombolysis to become effective and in those with thrombus within the right heart or in a patent foramen ovale.[10,11] Treatment failure of systemic thrombolysis is by no means a contraindication to SPE (and is often still an indication for pursuing surgery), although higher surgical site bleeding risk would be expected.[11,12] Meneveau and colleagues[13] demonstrated that surgical embolectomy after failure of thrombolysis yields better outcomes than repeating thrombolytic administration.

Although historically SPE has been used for the critically ill patient with no alternative options, this paradigm may be changing. In a single-center series of 115 patients receiving SPE, 49 patients (43%) had high-risk PE, 56 (49%) had intermediate-risk PE, and 10 patients had other indications for surgery (most commonly right atrial or ventricular mass). Of those with high-risk or intermediate-risk PE, 47% had contraindication to thrombolysis and 6% had failed thrombolysis or catheter-based interventions. The remaining 50 patients underwent SPE due to presence of significant RV dysfunction with central clot, without specific contraindications or preceding trials of other therapies.[14] In another single-center series, the classic indications for SPE, presence of intra-cardiac thrombus and contraindication to thrombolysis, were present in only 6 of 15 patients, with a majority of patients undergoing SPE in the setting of central thrombus with RV dysfunction.[15]

Surgical Technique

Today's SPE remains a straightforward procedure. After induction of general anesthesia, median sternotomy is performed with entry of the pericardium. Bicaval and ascending aortic cannulation are established and CPB initiated. If additional cardiac procedures (eg, extraction of intracardiac thrombus) are needed, cardioplegic arrest and aortic cross-clamping may be required; use of these practices for routine SPE is discouraged in some guidelines.[12] Intraoperative transesophageal echocardiography can assess for right atrial or ventricular thrombus at the time of surgery. Once CPB is established, a longitudinal incision is made in the main PA with extension to the proximal left PA. Clot is extracted using suction catheters, forceps, and/or Fogarty balloon catheters (**Fig. 1**A). A right PA incision also can be made for additional clot removal. The distal arteries may be further explored with videoscope assistance.[16] When sufficient thrombus has been removed, the arteriotomy is closed and CPB weaned. An inferior vena cava filter is often placed, although this is not based on current evidence or guidelines.[12,17]

Additional, more peripheral thrombi can be removed with bilateral thoracotomy and gentle manual compression of each lung to mobilize clot proximally, although this practice may increase bleeding complications.[18] Retrograde perfusion has also been used during surgery for a similar purpose and is effective in removing more thrombotic material.[19] In this approach, after conventional antegrade removal of thrombus, the pulmonary veins are exposed and cannulated with proximal clamping of the left atrium or alternatively accessed after creation of atrial septal defect.[19,20] Blood is infused, allowing retrograde flushing of thrombotic material into the more proximal pulmonary arteries.[19,21]

Outcomes of few cases of off-pump unilateral or bilateral embolectomy have been reported. Unilateral pulmonary arteriotomy is performed after proximal right or left PA clamping; the procedure is then repeated on the contralateral side, if needed.[22,23] A great majority of SPEs use CPB and this remains the appropriate surgical approach for most patients.[24]

Hemorrhage, hypoxemia, and residual RV failure may require additional management after SPE. Pulmonary hemorrhage, at times massive, with resulting severe hypoxemia may occur due to vascular injury from forceps or catheters or due to ischemia and reperfusion injury.[25] Management of hemorrhage is challenging given benefits of anticoagulation in these patients. Persistent cardiogenic shock from inadequate RV recovery can often be managed with inotropy or may require prolonged extracorporeal support.

Perioperative Extracorporeal Support

Given the clinical fragility of patients with high-risk PE, a role for rapid initiation of ECMO has emerged. With venoarterial (VA) ECMO, patients are provided oxygenation, carbon dioxide removal, and mechanical support, the last particularly critical in these patients with RV failure and shock. A venous cannula drains the right atrium or inferior vena cava, and oxygenated blood is returned to the descending aorta via a femoral

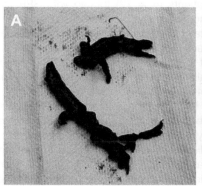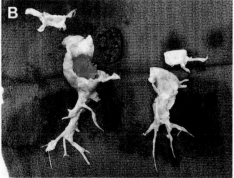

Fig. 1. (*A*) SPE specimen. Dark red clot is consistent with acute PE. (*B*) PTE specimen. White, fibrotic chronic embolic material is adherent to the vessel wall. The red proximal thrombus is subacute and the dark material is consistent with newer clot. As opposed to SPE, a PTE specimen must be dissected out to the distal segments and subsegments in order for the surgery to be successful and the pulmonary vascular resistance to normalize.

artery (or alternative cannulation site) after passing through the ECMO circuit. Anticoagulation is necessary to prevent clotting. Evidence for use of VA ECMO in PE is currently limited to case series and 1 systematic review.[26,27]

For critically ill PE patients, VA ECMO can be mobilized to provide life-sustaining support with a speed that cannot be matched by CPB and surgical embolectomy. VA ECMO, however, is a supportive tool that does little to address the underlying embolic burden. Thus, it is becomingly increasingly common to use ECMO as a stabilization strategy prior to definitive treatment with SPE.[26,28] ECMO has also been used as short-term mechanical support following SPE for those unable to wean from CPB.[29]

Outcomes

Mortality with early cases of SPE was high, likely related to imperfect surgical technique and periprocedural PE management, although patient selection was also a key factor. Kalra and colleagues[24] recently published a systematic review and meta-analysis of 1590 SPE procedures, finding overall in-hospital mortality of 26.3%. When studies were stratified by publication year, there were significantly worse outcomes in those published prior to 2000 compared with after. Recently, centers with high levels of surgical experience have found even lower mortality rates. Hartman and colleagues[30] reported on the outcomes of 96 SPE procedures at 3 tertiary care centers in New York City between 2003 and 2011, finding an overall 30-day mortality of 4.2%. Higher case volume was also associated with improved mortality in the meta-analysis.[24]

In patients with acute PE, outcomes from SPE are heavily influenced by the severity of illness leading up to surgery. Several studies have supported higher postoperative mortality rates in those with preoperative cardiac arrest. Stein and colleagues found a 3-fold increase in mortality among patients undergoing SPE when there was preoperative cardiac arrest.[31] A more recent analysis of 214 SPE procedures also demonstrated greater in-hospital mortality in the 13% of patients receiving preoperative cardiopulmonary resuscitation (32.0% vs 8.6%). This study also supported higher mortality amongst the group with high-risk PE versus intermediate-risk PE.[32]

In patients without contraindication, systemic thrombolysis is considered first-line therapy for high-risk PE and a treatment option for patients with intermediate-risk PE.[17] Lytic therapy, however, has been associated with an important risk of major bleeding, with intracranial hemorrhage of greatest concern.[17,33] There are no randomized clinical trials comparing thrombolysis to SPE for either high-risk PE or intermediate-risk PE, although observational data suggest SPE could be a worthy alternative. Lee and colleagues[34] analyzed data from New York State involving PE patients undergoing thrombolysis (n = 1854) or SPE (n = 257) and found no difference in survival at 30 days and at 5 years. Those receiving SPE had lower risks of stroke and need for reintervention but increased risk of major bleeding. Aymard and colleagues[35] compared the outcomes of 52 patients undergoing thrombolysis and 28 patients undergoing SPE; there was no difference in early mortality nor in mortality at mean follow-up of 63 months. Patients treated with SPE had less bleeding complications, although there was nonsignificant trend toward longer hospital stay. No differences in follow-up functional status or quality of life were detected. Azari and colleagues[36] compared the outcomes of 78 patients undergoing thrombolysis and 30 patients undergoing SPE in a similar study. Surgically managed patients showed nonsignificant trend toward improved mortality, and significant differences in RV dilation and functional class at 1 year were seen in favor of SPE. In a separate retrospective study, including 64 high-risk PE patients, those undergoing SPE had lower prevalence of abnormal perfusion scan and diffusion impairment at follow-up.[37]

With recognition of improving short-term and long-term outcomes of SPE, there has been increasing interest in this treatment strategy for hemodynamically stable but high-risk patients, particularly early in their clinical course. Of 56 hemodynamically stable patients undergoing SPE, Neely and colleagues[14] found operative mortality of 3.6%. In the analysis by Hartman and colleagues,[30] the subset of hemodynamically stable patients (n = 72) treated with SPE had 30-day mortality of 1.4% and mean postoperative hospital stay of 9.1 days. Proceeding to SPE early in a patient's PE course was emphasized in a small study of 15 patients, finding significantly increased mortality when surgery was delayed by more than 24 hours.[38]

Non–mortality-related safety outcomes have been less robustly described. The meta-analysis by Kalra and colleagues[24] found surgical site complications in 7%, pulmonary bleeding in 4%, gastrointestinal bleeding in 3%, and other bleeding complications in 10.6%. Of the 214 patients undergoing SPE in the observational study by Keeling and colleagues,[32] blood transfusion was required in 43.5%, and 8.4% required surgical re-exploration for bleeding. Stroke occurred in

4.7% of patients, and renal failure in 11.2%. In the other large (n = 257) multicenter series of SPE, blood transfusion occurred in 19.8% of patients, and 9% of patients were classified as having major bleeding. Stroke occurred in less than 1%, which was significantly less than in the comparison group receiving thrombolysis.[34]

One controversial area within PE management has been whether any of the more advanced interventions (systemic thrombolysis, SPE, or catheter-based therapies) can have an impact on the natural history of PE resolution. Prevention of future CTEPH is the goal, although it remains unclear if this is achievable. Recent follow-up data from the Pulmonary Embolism Thrombolysis study, the randomized clinical trial investigating the benefits of systemic thrombolysis in intermediate-risk PE, failed to show any differences in incidence of CTEPH, echocardiogram findings, or functional status between groups at long-term follow-up.[39] At this time it is unknown if similar outcomes will be expected with SPE.

PULMONARY THROMBOENDARTERECTOMY FOR CHRONIC PULMONARY EMBOLISM
Presurgical Evaluation

A diagnosis of CTEPH requires imaging to confirm and characterize the extent and location of thromboembolic disease. Due to high sensitivity, the ventilation-perfusion scan is the screening test of choice. Other conditions, however, can mimic CTEPH by perfusion scan, and thus additional evaluation is needed. Evolution in CT and magnetic resonance techniques have been promising and enhanced the role of these types of imaging in PTE evaluation. Most centers still rely, however, on standard catheter-based pulmonary angiography, at the time of hemodynamic assessment with right heart catheterization, to complete the presurgical evaluation.

Indications for Surgery

Evaluation for operability should be performed by a multidisciplinary team, including radiologists, cardiologists, pulmonologists, intensivists, anesthesiologists, and experienced surgeons.[40] The decision to operate depends on surgical accessibility of the obstructions, hemodynamics, and the severity of comorbidities. Currently there is no accepted algorithm to guide operability; this decision is based on center and surgical expertise. The international CTEPH registry found a large variation between countries and centers regarding the number of patients deemed operable. Low-volume centers reported 47% of patients evaluated as inoperable, whereas centers performing

greater than 50 PTEs a year found only 34% of patients inoperable.[41] Therefore, more experienced centers may operate on cases others would deem inoperable.

Asymptomatic patients found to have chronic PE but without significant PH generally do not require surgery but should be followed closely. Patients who are symptomatic, have significant PH, and have proximal or segmental obstructive disease without significant comorbidities should be considered surgical candidates. In most cases, if the disease is obstructing the main, lobar, or proximal segmental pulmonary arteries, PTE is feasible and likely successful. If the disease is limited to distal segmental and subsegmental branches, PTE is technically more challenging. Patients with distal disease and severe preoperative PH with RV dysfunction re the most difficult surgical cases. In some centers, this type of distal disease is considered inoperable and a second surgical opinion can be considered.[42]

Surgical Technique

PTE requires an experienced cardiothoracic surgical team and sophisticated postoperative care. An acute embolectomy alone, without a subsequent endarterectomy, is ineffective. The endarterectomy must be bilateral and complete. Techniques of this surgical procedure are well established and previously described.[43] To approach both pulmonary arteries, median sternotomy is performed and the pericardium is opened longitudinally. The superior vena cava, ascending aorta, and right and left pulmonary arteries are mobilized from under their pericardial reflections. Adequate visualization is accomplished using CPB and periods of circulatory arrest. This allows for a bloodless field by diverting pulmonary arterial blood flow and also reducing collateral flow. Periods of circulatory arrest, with cooling to 18°C to 20°C, are limited to 20 minutes at a time. Usually one 20-minute period on each side is enough for the dissection to be completed.

After CPB is instituted, small openings are made in the PA and left atrium to serve as vents. When the desired core temperature has been reached, the aorta is cross-clamped and cardioplegia is administered. The superior vena cava and aorta are retracted apart to expose the right PA. A longitudinal incision is made in the anterior wall and a suction catheter is placed distally to collect back bleeding from bronchial circulation and improve exposure of the interior of the PA. Good visibility is essential to initiate a correct endarterectomy plane. The plane should appear smooth and pearly white and lies between the intima and the media.

Although the endarterectomy specimen may be very thin at the initiation, it becomes thicker as more thrombotic material is approached distally. The specimen is dissected circumferentially and followed distally as far as possible. Each subsegmental branch is followed individually until it ends in a tail, which breaks off, beyond which an unobstructed area becomes visible (see **Fig. 1**B). Removal of all distal tails results in improved outcomes. Once the right side is completed, hypothermic reperfusion is reinstituted and the pulmonary arteriotomy is closed.

To provide better access to the left PA, the heart is retracted upwards and toward the right. A left pulmonary arteriotomy is made lateral to the pulmonary vent site, with caution not to injure the left phrenic nerve. Cardioplegia is renewed and the circulation is again arrested. The endarterectomy plane is initiated and the specimen followed into each segmental and subsegmental branch to ensure complete removal of thrombotic material. On completion of both sides, circulation is reinstituted and full rewarming is begun. If other cardiac procedures (closure of patent foramen ovale, coronary bypass, or valve repair) are needed, these are performed during the rewarming period. Pacing wires are placed, the right heart is deaired, the vents sites are repaired, and the aortic cross-clamp is released. When the patient is rewarmed, CPB is weaned and the patient is decannulated in the routine fashion.

A new surgical classification system describes 4 levels of disease based on the surgical specimen obtained. Level 0 describes having no evidence of CTEPH. In level I disease, obstructive material involves the main pulmonary arteries. When there is complete obstruction of a main PA, it is classified as IC. Level II disease denotes no disease in the main PA, with start of thrombotic material in lobar branches or after the takeoff of the upper lobe artery. In level III, the disease starts at the segmental branches; thrombotic material may not be obvious with the initial dissection. In level IV disease, obstructive material starts at the subsegmental level. Over the past several years, refinement of surgical instruments has allowed for successful resection of more distal disease, although level IV disease should only be operated on by experienced surgeons.[44]

Postoperative Care

Anticoagulation should be started as soon as feasible from a postsurgical hemostasis standpoint, usually the first night after surgery. Patients remain on anticoagulation for life.

Patients undergoing PTE suffer from postoperative complications similar to those of other cardiothoracic surgeries. Atrial fibrillation or flutter, pericarditis, atelectasis, and diaphragmatic dysfunction are managed as usual in an intensive care setting. Complications specific to PTE are reperfusion pulmonary edema and persistent pulmonary hypertension (PH). Reperfusion edema occurs in up to 40% of patients, of variable severity.[45] After PTE, areas of vasculature that were previously obstructed have a lower resistance than previously nonobstructed areas. A relative increase in blood flow to the newly endarterectomized lung creates hypoxemia from ventilation-perfusion mismatch; this can be exaggerated by postoperative atelectasis of the lower lobes, where most of the disease and reperfusion injury is. Severe reperfusion edema is associated with longer duration of mechanical ventilation and ICU stay.[46] Hypoxemia can last days to weeks and the treatment is primarily supportive. Reperfusion edema can be asymmetric and lateral decubitus positioning may improve oxygenation. Diuresis is used to reduce lung water and high flow oxygen can be used for earlier extubation. A small, randomized single-center trial found that a low tidal ventilation strategy does not reduce the incidence of reperfusion lung injury nor improve clinical outcomes.[45] In severe cases, venovenous ECMO can provide support for refractory hypoxemia as a bridge to recovery.[47]

Approximately 11% to 35% of patients have residual thromboembolic PH after PTE; this is a predictor of postoperative mortality.[42,48] Irreversible PH is usually a sign of nonthrombotic small vessel vasculopathy or very distal thromboembolic disease that was not cured by the endarterectomy. Treatment of PH and RV dysfunction can be difficult in the immediate postoperative period. Inotropic support can support RV function, and vasopressors should be used to avoid hypotension and resulting RV ischemia. Pulmonary vasodilators may be associated with systemic hypotension and should be avoided until the patient is hemodynamically stable. Inhaled nitric oxide or inhaled epoprostenol may reduce pulmonary vascular resistance without an associated reduction in blood pressure.[49] In severe cases of RV failure with inability to wean from CPB, VA ECMO has been used with some success.[50]

Outcomes

After PTE, most patients have improvements in hemodynamics, functional status, and exercise capacity.[51] In-hospital mortality in experienced PTE centers approaches that of other routine cardiac

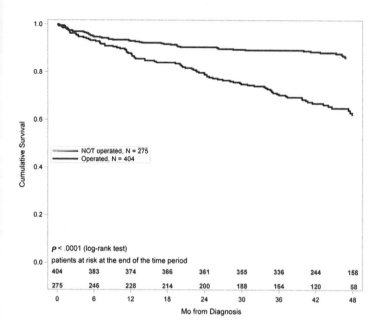

Fig. 2. Estimated survival from the time of diagnosis in operated and nonoperated patients with CTEPH. (*From* Delcroix M, Lang I, Pepke-Zaba J, et al. Long-term outcome of patients with chronic thromboembolic pulmonary hypertension: results from an international prospective registry. Circulation 2016;133(9):865; with permission.)

surgeries. The University of California San Diego group, which has the largest cohort, published their in-hospital mortality at 4.4% in their initial 1500 patients[48] and 2.2% for their most recent 500 patients.[44] Estimated 6-year survival is 75%, with 93% of surviving patients being New York Heart Association functional class I or class II.[52] A large UK cohort of 469 patients found overall survival at 3 years of 76%, with 90% 3-year survival for those who survived the initial 3 months. Almost all patients were functional class I or class II 1 year after surgery.[53] In a large European registry, patients who underwent PTE had an 89% 3-year survival compared with 70% for patients who did not have surgery and were medically managed (**Fig. 2**).[54]

Outcomes of those with residual PH after PTE are also good. Freed and colleagues[55] found residual PH in 31% of patients at 3 months. Residual PH significantly compromised symptom status and functional capacity but did not affect survival at 5 years. Additionally, medical therapies for these patients are evolving. A large randomized clinical trial found that riociguat improved exercise capacity in patients with residual PH after PTE.[56]

SUMMARY

Surgical therapy for PE requires a keen understanding of the acuity of the thrombotic disease. In cases of acute PE, timely SPE can be lifesaving by preventing RV-mediated cardiovascular collapse. SPE is now experiencing a renewed attractiveness for varied populations of intermediate-risk and high-risk PE patients, with greatly improved outcomes. For patients with CTEPH, PTE remains the therapy of choice. In experienced centers and in appropriately selected patients, PTE is safe and associated with good long-term prognosis.

REFERENCES

1. Office of the Surgeon General (US), National Heart, Lung, and Blood Institute (US). The Surgeon General's call to action to prevent deep vein thrombosis and pulmonary embolism. Rockville (MD): Office of the Surgeon General; 2008.
2. Kucher N, Rossi E, De Rosa M, et al. Massive pulmonary embolism. Circulation 2006;113(4): 577–82.
3. Becattini C, Agnelli G, Pesavento R, et al. Incidence of chronic thromboembolic pulmonary hypertension after a first episode of pulmonary embolism. Chest 2006;130(1):172–5.
4. Pengo V, Lensing AW, Prins MH, et al. Incidence of chronic thromboembolic pulmonary hypertension after pulmonary embolism. N Engl J Med 2004; 350(22):2257–64.
5. Meyer JA. Friedrich Trendelenburg and the surgical approach to massive pulmonary embolism. Arch Surg 1990;125(9):1202–5.
6. Sharp EH. Pulmonary embolectomy: successful removal of a massive pulmonary embolus with the support of cardiopulmonary bypass. Case report. Ann Surg 1962;156:1–4.
7. Cooley DA, Beall AC Jr. A technic of pulmonary embolectomy using temporary cardio-pulmonary

bypass. Clinical and experimental considerations. J Cardiovasc Surg (Torino) 1961;2:469–76.

8. Couves CM, Sproule BJ, Fraser RS. Acute pulmonary embolism: successful embolectomy using cardiopulmonary bypass. Can Med Assoc J 1962;86:1056–60.

9. Beall AC Jr, Cooley DA, Debakey ME. Surgical management of pulmonary embolism: experimental and clinical considerations. Dis Chest 1965;47:382–91.

10. Guyatt GH, Akl EA, Crowther M, et al. Executive summary: antithrombotic therapy and prevention of thrombosis, 9th ed: American college of chest physicians evidence-based clinical practice guidelines. Chest 2012;141(2 Suppl):7S–47S.

11. Jaff MR, McMurtry MS, Archer SL, et al. Management of massive and submassive pulmonary embolism, iliofemoral deep vein thrombosis, and chronic thromboembolic pulmonary hypertension: a scientific statement from the American Heart Association. Circulation 2011;123(16):1788–830.

12. Konstantinides SV, Torbicki A, Agnelli G, et al. 2014 ESC guidelines on the diagnosis and management of acute pulmonary embolism. Eur Heart J 2014;35(43):3033–69, 3069a–k.

13. Meneveau N, Seronde MF, Blonde MC, et al. Management of unsuccessful thrombolysis in acute massive pulmonary embolism. Chest 2006;129(4):1043–50.

14. Neely RC, Byrne JG, Gosev I, et al. Surgical embolectomy for acute massive and submassive pulmonary embolism in a series of 115 patients. Ann Thorac Surg 2015;100(4):1245–51 [discussion: 1251–2].

15. Greelish JP, Leacche M, Solenkova NS, et al. Improved midterm outcomes for type A (central) pulmonary emboli treated surgically. J Thorac Cardiovasc Surg 2011;142(6):1423–9.

16. Pawale A, Seetharam K, Oswald E, et al. Video assistance for surgical pulmonary embolectomy. Eur J Cardiothorac Surg 2017;52(5):989–90.

17. Kearon C, Akl EA, Ornelas J, et al. Antithrombotic therapy for VTE disease: CHEST guideline and expert panel report. Chest 2016;149(2):315–52.

18. He C, Von Segesser LK, Kappetein PA, et al. Acute pulmonary embolectomy. Eur J Cardiothorac Surg 2013;43(6):1087–95.

19. Zarrabi K, Mollazadeh R, Ostovan MA, et al. Retrograde pulmonary embolectomy in 11 patients. Ann Thorac Surg 2008;85(4):1471–2.

20. Zarrabi K, Zolghadrasli A, Ali Ostovan M, et al. Residual pulmonary hypertension after retrograde pulmonary embolectomy: long-term follow-up of 30 patients with massive and submassive pulmonary embolism. Interact Cardiovasc Thorac Surg 2013;17(2):242–6.

21. Hussain ST, Bartholomew JR, Leacche M, et al. Retrograde pulmonary embolectomy for acute pulmonary embolism: a simplified technique. Ann Thorac Surg 2017;103(5):e473–4.

22. Ashrafian H, Kumar P, Athanasiou T, et al. Minimally invasive off-pump pulmonary embolectomy. Cardiovasc Surg 2003;11(6):471–3.

23. Sa YJ, Choi SY, Lee JH, et al. Off-pump open pulmonary embolectomy for patients with major pulmonary embolism. Heart Surg Forum 2007;10(4):E304–8.

24. Kalra R, Bajaj NS, Arora P, et al. Surgical embolectomy for acute pulmonary embolism: systematic review and comprehensive meta-analyses. Ann Thorac Surg 2017;103(3):982–90.

25. Garvey JW, Wisoff G, Voletti C, et al. Haemorrhagic pulmonary oedema: post-pulmonary embolectomy. Thorax 1976;31(5):605–9.

26. Yusuff HO, Zochios V, Vuylsteke A. Extracorporeal membrane oxygenation in acute massive pulmonary embolism: a systematic review. Perfusion 2015;30(8):611–6.

27. Weinberg A, Tapson VF, Ramzy D. Massive pulmonary embolism: extracorporeal membrane oxygenation and surgical pulmonary embolectomy. Semin Respir Crit Care Med 2017;38(1):66–72.

28. Lodewyks CL, Bednarczyk JM, Mooney OT, et al. Extracorporeal membrane oxygenation, pulmonary embolectomy, and right ventricular assist device for massive pulmonary embolism. Can J Cardiol 2017;33(7):950.e7-9.

29. Edelman JJ, Okiwelu N, Anvardeen K, et al. Surgical pulmonary embolectomy: experience in a series of 37 consecutive cases. Heart Lung Circ 2016;25(12):1240–4.

30. Hartman AR, Manetta F, Lessen R, et al. Acute surgical pulmonary embolectomy: a 9-year retrospective analysis. Tex Heart Inst J 2015;42(1):25–9.

31. Stein PD, Alnas M, Beemath A, et al. Outcome of pulmonary embolectomy. Am J Cardiol 2007;99(3):421–3.

32. Keeling WB, Sundt T, Leacche M, et al. Outcomes after surgical pulmonary embolectomy for acute pulmonary embolus: a multi-institutional study. Ann Thorac Surg 2016;102(5):1498–502.

33. Meyer G, Vicaut E, Danays T, et al. Fibrinolysis for patients with intermediate-risk pulmonary embolism. N Engl J Med 2014;370(15):1402–11.

34. Lee T, Itagaki S, Chiang YP, et al. Survival and recurrence after acute pulmonary embolism treated with pulmonary embolectomy or thrombolysis in New York State, 1999 to 2013. J Thorac Cardiovasc Surg 2017;155(3):1084–90.e12.

35. Aymard T, Kadner A, Widmer A, et al. Massive pulmonary embolism: surgical embolectomy versus thrombolytic therapy–should surgical indications be revisited? Eur J Cardiothorac Surg 2013;43(1):90–4 [discussion: 94].

36. Azari A, Beheshti AT, Moravvej Z, et al. Surgical embolectomy versus thrombolytic therapy in the management of acute massive pulmonary embolism:

short and long-term prognosis. Heart Lung 2015; 44(4):335–9.

37. Lehnert P, Moller CH, Mortensen J, et al. Surgical embolectomy compared to thrombolysis in acute pulmonary embolism: morbidity and mortality. Eur J Cardiothorac Surg 2017;51(2):354–61.

38. Ahmed P, Khan AA, Smith A, et al. Expedient pulmonary embolectomy for acute pulmonary embolism: improved outcomes. Interact Cardiovasc Thorac Surg 2008;7(4):591–4.

39. Konstantinides SV, Vicaut E, Danays T, et al. Impact of thrombolytic therapy on the long-term outcome of intermediate-risk pulmonary embolism. J Am Coll Cardiol 2017;69(12):1536–44.

40. Fedullo PF, Auger WR, Kerr KM, et al. Chronic thromboembolic pulmonary hypertension. N Engl J Med 2001;345(20):1465–72.

41. Pepke-Zaba J, Delcroix M, Lang I, et al. Chronic thromboembolic pulmonary hypertension (CTEPH): results from an international prospective registry. Circulation 2011;124(18):1973–81.

42. Madani M, Mayer E, Fadel E, et al. Pulmonary endarterectomy. patient selection, technical challenges, and outcomes. Ann Am Thorac Soc 2016;13(Suppl 3):S240–7.

43. Jamieson SW, Kapelanski DP. Pulmonary endarterectomy. Curr Probl Surg 2000;37(3):165–252.

44. Madani MM, Auger WR, Pretorius V, et al. Pulmonary endarterectomy: recent changes in a single institution's experience of more than 2,700 patients. Ann Thorac Surg 2012;94(1):97–103 [discussion: 103].

45. Bates DM, Fernandes TM, Duwe BV, et al. Efficacy of a low-tidal volume ventilation strategy to prevent reperfusion lung injury after pulmonary thromboendarterectomy. Ann Am Thorac Soc 2015;12(10):1520–7.

46. Duwe BV, Kerr K, Fedullo PF, et al. Clinical impact of reperfusion lung injury on patients undergoing pulmonary thromboendarterctomy. Am J Respir Crit Care Med 2009;179:A4628.

47. Thistlethwaite PA, Madani MM, Kemp AD, et al. Venovenous extracorporeal life support after pulmonary endarterectomy: indications, techniques, and outcomes. Ann Thorac Surg 2006; 82(6):2139–45.

48. Jamieson SW, Kapelanski DP, Sakakibara N, et al. Pulmonary endarterectomy: experience and lessons learned in 1,500 cases. Ann Thorac Surg 2003; 76(5):1457–62 [discussion: 1462–4].

49. Abe S, Ishida K, Masuda M, et al. A prospective, randomized study of inhaled prostacyclin versus nitric oxide in patients with residual pulmonary hypertension after pulmonary endarterectomy. Gen Thorac Cardiovasc Surg 2017;65(3):153–9.

50. Nierlich P, Ristl R. Perioperative extracorporeal membrane oxygenation bridging in patients undergoing pulmonary endarterectomy. Interact Cardiovasc Thorac Surg 2016;22(2):181–7.

51. Mayer E, Jenkins D, Lindner J, et al. Surgical management and outcome of patients with chronic thromboembolic pulmonary hypertension: results from an international prospective registry. J Thorac Cardiovasc Surg 2011;141(3):702–10.

52. Archibald CJ, Auger WR, Fedullo PF, et al. Long-term outcome after pulmonary thromboendarterectomy. Am J Respir Crit Care Med 1999;160(2): 523–8.

53. Condliffe R, Kiely DG, Gibbs JS, et al. Improved outcomes in medically and surgically treated chronic thromboembolic pulmonary hypertension. Am J Respir Crit Care Med 2008;177(10):1122–7.

54. Delcroix M, Lang I, Pepke-Zaba J, et al. Long-term outcome of patients with chronic thromboembolic pulmonary hypertension: results from an international prospective registry. Circulation 2016;133(9): 859–71.

55. Freed DH, Thomson BM, Berman M, et al. Survival after pulmonary thromboendarterectomy: effect of residual pulmonary hypertension. J Thorac Cardiovasc Surg 2011;141(2):383–7.

56. Ghofrani HA, D'Armini AM, Grimminger F, et al. Riociguat for the treatment of chronic thromboembolic pulmonary hypertension. N Engl J Med 2013; 369(4):319–29.

Moving?

Make sure your subscription moves with you!

To notify us of your new address, find your **Clinics Account Number** (located on your mailing label above your name), and contact customer service at:

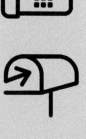

Email: journalscustomerservice-usa@elsevier.com

800-654-2452 (subscribers in the U.S. & Canada)
314-447-8871 (subscribers outside of the U.S. & Canada)

Fax number: 314-447-8029

Elsevier Health Sciences Division
Subscription Customer Service
3251 Riverport Lane
Maryland Heights, MO 63043

*To ensure uninterrupted delivery of your subscription, please notify us at least 4 weeks in advance of move.

ELSEVIER

Printed and bound by CPI Group (UK) Ltd, Croydon, CR0 4YY

08/05/2025

01864726-0001